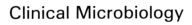

Clinical Microbiology

DR. GANSHAM SINGH
GUYANA

Clinical Microbiology

Sixth Edition

E. Joan Stokes
MB, FRCP, FRCPath
Consulting Clinical Bacteriologist, University College Hospital, London

G. L. Ridgway
MD, BSc, MRCPath
Consultant Clinical Microbiologist, University College Hospital, London

Foreword by
Sir Ashley Miles CBE, MD, FRCP, FRCPath, FRS

Edward Arnold

© E. Joan Stokes and G.L. Ridgway 1987

First published in Great Britain 1955 as Clinical Bacteriology by
Edward Arnold (Publishers) Ltd, 41 Bedford Square, London WC1B 3DQ

Edward Arnold (Australia) Pty Ltd, 80 Waverley Road, Caulfield East,
Victoria 3145, Australia

Edward Arnold, 3 East Read Street, Baltimore, Maryland 21202, U.S.A.

Second Edition 1960
Reprinted 1962
Third Edition 1968
Reprinted 1970
Fourth Edition 1975
Fifth Edition 1980
Reprinted 1983
Sixth Edition 1987

British Library Cataloguing in Publication Data

Stokes, E. Joan
   Clinical microbiology.——6th ed.
   1. Medical microbiology
   I. Title   II. Ridgway, G.L.   III. Stokes, E. Joan. Clinical bacteriology
   616'.01   QR46

ISBN 0 7131 4532 3

Whilst the advice and information of this book is believed to be true and
accurate at the date of going to press, neither the authors nor the publisher can
accept any legal responsibility or liability for any errors or omissions that may
be made.

Text set in 10/11 pt English Times Compugraphic
by Colset Private Ltd, Singapore.
Printed and bound in Great Britain
by Butler & Tanner Ltd, Frome and London.

Foreword to the First Edition

Of the many disciplines in clinical pathology, bacteriology is perhaps the least easy to codify in fixed routines. Every patient with a suspected infection is a new biological problem that both the clinician and the bacteriologist can solve only by following their noses wherever their investigations lead them; and any attempted identification of the infecting microbe in the laboratory may lead the bacteriologist along unexpected paths. Clinical bacteriology is an exploratory art that demands flexibility of mind and technique, and the latest methods are less important to the (would-be) practitioner than a set of uniformly good procedures with which to explore the common and the not-too-rare infections of man, and with which he stands a reasonable chance of discovering new ones.

The methods in this book will go far to meet these requirements. They are well tried. Many indeed had their beginning in 1940–44 in the work of Dr Stokes and other former colleagues of mine in the Emergency Pathological Services of the London Sector 4, and much has been added to keep pace with advances in post-war medicine; and they have an added merit in being subordinated to an all round picture of the practice of clinical bacteriology in a hospital department.

The work of those war years, when the treatment of war wounds and the difficulties of epidemic control in the emergency hospitals stimulated the study of cross-infection, also bears fruit in an innovation – Chapter on Hospital Epidemiology. The inclusion of such a chapter very properly implies that the hospital bacteriologist today must be more than the explorer of each single clinical problem as it arises; as a watchdog in hygiene and as a hospital epidemiologist, he has a function that is almost equally important.

Dr Stokes insists a little on the academic approach. If it is academic to bear in mind the better established principles of bacteriology and immunology and to define the limits of, and justifications for, the hodge-podge of techniques that make up the practice of those sciences, then in attempting to do these things the book may be said to have an academic background; but to my mind they are equally the hallmarks of good practice.

A.A. Miles.

Preface

During the last five years diagnostic procedures in hospital microbiology laboratories have changed greatly. The number of specimens processed is now very large, partly due to the concentration of expertise in fewer laboratories. In the past almost all infections diagnosed in British hospitals were caused by bacterial pathogens but now a comprehensive microbiology service is needed. Viruses, fungi and protozoa must often be sought, whether or not the clinician requests such investigations. Specimens arriving in hospital laboratories do not advertise the nature of the pathogen; it may not be bacterial.

The aim of this book is to help those responsible for laboratory diagnosis of infection by describing techniques which have been found satisfactory in the authors' laboratory and by pointing out problems likely to arise and how they have been dealt with. The reason the title has been changed from *Bacteriology* to *Microbiology* is the inclusion of two new chapters: one on mycology and one on parasitology.

Fungal infections are often seen in those undergoing antimicrobial or immunosuppressive treatment. The speed and the frequency of intercontinental travel, have led to the possibility of infection in non-travelling Britons by microbes common in Asia and Africa. Protozoal infections can no longer be regarded as 'tropical'. Our expertise in these fields is limited because we are able to send specimens to expert laboratories near at hand. We have therefore invited our colleagues Dr R.J. Hay of the Mycology Department of the London School of Hygiene and Tropical Medicine and Mr A.H. Moody of the Parasitology Department of the Hospital for Tropical Diseases to indicate the circumstances in which fungal or protozoal infections should be sought, to recommend methods suitable for non-specialist laboratories and to indicate at what stage specialist help should be requested. We have limited the diagnostic techniques for viruses to those which can be performed in a bacteriology laboratory without special equipment. They are sufficient for the diagnosis of most viral infections in hospital patients. The text of the last (5th) edition of *Clinical Bacteriology* has been completely revised; most of it is new. Methods no longer in routine use have been deleted.

The introduction of kits and mechanization in order to process very large numbers of specimens (the majority of which will prove negative) may lead to mechanization of the minds of the investigators and to the belief that when a routine procedure is completed the result will be of value; this is not necessarily so. To use kits properly needs skill and judgement, to take short cuts is courting disaster. We hope that discussion of the problems we have encountered will alert the reader to the continuing need for good basic technique and encourage the recognition and avoidance of false results.

To write a comprehensive guide to techniques available for the diagnosis of microbial disease would be a daunting task. We think it is more useful to describe only methods we have tested and found to be reliable. They are necessarily limited to the best and most cost-effective we have been able to discover for the population we serve. However, whatever methods are chosen, the fundamental approach to the problems of laboratory diagnosis of microbial disease, and the ways in which clinical microbiologists can contribute to the treatment and prevention of infection, is the same in all parts of the world. Understanding of the purpose of investigations and their limitations is as essential as careful performance of reliable methods. We aim to deal with both these aspects of clinical microbiology.

We hope this account will help hospital microbiologists to apply their academic training to the needs of rapid diagnosis without sacrificing scientific principles. We were fortunate to be shown the way by the teaching of Sir Ashley Miles, to whom we are very grateful. It also explains to clinicians what can be expected of a diagnostic laboratory and how they can gain most from collaboration with it.

We wish to thank all the laboratory staff who have participated in testing and introducing new methods. We are particularly grateful to Mr D. Felmingham for assistance with Chapter 9, and to Mr A.W.F. Cremer and Mr D. Castle for checking sources of materials and supervising new methods. Professor J.R. Pattison and Mr B.J. Mellars gave invaluable advice and details of virological methods. Contributions from Miss M. O'Hare, and Mrs M. Robbins are gratefully acknowledged. Finally we thank Mr P. Luton for the new photographs in Chapters 9 and 10, and Mrs A. Luton for typing interminable drafts.

EJS
GLR

1987

Contents

1

The Practice of Clinical Microbiology

Clinical microbiology is no longer the study simply of specimens received from patients suffering from infections. Whilst the laboratory identification of potential pathogens remains paramount, the microbiologist is more and more called upon to advise on the interpretation of results, further management of therapy and control of the spread of infection to other persons. In an age of rapidly advancing technology it is all too easy for the busy microbiologist to forget the basic principles on which his craft is based. For over thirty years the arguments put forth in this chapter have remained unchanged and we make no apologies for reiterating them because they are perhaps even more relevant today.

Organisms identified or demonstrated in specimens from patients are of two types. Either they reflect the normal microbial flora or they are unlikely to be normal residents and must therefore be considered as possible pathogens. However, even if the organisms are normally resident they may still cause disease if their distribution is abnormal. For example, *Escherichia coli* and *Clostridium perfringens* are both normally found in the bowel, but when the former is isolated from bladder urine of a patient with symptoms of urinary infection or the latter from a wound swab from a patient with gas gangrene, they are likely pathogens because they have been shown to be the cause of these infections on numerous previous occasions. Conversely, simply because an organism is found in an abnormal site does not imply that it must be causing disease; commensals often contaminate specimens.

The carrier state must not be overlooked. *Streptococcus pyogenes* is a common bacterial cause of sore throat, yet it may also occur in healthy carriers. Thus the finding of the organism in the throat of a patient with symptoms may either mean it is the cause, or that another organism (e.g. *Corynebacterium diphtheriae* or adenovirus), yet to be identified, is responsible in an incidental *Str. pyogenes* carrier.

The distinction between a pathogenic organism and a non-pathogen (commensal or saprophyte) is thus imprecise. The presence of a potential pathogen in human tissue results in a variety of conditions ranging from healthy carriage to a moribund state. Other less well understood factors will determine at what stage the equilibrium between host and parasite is reached; for example, immunological competence, nutritional state and underlying disease. The unstable balance between pathogen and non-

1

pathogen has been highlighted by the appreciation that coagulase-negative staphylococci may cause severe infection in the immunocompromised patient. The response of a patient to invasion by a microbe depends on his immune state, both general and specific for the invader. It also depends on the ability of the microbe to multiply (an anaerobe, for example, needs special conditions to do so) and on the 'virulence' of the strain. This leads to the adoption of two basic rules in microbiology:

1. Never without good reason dismiss a microbe as a contaminant because it is not an 'accepted' pathogen.

2. Never without good reason accept a microbe as the *necessary* cause of a disease merely because it is an 'accepted' pathogen.

Koch's postulates in clinical microbiology

The cause and effect relationship between a microbe and a disease may be further illuminated by the application of Koch's postulates:

1. The microbe should be found in all cases of the disease, distributed in the body according to the lesions observed.

2. The microbe should be grown artificially in pure culture for several subcultures.

3. The pure culture should reproduce the disease in a susceptible animal.

Postulate 1 must be modified for the single case to read, 'The microbe should be constantly found associated with the lesions during the course of the disease'.

Postulate 3 is often impossible to carry out because many human infections cannot be reproduced in animals. It may be possible to show that animal serum containing a high level of antibody will specifically protect against infection by the microbe. Testing patient's serum for antibody may contribute further evidence, particularly if a rise in titre during infection and a fall in titre after recovery can be demonstrated. A positive result indicates current or previous exposure to the antigen. A negative result will not exclude a causal role, as antibody production may be delayed or absent. Similarly, presence of antibody in a serologically virgin population may be of significance on its own, whereas antibody levels to microbes common in the community will be of significance only if a change in level can be demonstrated in serial blood samples during the course of the illness. There are in addition many examples of cross-reacting antigens, of which the positive proteus agglutination with serum from patients with rickettsial infections is a well known example. Evans (1976) discussed modification of Koch's postulates to include newer techniques for establishing causation.

Two types of evidence

There are two types of evidence which may be gained from laboratory investigation. First, simple tests may be made which in themselves are of little significance but which, when taken into consideration with the history and physical signs, may help to establish the diagnosis. If urine from a patient with symptoms of renal tract infection contains acid-fast bacilli it is probable that the patient has renal tuberculosis, and demonstration of the bacilli adds weight to the diagnosis. Similarly, if Gram-negative diplococci are found in a smear from the urethra of a man with acute urethritis, the finding adds weight to the diagnosis of gonorrhoea. But neither of these findings when considered alone has much significance because they may be seen in specimens taken from healthy people. The diagnosis in these cases is essentially a clinical one. A further example is the demonstration of a specific antigen in a specimen which may strongly indicate that a particular pathogen is present, but it does not *prove* that this is so because of the overlap of antigens between species. A variety of commensals may be present, one of which could account for the reaction; moreover, the pathogen, if present, may be dead. Positive direct-antigen tests make a presumptive diagnosis quickly and are particularly helpful when culture is slow or costly (e.g. for *Chlamydia trachomatis* and viruses), but diagnosis depends on knowledge of the patient's condition and again the evidence is essentially clinical.

The second type of evidence is based on isolation in pure culture and identification of the organism concerned. In the first case just considered this could be reported not as 'acid-fast bacilli seen' but as *'Myco. tuberculosis* present'. This is a piece of evidence which is significant by itself without the support of clinical findings, and even if the patient has no other signs of tuberculosis the presence of the organism still needs an explanation.

Circular arguments

It is very important that there be no confusion between the two types of evidence; 'acid-fast bacilli seen' is never synonymous with *'Myco. tuberculosis* present'.

The first type of evidence is often useful in the initial diagnosis of infection in an individual. However, unless its limitations are clearly understood, its use may lead to confusion of thought. The clinician thinks a particular pathogen is likely and, when the laboratory finds an organism resembling this, pressure of work (and a desire to please his colleague by rapid diagnosis) may lead the microbiologist to report without necessary laboratory confirmation; this will inevitably lead to false diagnosis in some cases. A more subtle error is to allow oneself to be influenced by knowledge of the patient's symptoms in assessing the significance of low antibody titres. Laboratory evidence is useless unless it is impartial. Laboratory tests are often repeated when the results fail to fit the clinical findings but very seldom when they satisfy clinical expectations. It is illogical to use a test for diagnosis of a particular infection and *at the same time* use the clinical findings to gauge its reliability.

Before tests are adopted for routine use they should be extensively tried out on *known* positive and negative material and their value and limitations established. When this has been done the experimental stage is over and it then remains for the microbiologist to see that the conditions of the test are observed and that proper controls are included. If there is any doubt about its reliability when handled in a routine laboratory, duplicate tests should be set up in *all* cases, irrespective of clinical findings; if this reveals variation in results which cannot be overcome the test is useless and must be discarded.

Another false argument encountered is the premise that, because a microbe is usually found in a specific site, an isolate from that site which resembles it is therefore that microbe. The clinical microbiologist must recognize changes in the distribution of the human flora and not assume that there is no change without proof.

Legitimate use of clinical findings

It may now seem that it would be better if the microbiologist were to have no knowledge at all of the clinical condition so that he was not in a position to be biased, but information about the patient's clinical state is very valuable when legitimately used. When laying down rules for routine investigation they should be made to cover, as far as possible, all known eventualities and, no matter what the clinical findings, nothing should be omitted from this routine. If, however, the patient's condition suggests infection by a certain group of organisms, special methods may be employed from the outset which may make it possible to isolate and identify the pathogen more quickly than by the routine method alone; for example, primary inoculation of a Nagler plate when *Cl. perfringens* is suspected. In addition, the use of direct antigen methods, such as gas-liquid chromatography, or specific immunological techniques, too costly for routine use, may be considered.

Avoidance of false reasoning

False reasoning along the lines indicated may be avoided either by fully identifying all the microbes found, which is not usually practicable in a hospital laboratory, or by adopting the following procedure. All bacteria isolated from sites which are normally sterile are assigned to their genus on laboratory evidence alone; when it is useful to proceed further the species is also named. If the laboratory identification has stopped short at the genus this is made plain in the report. For example, a microbe identified by colonial and microscopic morphology and by a positive oxidase test is reported as '*Pseudomonas* species'. When necessary, further biochemical tests may be performed and the species fully identified, but this will delay the report and often (e.g. in repeat urine samples) serves no useful purpose. Haemolytic streptococci, on the other hand, must be fully identified and grouped because the result is important both in the prognosis and treatment of the individual patient and from the point of view of hospital epidemiology; they are therefore reported by name.

Specimens from sites which have a normal flora are treated somewhat differently. It is rarely necessary to identify all the microbes cultured. The routine procedure is to exclude all known pathogens, using the best selective methods available, and reports are sent which make it clear that this has been done. For example, the report of a faeces culture may read. 'No *Salmonella*, *Shigella* or *Campylobacter* isolated'. This tells the clinician what he needs to know without giving him any misleading information and is preferred to the type of report which reads 'Cultures yield *Esch. coli*, *Str. faecalis* and *Proteus vulgaris*'. Naming the species is at first sight impressive. However, full identification cannot be made without delay and may mislead the clinician into giving unwarranted importance to the isolate. Identification of the organism to genus or species level may be carried out to exclude a pathogen, or for other purposes (e.g. epidemiological markers or research); in such cases it is reasonable to suppress information irrelevant to clinical management from the report returned to the clinician. 'No pathogen isolated' or 'Cultures yield normal flora only' are common variations. Such reports are imprecise and give no indication of what has *not* been excluded – for example, *Vibrio cholerae* in a faeces sample. Moreover, it is unwise to assume that we know what 'normal flora' is under all circumstances. These reports are therefore undesirable.

The amount of work necessary for satisfactory identification of the microbes frequently encountered in clinical microbiology and the way in which different investigations may be reported will be considered later, but the guiding principles for avoiding unsound reasoning in diagnostic work are the same in all cases and may be stated thus:

1. The report must be based on laboratory evidence only.

2. All microbes named must either be isolated in pure culture and identified by biochemical or serological tests or be unequivocally demonstrated by reliable direct detection methods.

3. When identification has proceeded only as far as the genus this must be made clear.

4. When identification falls short of the genus in the examination of cultures from sites with a normal flora, the microbe is considered to be insufficiently important for identification and is not mentioned in the report which concerns known pathogens only.

The need for speed

It may appear that the second of these rules is incompatible with speed and that it is more valuable for the experienced microbiologist to use his 'clinical' judgement of the appearance of microbes to send a quick report because, it may be argued, he will fail to identify only atypical strains which are infrequent and, from a practical point of view, do not matter since they are probably of low virulence. Speed in clinical microbiology is, of course, very important and it is perfectly legitimate for the microbiologist to use his experience of morphological appearances to give a quick *preliminary* report, which may be very valuable in indicating lines of treatment or the need for isolation, but the investigation must never be allowed to stop at this stage. The idea that strains which appear atypical are comparatively harmless is unsound, and epidemics have arisen because such strains have not been recognized. The preliminary report must therefore be checked to avoid this risk and also to ensure that neither the clinician nor the microbiologist puts too much faith in it. The great variation in appearance that occurs between different strains of the same species, and the unreliability of colonial and microscopical morphology as a final test of identity, can be appreciated only if it is checked by biochemical or serological methods. Atypical strains will continue to be thought rare if these are omitted.

Direct antigen tests can give rapid and reliable results but may mislead when they are used on unsuitable specimens. For example, a positive result showing gonococcal or chlamydial antigen in a urethral swab from an infected patient is reliable because other microbes are absent or too scanty to be visible microscopically, but a positive result from a rectal swab cannot be relied on because numerous other microbes will be present and antigenic cross-reactions cannot be excluded.

If microbiological reports based on inadequate tests are entered in the case records, much harm may be done. Because the report came from the laboratory, it may be regarded by the clinician as accurate in the same way that a chemical estimation is thought to be accurate, and the records with the microbiological findings may be included in a survey of cases for research purposes, with very misleading results. If the principles of reporting investigations, listed above, are followed there is no danger of a misunderstanding about the value of the findings.

The clinical microbiologist

It is often erroneously considered that the clinical microbiologist needs only to be aware of techniques which allow the rapid identification of medically important micro-organisms; this is not so. Microbiology is a science and it is particularly important that high standards are maintained. If the microbiologist in day to day contact with specimens is insufficiently trained, or fails to apply scientific principles, he will fail to recognize departures from the expected behaviour of host and parasite. Whilst such observations may be of little value in the treatment of individual patients, it is on them that increased knowledge of infectious disease depends.

The standard of training achieved by non-medical scientists in microbiology is high. No longer should the clinical microbiologist feel tied to the bench for lack of technical expertise to help him. It remains for him to ensure that tests relevant to the clinical problem are carried out efficiently and economically, and that the clinical interpretation of the results is valid. To this end he should be readily available to his clinical colleagues for advice and consultation, acting as an intermediary between the bedside and the bench. Lack of clinical information is a perennial complaint of laboratory-based practitioners; the clinical microbiologist must therefore visit the wards to supplement this information. Such visits may be on a regular basis to problem areas (e.g. intensive therapy units) or in response to individual requests. It is our experience that once a consultation service is offered it will, in general, become popular and widely used. However, medical problems may occur at any time, day or night, and it is therefore necessary to provide full cover if one is to expect full clinical liaison. The competence of the clinical microbiologist at the bench must not be allowed to suffer by this increased clinical involvement. Lack of familiarity with tests will make him unable to judge their relative efficacy.

The optimal use of antibiotics is of paramount importance for a number of reasons: the patient needs effective treatment, the spread of resistant microbes must be prevented in both hospital and community, and unnecessary cost must be avoided. The number and range of antibiotics available are bewildering, and the clinical microbiologist has an important role to play in guiding clinical colleagues in their use. The hospital pharmacist can help by providing a list of patients daily for whom antibiotics have been prescribed. If it is agreed that the clinical microbiologist can visit them without a formal request, much time will be saved. In our experience, junior clinical staff welcome advice on the appropriateness of treatment in the light of laboratory findings and the response to treatment. Advice on dosage and the need for monitoring antibiotic levels in serum is also helpful to them. The clinical microbiologist also gains because it enables him to ensure that laboratory investigations are relevant to clinical problems. This close co-operation leads to better treatment at less cost.

In many hospitals the consultant clinical microbiologist will also be designated infection control officer. Ward visits will allow recognition of problems, particularly where patients under the care of more than one consultant are involved. Visits to other areas, such as operating theatres, kitchens and domestic areas, are also necessary as part of his work.

There are a number of pitfalls to be avoided in this interactive role. Clinical diagnosis should not influence the interpretation of laboratory tests. Involvement in direct patient care should be regarded as a privilege; it is the consultant in charge of the patient who must face the consequences of therapy, not the microbiologist. Advice should be written in the case notes, when necessary, and standing orders never altered by the microbiologist. One piece of bad advice can undo years of carefully built up confidence.

Recognition of a need for advice in antimicrobial chemotherapy implies no criticism of the expertise of clinicians. The time is long past when any clinical doctor can be self-sufficient; the consultant in charge of the patient carries the ultimate responsibility for treatment but others with medical training should be prepared to advise and *they* have the responsibility of ensuring that their advice is good.

Reference

Evans, A.S. (1976) *Yale Journal of Biology and Medicine* **49**, 175

2

General Procedure

Speed tempered with accuracy is essential for the diagnosis of acute infection. Delay will have consequences not only for the patient (who may be receiving inappropriate or no therapy) but also for staff and other patients exposed for an unnecessarily prolonged period to the risk of infection. However, the results obtained from the investigation of potentially infected material reflect not only the ability of the laboratory but also the standards of specimen collection and transport. The sampling of fluids normally sterile (e.g. urine, cerebrospinal fluid) requires greater care than surgical aseptic technique procedures. Air-borne contamination by saprophytes has little consequence to operative procedures in most circumstances, but may ruin the suitability of a specimen for microbiological investigation. Less stringent caution will apply to specimens contaminated by the patient's normal flora, but, even here, exclusion of extraneous material is important to prevent misinterpretation. Delay in the transport of specimens will allow saprophytes to multiply at room temperature, or result in an overgrowth by normal flora obscuring pathogens present in small numbers.

Collection of specimens

If reliable results are to be obtained, the following guidelines for taking specimens should be observed:

1. All specimens must be labelled with the patient's name and the date and time of sampling, and must be accompanied by a signed form which states the name and age of the patient, the ward or department, the nature of the specimen and the site from which it was taken, the clinical diagnosis and duration of the illness, the examination required and the nature of any recent, current or proposed antibacterial treatment. Without this information, interpretation may be impossible or misleading. Moreover, full information may suggest to the laboratory further tests, not requested by the clinician, which will hasten the laboratory diagnosis.

2. Specimens for culture must never be in contact with antiseptics or disinfectants. If the site must be cleaned, a dry sterile swab moistened with sterile saline and held in sterile forceps should be used, and the site should be dried before sampling.

3. All specimens for culture must be sent to the laboratory on the day of

collection and with as little delay as possible; speed is essential in the following investigations:

(a) *Neisseria meningitidis* and *N. gonorrhoeae* are very sensitive to exposure to air in the cold. Cerebrospinal fluid from patients with signs of meningitis must arrive warm and be incubated immediately. Negative results from specimens which have cooled are valueless. Swabs for the culture of *N. gonorrhoeae* should be seeded on warm blood agar at the bedside unless special medium for transport is available (page 311).

(b) *Eye swabs.* Lachrymal secretion contains lysozyme, an enzyme which rapidly kills bacteria; therefore swabs should be plated at the bedside.

4. *Urine.* Catheterization is no longer considered justifiable simply for urine culture; therefore, most samples are clean midstream specimens inevitably contaminated with a few bacteria, among which are likely to be common urinary pathogens which will multiply in warm urine. It is therefore essential that either the specimen be cultured within an hour of voiding or that it be refrigerated forthwith (4°C) to prevent bacterial growth.

5. *Faeces.* Bedpans for collecting specimens for culture should be heat treated to prevent accidental contamination by bacteria from another sample of faeces. Part of the specimen containing any abnormal material such as pus or mucus is placed in a clean screw-capped bottle or waxed carton. A warm specimen freshly passed into a warmed bedpan is necessary for examination for amoebae. Rectal swabs are taken by passing the swab through the anal canal while the patient 'bears down'. They are very satisfactory for the culture of dysentery bacilli, provided they arrive in the laboratory while still moist. It is helpful to moisten the swab in sterile water before sampling.

6. *Sputum* for culture should be collected into a sterile screw-capped bottle when the patient first wakes in the morning. If there is very little of it, it may be possible to collect a satisfactory sample by placing the patient comfortably so that his head and shoulders are lower than his chest. If he remains thus for about 10 minutes, sputum may drain into the trachea and then he will be able to cough it into a conveniently placed container. Specimens for microscopic examination should be taken into disposable containers; they should be clean and dry, and need not be sterile.

7. *Serous fluids*: pleural, pericardial, synovial, ascitic. Specimens should be sent in sterile screw-capped bottles for culture. Additional specimens may be required for cytological studies, including cell count. If culture for *Myco. tuberculosis* is required, a large volume of fluid (200 ml if possible) should be obtained.

8. *Cerebrospinal fluid.* Two samples are sent in sterile bottles, about 3 ml each: one for culture (see guideline 2, page 5), the other for cell count and chemical analysis.

9. *Blood*

(a) For culture: full aseptic technique is essential to prevent contamination by skin organisms (see page 27).

(b) For serology: whilst, theoretically, serological tests can be performed on unsterile specimens, this is to be avoided. Contamination of the sample may lead to haemolysis of the specimen, making testing difficult. Furthermore, modern serological techniques utilize highly sensitive reagents; contaminated specimens may contain components that cause misleading cross-reactions. The venesector should avoid direct contact with the patient's blood at all times, to prevent the risk of accidental infection.

10. *Tissue.* Biopsy or autopsy specimens should be sent in a *dry* sterile container. They must not be allowed to dry, therefore small samples are sent without delay; saline and water are to some extent bactericidal and should not be added.

11. Whenever possible specimens should be sent early in the day so that there is time to examine them during normal working hours. When an investigation is required which needs immediate attention notice should be given at least an hour before the specimen is taken.

12. All specimens from patients, whether for culture or for other investigations, are potentially dangerous to persons who handle them. This applies even if known risks (e.g. hepatitis or HIV infection) have been excluded. Leaking containers should be destroyed by incineration or autoclaving, and a repeat sample obtained. In the rare instance when this is not possible, a senior member of the laboratory staff should process the specimen, wearing protective clothing and using an exhaust protective cabinet (Class I or III).

Macroscopic examination

Unsuitable specimens

When a specimen is received in the laboratory it is usually assumed that the guidelines listed above have been followed; nevertheless, it is as well to look out for signs of a badly taken specimen – the swab that smells of antiseptic, the leaking urine jar and the small watery specimen of 'sputum' that is really saliva. Information about some specimens can be gained from the presence of normal flora. Clearly something is wrong if a throat swab or a sample of faeces is sterile, and the examination must be repeated. It is important that at least one original culture medium show the normal flora. When faeces or swabs for diphtheria are seeded on highly selective media only, it is impossible to judge if the specimen has been contaminated with disinfectant, because sterile cultures may be due to the efficiency of the method of selection. When large numbers of specimens from an epidemic are to be examined it is reasonable to take one or two plates containing non-selective medium, mark them in small squares and seed each specimen first on one of these squares and then on to the appropriate medium for the selection of pathogens. In this way unsatisfactory specimens will be recognized without an extravagant use of medium.

Selection of material for examination

It is possible, as a routine, to examine only a very small part of the specimen; the chance of a positive result is increased by careful selection. Note any pus or blood in the specimen and whenever possible choose a purulent part for culture.

Microscopic examination

Examination of stained films or of a wet preparation should precede culture. The purpose of the examination is twofold. First it is a guide to further procedures; for example, if fungi are seen in the film a culture is made in conditions favourable for their growth in addition to the routine method for the cultivation of bacteria. Secondly it is the most valuable indication of the proportion of different species in the specimen. Sometimes bacteria seen in the film fail to grow; this may be either because they are dead or because they have not been cultured under favourable conditions. It must be remembered that death of bacteria frequently alters their staining properties such that Gram-positive organisms appear Gram-negative, and also that the morphology of a bacterium in a pathological fluid may undergo a profound change when cultured on artificial media.

Mechanization of the Gram-stain results in more regularly stained slides and releases skilled staff for other work. Proper maintenance of stain containers is essential to prevent growth of air-borne contaminants in the stain. A clean, freshly filled set is required each morning. The method can also be used for acid-fast bacilli (see Heimer et al., 1978).

Urine deposits, faeces and mucous discharges are examined wet for cells, fungi, protozoa and helminths. Dark-ground or phase-contrast microscopy is needed to find spirochaetes in blood, urine or tissue fluids.

Specimens may be concentrated before examination. This is easily done by centrifuging liquid specimens such as cerebrospinal fluid, urine and unclotted serous fluids, but the procedure is rather more complex for specimens such as faeces and sputum which must be homogenized before they can be satisfactorily concentrated (see chapters 4 and 6).

Routine and selective methods of culture

It is impossible to lay down a strict routine for all specimens because each investigation develops individually according to the findings at each stage. Broadly, however, all specimens from sites normally sterile are seeded on blood agar and incubated in air plus 5–10% CO_2, and anaerobically plus about 10% CO_2, because the majority of medically important bacteria will grow under these conditions within 48 hours. A negative result may be as important as a positive one; therefore, when primary cultures are sterile and yet from the clinical findings and microscopy infection seems likely, another sample, as large as possible, is concentrated by centrifugation when applicable and cultured immediately in air, in air plus 5–10% CO_2 and anaerobically plus about 10% CO_2. A variety of highly nutrient liquid and solid media are employed, suitable for the growth of all known human pathogens. Incubation of solid media should be continued for at least a week, and liquid media are subcultured at frequent intervals for up to a month before they are discarded.*

Animal inoculation is now seldom required for diagnostic purposes, with the exception of Corynebacterium diphtheriae.

It is not practicable in a clinical laboratory to incubate plates longer

*A more detailed account of the method will be found in Chapter 3.

than 48 hours as a routine; therefore, if no colonies are visible after this time they are reported as 'sterile after 48 hours' incubation'. The prolonged investigation outlined above is made only when the establishment of a negative result is of prime importance, and is particularly applicable to suspected anaerobic infections.

Primary cultures should not be discarded until the end of the investigation when the report has been sent. It is convenient at the end of each day to collect plate cultures, which are not to be reincubated, in a wire basket with a dated label so that they can easily be found when necessary.

Routine primary seeding on MacConkey's bile salt agar is not essential but it is often time-saving. Ability to grow on this medium is often a guide to identity and, since swarming is inhibited, it may be possible to obtain pure cultures more quickly from colonies on the MacConkey plate when swarming obscures all growth on blood agar.*

Selective culture greatly increases the chance of recovering known pathogens from sites with a normal flora. There are several methods of selection. The atmosphere, the composition of the medium and the incubation temperature may all be varied to favour the growth of the species to be selected, and antibiotics may be spread on the surface of solid media or incorporated in it to inhibit the growth of contaminating organisms. An example of selection by atmosphere is the isolation of haemolytic streptococci from throat swabs by incubating the cultures anaerobically. Although haemolytic streptococci are aerobes, they grow well under anaerobic conditions and many strains produce large colonies and more marked haemolysis when cultured thus. Moreover, the growth of many commensals, staphylococci, neisseria and diphtheroids is inhibited so that they form very small colonies. This is an efficient method because not only are many unwanted bacteria inhibited but also the growth of the selected species may be enhanced.

Most selective media contain chemicals which inhibit the growth of contaminating organisms efficiently but also to some extent inhibit the growth of the species selected. Such media may be invaluable for the recovery of pathogens from contaminated specimens but should be used solely for this purpose. If a bacterium is sought in a body fluid which is normally sterile (e.g. blood or urine) it is better to use good nutrient media such as blood agar and broth, which have no inhibitory effect. Examples of media which select by differential inhibition include tellurite blood agar for *C. diphtheriae* and desoxycholate citrate agar for the shigella and salmonella groups. The inhibiting effect of a given batch of medium can be demonstrated by comparing surface viable counts of a pure culture of the selected organism on blood agar and on the medium. After 24 hours' incubation the count on blood agar will be higher, sometimes as much an hundredfold higher, and although after further incubation more colonies may appear on the selective medium the count never reaches that on blood agar. Selection by these media can therefore never approach perfection because they are incapable of supporting the growth of very small inocula. Tellurite cultures are always incubated for 48 hours before they are discarded. Occasionally

*For prevention of swarming on blood agar see page 120.

colonies appear on the second day when the overnight culture was negative. Tetrathionate broth, which selects paratyphoid bacilli and other salmonellae, differs from these because the selected bacteria can metabolize tetrathionate, and most strains grow in the medium at least as well as they grow in a good nutrient broth; it is therefore reasonable to use it for urine cultures.

In later chapters various selective media will be recommended for particular purposes; they are by no means the only ones available. It is better to become technically expert with a good medium rather than to change continually to media which are said to be superlative. It is therefore advisable to choose a medium, not necessarily the one described, and gain experience with it until there is good reason for making a change. Most highly selective media are variable and each new batch of the inhibiting substance should be tested before it is used to make media for routine work.

Antibiotics may be incorporated in media to select pathogenic bacteria from commensals. There are many examples in modern microbiology; for example, the use of polymyxin, nystatin and vancomycin in selective media for *N. gonorrhoeae*. The amount of antibiotic used must be carefully calculated because even relatively resistant organisms may not grow in high concentrations of antibiotic.

Selection of bacteria by alteration of incubation temperature is less widely used. Incubation at 43°C for campylobacter also selects faecal organisms from soil commensals in water. A low temperature (4°C) will select *Listeria monocytogenes* and *Yersinia enterocolitica* from commensal bacteria.

In recent years there has been a proliferation of commercially produced kits for the detection and identification of bacteria in clinical material; there is no doubt that they represent a significant advance in diagnostic bacteriology. In general, they are expensive and they do not replace the need for basic bacteriological skills. It is important that kits are properly evaluated by users and their limitations discovered before more traditional methods are discarded. It is not sufficient to rely solely on evidence supplied by the manufacturer. Our choice of the numerous kits available is based partly on published evidence (e.g. Holmes *et al.*, 1977), on the results of their performance in quality control assessment (UKEQAS, see page 22) and on our own laboratory experience. The tendency of the inexperienced to place reliance on kit results out of all proportion to the performance capability of the method must be resisted.

Centralization of laboratories, increasing workload and decreasing budgets have encouraged the development of automation in the clinical laboratory. Bacteriology does not readily lend itself to such methods. The same reservations apply to automation as to kits. Economy, reliability and specificity must be clearly established before they are accepted into routine use.

Antagonists of antibacterial substances

Sometimes an infection must be investigated during antibacterial treatment. In such cases the chance of obtaining positive cultures is reduced, but if the antibacterial drugs in the specimen are neutralized by antagonists, a positive result may yet be obtained. Sulphonamides act by depriving the bacteria of an essential growth factor, para-aminobenzoic acid. The effect is easily neutralized by adding 0.1 per cent of a saturated solution of para-aminobenzoic acid to broth.

Beta-lactamases are enzymes produced by many bacteria which neutralize penicillins and cephalosporins. They can be spread on the surface of media or incorporated in it to neutralize the effect of these drugs on sensitive bacteria. A suitable sterile preparation can be obtained commercially (Genzyme Biochemicals Ltd).

Sampling before these drugs are given is much better than relying on neutralization because the preparation, being a product of bacterial metabolism, may contain small amounts of substances inhibitory to some bacteria. Moreover, there is a risk of contamination from the preparation which cannot be filtered without very considerable loss in potency (Hamilton-Miller and Brumfitt, 1974).

No satisfactory antagonists are available, so far, for the newer antibiotics. Antimicrobial-removing resins are available. We have had limited experience of their use, but their advantages have been less than was hoped.

Records

It is impossible to lay down hard and fast rules for the treatment of specimens because each one must be considered separately. It is, however, very valuable to have a rigid routine for recording results so that anyone working in the same laboratory can take over an investigation at a moment's notice and follow clearly what has already been done. Good records have the added advantage that they are available for research, and if there is an inquiry about the validity of bacterial diagnosis in a court of law or elsewhere it is possible to refer to the actual methods of identification and the results obtained. Without them it is impossible for the microbiologist to keep in touch with the work done in his laboratory. The following method has been found satisfactory.

Each specimen, as it comes into the laboratory, is given a number which is stamped with a duplicate numbering machine on the front of the two-part request form where the report will be entered. The under copy serves as a record card and receives the same number; 12.5 cm × 20 cm is a suitable size. The name, ward, date, the nature of the specimen and the examination required are entered on the card and in the laboratory register. The request form remains in the office to await the report and the specimen with its card enters the laboratory. The card, being a duplicate of the request form, has on it any clinical information available which can be referred to without difficulty during the investigation. Cultures are made, the plates and tubes being labelled with the number of the specimen and the date, and a note is made on the back of card of the media used and the atmosphere in which the cultures were incubated. Results of the direct examination, macroscopic and microscopic, are entered on the front of the card to be included in the report. After overnight incubation the cultures are examined by the naked eye, and with a hand lens having a focal length of approximately 7–8 cm. Each different type of colony is noted and, working in order of predominance of growth, is labelled with small letters *a, b, c,* etc. The degree of predominance is denoted by plus signs: $+ + + =$ profuse growth, $+ + =$ several hundred colonies, $+ =$ about a hundred colonies, $\pm = $ 10–50 colonies; if there are fewer than ten the actual number is entered. The approximate diameter, measured in millimetres, of an isolated colony of each type is noted, followed by a sufficient description of the colony to enable anyone looking at the culture later to be able easily to distinguish it from the others present. Next, smears are made from single colonies of each type from all the plate cultures and Gram-stained (see page 85); the result of microscopic examination is entered on the card.

At this stage the record of a 24-hour aerobic blood agar (BA/O$_2$) culture from, say, a wound swab No. 493 might be:

No. 493 WOUND SWAB.

$\quad$ BA/O$_2$

$\quad$ (*a*) $+ + +$ $\quad$ 2 mm β-haemolytic yellow; G $+$ cocci in clusters.

$\quad$ (*b*) $+ +$ $\quad$ 0.2 mm transparent non-haem. Showing satellitism to *a*; G $-$ pleomorphic bacilli.

$\quad$ (*c*) $\pm$ $\quad$ 0.5 mm β-haem.; G $+$ short chain strep.

The same procedure is followed for each plate culture, the small letters being continued for colonies on the anaerobic plate (BA/AnO$_2$) thus:

$\quad$ BA/AnO$_2$

$\quad$ (*d*) $+ + +$ $\quad$ 0.5 mm β-haem.; G $+$ strep. (as *c*).

$\quad$ (*e*) $+ +$ $\quad$ 0.2 mm non-haem.; G $+$ cocci in clusters (as *a*).

$\quad$ (*f*) $+ +$ $\quad$ 0.1 mm transparent non-haem.; G $-$ bacilli (as *b*).

It is now possible to decide what further tests are necessary for final identification of these organisms. 493*a* is a staphylococcus and must be tested for coagulase production; *b* is a haemophilus, and in most cases it need not be tested further; *c* is a haemolytic streptococcus and must be subcultured for Lancefield grouping. Single colonies are transferred to the appropriate media for these tests and a note is made; the results will be entered next day.

$\quad$ (*a*) coagulase $+$

$\quad$ (*c*) Lancefield grouping $\;$ A B C D F G

$\qquad\qquad\qquad\qquad\qquad\quad$ $+ - - - - -$

The final report will read as follows:

$\quad$ Direct examination: Numerous pus cells and Gram-positive cocci, a few Gram-negative bacilli.

$\quad$ Cultures yield: *Str. pyogenes, Staph. aureus* and a Haemophilus sp.

The card is returned to the office, the report which has been entered on the front of it is typed on the request form and signed, and the card is filed. (See also page 21.)

Sometimes when a colony which is present in the pool of inoculum on the primary plate is spread out on another plate to obtain isolated colonies it proves to be mixed with another microbe not previously noted, or sometimes what was thought to be a single colony is actually a mixture. This often happens with anaerobes and leads to confusion unless a rule of notation is strictly followed. Let us take part of the record of another specimen to illustrate how this difficulty is overcome:

No. 832 PUS SWAB from postpartum uterus.
Day 1. BA/CO_2
   (*a*) ±   1 mm non-haem.; G + diphtheroid bacilli.
   BA/AnO_2
   (*b*) + + + 1 mm non-haem, moist; G + strep., a few G − bacilli.
   (*c*) ±   0.5 mm matt non-haem.; G + diphtheroid as *a*.
   (*b*) subcultured to blood agar CO_2 and AnO_2

Day 2.
  (*b*) BA/CO_2 sterile 24 hours.

   BA/AnO_2
   (*ba*) + + + 0.1 mm non-haem. moist; G + strep.
   (*bb*) + + minute non-haem.; G − slender bacilli.

It occasionally happens, particularly in isolating clostridia, that a strain labelled (*bb*) is still mixed; in that case the two strains are labelled (*bba*) and (*bbb*).

So far in the examples quoted it has been necessary to identify all the bacteria found because the specimens have come from sites normally sterile. When selective methods are used to recover known pathogens from sites with a normal flora, this method of recording cultures is modified. An example of a throat swab culture record will serve to illustrate the modification.

No. 262 THROAT SWAB – tonsillitis.
Day 1. BA/AnO_2
   (*a*) + + 0.5 mm translucent β-haem.; G + strep.
   + + + 0.2 mm α-haem.
   +   0.5 mm non-haem.
   Tellurite.*
    Sterile, reincubated.
   (*a*) to glucose broth for grouping.

Day 2. Tellurite.
   (*b*) ± 0.5 mm black moist; cocci.
   (*a*) Lancefield group A C G
       + − −

Report.
 Cultures yield *Str. pyogenes. No C. diphtheriae isolated.*

Reports

In order to avoid confusion there should be uniformity of reports sent

*Hoyle's blood tellurite agar.

from the laboratory. There is unfortunately a very wide choice of names for most of the common bacteria and, although it is a mistake to cling to the old-fashioned names solely because they are popular with physicians and surgeons who learned them many years ago, it is unnecessarily confusing if new names are continually being introduced in an effort to keep up to date. Advances in the classification of bacteria have benefited both clinician and microbiologist. It is therefore important that the correct generic and specific names be generally adopted. The terminology used in this text is based on the seventh edition of *Topley and Wilson's Principles of Bacteriology, Virology and Immunity* (Wilson, *et al.*, 1983).

When reporting mixed cultures some indication should be given, whenever possible, of the most important pathogen. This is often done by stating the amount of growth – heavy, moderate or scanty – of each type of microbe, hoping that from this the clinician will be able to gauge their importance. Unfortunately the unjustified assumption is often made that the proportion of each type of bacterium in the culture accurately reflects the proportion of each in the lesion. Many highly pathogenic bacteria which flourish in the tissues, as judged by their numbers in the stained film, and grow fairly well in pure culture may be outgrown in mixed culture; moreover, even if the bacteria flourish both in tissues and on artificial media, since the oxygen tension in the wound is unknown, it is clearly impossible to judge which culture results reflect best the conditions in the wound when the proportion differs on the aerobic and anaerobic plates. The futility of assessing the proportion of different microbes in a wound from the culture of a single swab may be demonstrated by taking several swabs from different areas in the same wound on the same occasion, when, even if the wound is small, there is commonly a marked difference in the proportion of different types of bacteria found in the cultures.

It is clear then that there are many factors, some outside the microbiologist's control, which influence the relative number of colonies of different types in mixed cultures. Therefore, the amount of growth of each type is not routinely reported; instead the bacteria are named in order of their importance as judged from the stained film, the plate culture and their reputation as pathogens. When, however, a series of cultures is made in an attempt to assess the results of treatment, for example in a streptococcal carrier, it may be useful to report the amount of growth of the pathogen, but in this case the specimens should be taken and the cultures made by the same person under the same conditions on each occasion.

Interpretation of results

The microbiologist is often called upon to assess the significance of positive and negative results, particularly in specimens from carriers. Each case of this kind must be judged on its own merits, but the first thing to decide is how far the culture results represent conditions in the infected area. It is never possible to give a reliable opinion on results from a single specimen. If, when a series of, say, three throat swabs have been taken by an experienced sampler and have been seeded without delay, they have consistently yielded a few colonies only of the pathogen, it is reasonable to assume that there are only a few of them in the throat.

Negative results from faeces depend to a very great extent on the type of normal flora present. If they are mainly lactose fermenters and grow poorly on the selective media used, it may be possible to isolate the pathogens when there are only 30–50/ml of faeces suspension cultured, but if there are many non-lactose fermenters including *Proteus* and *Pseudomonas* which flourish in these media it may be impossible to detect pathogens unless they are present in the order of 10^8 viable bacteria per ml of suspension.

Although this difficulty does not arise in cultures of material which is normally sterile it may yet be difficult to assess the significance of positive and negative results. It is impossible to prove, in the logical sense, the absence of bacteria. By a negative result we may mean that routine aerobic and anaerobic cultures are negative after 48 hours' incubation. If the specimen has been efficiently taken from an untreated patient this excludes acute infection by the common pathogens, which may be all that is required; but investigations lasting many weeks are necessary before it is possible to give an opinion that a lesion is not caused by bacterial infection, and this can never be certain until an alternative diagnosis is established. The significance of a positive result must be judged in relation to the patient's tissue response, and to the presence or absence of specific antibodies to the bacterium isolated. The presence of a bacterium in a normally sterile specimen does not necessarily imply infection by it; the microbe may have entered the specimen during or after sampling. If the cultures were made in liquid medium it is impossible to judge the weight of original infection because heavy growth after overnight incubation may result from the presence of one viable contaminating organism. When, however, the same microbe is repeatedly found in pure culture in material from the same site sampled with due care, it may be assumed to be present in the specimen before sampling and, if there are signs of inflammation, pus cells, swelling and fever, it is probable that the bacterium is the cause of the infection; but even if all these signs are present it may still be only a secondary invader masking infection by a microbe such as *Myco. tuberculosis* or *Actinomyces bovis* which grow on artificial media with comparative difficulty. Suitably stained films may reveal the hidden pathogen, but in some cases it is discovered only later when elimination of the secondary invader has failed to cure the infection.

Computer aid for bacteriology records

Computers are essential for processing the heavy workload in large chemical pathology and haematology laboratories. The capital cost of such equipment means that there is pressure on other pathology disciplines to share the equipment. Diagnostic microbiology does not readily lend itself to computerization, as the bench work is not easily automated. Nevertheless, a computer can be very helpful for processing the data obtained from the bench.

Systems designed for the processing of numerical data (as, for example, chemical pathology results) are not suitable for microbiology. Many reports can be stylized to take advantage of rapid processing methods. However, flexibility must be a feature of the system to allow for interpretative reports involving human judgement. The report produced must therefore be as good as a manually produced one. When computer processing of microbiological data is introduced it is for the consultant microbiologist to insist that the computer serves the laboratory, and not the reverse. Modern data processing methods should allow data input using conventional typewriter keyboards and visual display units (Ridgway *et al.*, 1980). There is no need for staff to learn numerical codes or to become punch-type operators. Laboratories in Britain usually have a high turnover of staff, and this must be taken into account. The system must be easily and rapidly mastered by all laboratory staff. In addition to the processing of reports, computers can be used for calculations and statistical correlations. These functions may either be incorporated into the mainframe system or be carried out by microcomputers. However, where reporting is essentially manual, the use of a microcomputer, whilst useful for analysis of laboratory data, may result in a considerable increase in secretarial workload, owing to the need to put the data on computer file in addition to producing a report manually.

Advantages

The following advantages should be gained.

1. All specimens recently received can be listed according to the first letter of the patient's surname, enabling staff to answer telephone enquiries easily. When a report is already on its way, it will appear on the list and no search of the files is required; when it is being worked on, the laboratory number and type of specimen will enable the secretary to locate the member of staff dealing with it so that he can comment. When no record is found on the list the specimen had not been dealt with before the list was made. No day book is required and lists can be produced twice daily. The use of visual display units in addition to printed lists greatly facilitates the answering of enquiries.

2. The staff can easily check from the lists that reports have gone at the time expected and will investigate the cause of unusual delay.

3. Laboratory reports are produced automatically. Bacterial names are standardized and are clearly written; nevertheless, flexibility of reporting must be maintained.

4. Transcription between the microbiologist's report and the typed report is automatic and less liable to error.

5. Laboratory statistics including a weighting system for work done can be calculated automatically.

6. Lists can be prepared on a weekly, monthly and annual basis of positive results. These allow the infection control staff to investigate such infections as early as possible, and also to monitor trends within both hospital and community.

7. Information required for research can be stored and produced when required. Accidental omission of such information is virtually excluded.

Essentials specific for microbiology

1. The clinical information on the request form must be constantly available to the person handling the specimen.

2. Specimens arriving late should not be held up pending the requirement for secretarial staff to input details onto the computer.

3. Culture procedure depends on the number and kind of species isolated, and human judgement is repeatedly necessary. Some form of work sheet or card for recording the tests made at each stage is therefore mandatory; records as described earlier in this chapter cannot be dispensed with. The report is automatically recorded but not the evidence which led to it.

Some systems attempt to include media inoculated and results of identification tests, and, to a limited extent, this is reasonable but the need to have great flexibility if all culture specimens are to be included makes the system expensive; moreover, media and tests often change as improvements are discovered. Although rules are made for the basic procedures of primary culture nothing should be done to inhibit the laboratory worker from amplifying them in the light of clinical information or of the results of microscopic examination. Systems which include media to be inoculated and identification tests to be performed may succeed when known pathogens are to be excluded from samples such as faeces but will tend to be over-restrictive when an open mind is needed about bacteria isolated from specimens which are normally sterile.

4. The report must be checked before reaching the ward. This is best done before printing. Laboratory errors must be discovered as early in the day as possible to allow time for tests to be repeated. After printing, a rapid check can be made by the secretary because faults in print-out are almost always nonsensical and obvious.

5. Cumulative reports showing changes in normal values are one of the important advantages brought by computers. In microbiology, however, cumulative reports are not as important as they are in other disciplines because they deal not with normal values, which reflect closely the progress of the disease and the effect of treatment, but with the presence of pathogens which may indicate either failure of treatment, hospital infection during treatment, or failure to isolate or identify correctly at a previous attempt. There is usually no possibility of checking previous results because, unlike blood samples for chemistry or haematology, specimens for culture cannot usually be kept for long periods. Nevertheless, a system which enables the clinical microbiologist to see all previous reports on each patient when checking current results is of great value. It will enable him to check current work, when necessary, and may bring to light hospital infection in individual patients. The tendency to disregard results which cannot be checked and are 'not consistent with previous results' must be resisted unless there is good reason to suspect they were

false (see 'Circular arguments' in Chapter 1). In the treatment of syphilis, serological results indicate progress and cumulative reports should be provided when possible. A chronological list of all microbiological results is also useful when summarizing the patient's record at the end of an infectious illness.

6. When the computer is to be used to process results of a clinical research investigation a further check is usually needed. It cannot safely be assumed that information on the request form is correct, and when it is to be included in the programme it must be verified. Further tests may be needed, for example, to check sensitivity to antibiotics not needed in treatment, or to identify in more detail microbes relevant to the investigation but not to the patient's illness.

Problems common to all disciplines

1. Provision must be made for processing specimens from patients before they have received their hospital identification number.

2. The laboratory should not be tied to specific times for using the computer. To obtain maximum benefit, with minimum inconvenience, the system should be available day and night, including weekends. File copying and essential maintenance will be necessary, but can be organized outside peak user times.

3. Any part of the mechanical process may break down and although every effort to restore the service will be made an alternative reporting system is essential for emergency use. Computer staff must be available whenever the laboratory is open (usually daily throughout the year) because once a successful computer reporting system is in use reversion to a manual system puts a severe strain on the laboratory staff and is acceptable only for short periods of mechanical breakdown.

Reporting without the computer

Reports can be quickly made without secretarial or computer help by using pre-printed self-adhesive stickers applied to the top copy of a duplicate no-carbon-required (NCR) request form. Details of such a system are to be found in the previous edition of this book (Stokes and Ridgway, 1980).

Quality control

There is no longer any doubt that quality control is essential for the maintenance of high standards in laboratory diagnosis. The assessment of performance in microbiology is not easy because many of the specimens contain living microbes. Those of medical interest are often fragile and liable to die before they can be identified, especially when the specimen contains antimicrobial drugs. Other commensal or contaminating bacteria tend to be more robust and are liable to outgrow the pathogens. When no pathogen is isolated, it is therefore easy to assume none was present or that they were killed by treatment. False identification will not be suspected without some form of monitoring.

Serum samples for estimation of antibody or antigen are more stable, but human serum containing them is difficult to obtain and antibody artificially prepared in animal serum is not a satisfactory substitute. Test material for assessment in hospital microbiology laboratories is therefore difficult to provide. Quality control is of two kinds, internal and external.

Internal quality control

To ensure that equipment is properly maintained and working satisfactorily is a basic need of all laboratories. This routine task may lapse unless a check-list is made and attended to daily. In microbiology this will include temperature checks on all incubators and waterbaths. Anaerobic jars and incubators need daily checking. Chemical indicators of anaerobiosis are helpful but a biological test is also needed; the simplest is to show lack of growth of a strict aerobe (e.g. *Pseudomonas* species) but a demonstration of ability to sustain the growth of a strict anaerobe (e.g. *Cl. novyi (oedematiens)*) is a better indicator. Poor results are often caused by inferior culture medium, which may be because the ingredients were inferior, preparation was faulty or there was contamination by microbial inhibitors. All bench workers must be constantly on the lookout for evidence of these faults but tests for them are time consuming and not easily carried out. Ability to support growth of a stock laboratory strain of a pathogen when heavily inoculated is not good evidence that the medium will yield growth of the pathogen in a specimen when present in small numbers, growing *in vitro* for the first time and perhaps competing with less fragile commensals. Selective media are particularly likely to be faulty and there may be plate-to-plate variation when the ingredients have been insufficiently mixed. Regular checks of such media to test adequate growth of the pathogens and inhibition of likely commensals are too laborious to be undertaken by most laboratories, but faults will come to light if simulated 'specimens' containing known pathogens are regularly examined.

External quality control or quality assessment

The preparation and distribution of simulated 'specimens' is a laborious and highly skilled task. In Britain the United Kingdom External Quality Assessment Scheme (UKEQAS) has been set up to undertake this task and to assess the results. It is believed that all UK laboratories receiving specimens from patients participate, including those outside the National Health Service. Laboratories serving the armed forces overseas also participate and some laboratories outside the UK. Participation is voluntary.

The main purpose of the scheme is educational. It enables laboratories to assess their performance in comparison with all other participants. The 'specimens' distributed may contain important but rare pathogens such as *C. diphtheriae*, *Salm. typhi* or *Vib. cholerae*, which helps them to ensure that their technique is adequate when the need arises. 'Specimens' contain varying numbers of pathogens, as they would in practice. The same strain is sometimes distributed on more than one occasion; when a laboratory fails to achieve the same result on both occasions faulty technique is obvious. Negative 'specimens' containing only commensals are also sent.

Most 'specimens' are lyophilized and no attempt is made to disguise them as true specimens. To ensure that the examination is relevant a brief clinical statement is included as might be received on a properly completed request form. Results arriving after the expiry of a short time limit are not scored; in practice they would be useless. After the expiry date participants receive a notice of the intended results to enable them to request a culture of any pathogen they failed to isolate, or identify correctly, and to help them investigate the cause of failure without undue delay. A computer print-out of the scores arrives as soon as possible.

These distributions of simulated specimens and assessment of all the results comprise a tool to enable participants to monitor and improve their performance; it is not a competition. Laboratories who examine these 'specimens' more meticulously than normal are misusing the tool. We think the most useful procedure on receiving quality assessment specimens is to examine them exactly as if they were normal specimens by whoever would do so on that day. In addition, if a senior member of staff also examines them, a correct result may be obtained when the routine method fails. This teaches junior staff and encourages them to achieve good technique and maintain a high routine standard. When the junior succeeds and the senior fails, lack of judgement or expertise is unlikely and the reason may be traced to faulty medium preparation, especially plate-to-plate variation of a selective medium (see above).

Time should be set aside to discuss quality control results and perhaps the need to change technique. A laboratory performing badly and showing no evidence of improvement receives confidential notification that this is so and will be offered help from senior colleagues appointed by professional bodies to undertake this task. Only these helpers will know which are the poor performers, confidentiality being achieved by a numerical code of the participants.

An additional advantage of UKEQAS is the ability to relate methods to results in the field. A comparison of methods under standard conditions in a single, or a few, specialist laboratories is valuable, but the best methods emerging from such tests are not necessarily the best when performed by less specialized staff under routine conditions. The need to change technique is much more forcefully demonstrated when a good technique consistently achieves the best results in the examination of simulated specimens in nation-wide distributions. Sometimes a technique seldom performed and needing special materials shows a widespread lack of expertise when tested by UKEQAS. Two examples are the Vi antibody test and toxicity tests for *C. diphtheriae*. It is then apparent that it would be better and more cost-effective for these tests to be performed only in reference laboratories. When the committee of microbiologists who advise UKEQAS is satisfied that assessment of methods related to results is valid, they are published. Results of diphtheria toxin production from distributed cultures of *C. diphtheriae* (Snell *et al.*, 1984b) and a comparison of antibiotic susceptibility test methods (Snell *et al.*, 1984a, c) are completed assessments so far. Reed *et al.* (1985a, b) give an account of methods of organizing and assessing distributions for virology.

References

Hamilton-Miller, J.M.T. and Brumfitt, W. (1974) *British Medical Journal* iii, 410

Heimer, G.V., Joseph, N. and Taylor, C.E.D. (1978) *Journal of Clinical Pathology* 31, 185

Holmes, B., Willcox, W.R., Lapage, S.P. and Malnick, H. (1977) *Journal of Clinical Pathology* 30, 381

Reed, S.E., Gardner, P.S., Snell, J.J.S. and Chai, O. (1985a) *Journal of Clinical Pathology* 38, 534

Reed, S.E., Gardner, P.S. and Stanton, J. (1985b) *Journal of Clinical Pathology* 38, 542

Ridgway, G.L., Batchelor, J.G., Luton, A.L. and Barnicoat, M.J. (1980) *Journal of Clinical Pathology* 33, 744

Snell, J.J.S., Brown, D.F.J. and Gardner, P.S. (1984a) *Journal of Clinical Pathology* 37, 321

Snell, J.J.S., Damello, J.V., Gardner, P.S., Kwantes, W. and Brooks, R. (1984b) *Journal of Clinical Pathology* 37, 769

Snell, J.J.S., Danvers, M.V.S. and Gardner, P.S. (1984c) *Journal of Clinical Pathology* 37, 1059

Stokes, E.J. and Ridgway, G.L. (1980) *Clinical Bacteriology*, 5th edn. Edward Arnold, London

Wilson, G.S., Miles, A.A. and Parker M.T. (Eds.) (1983) *Topley and Wilson's Principles of Bacteriology, Virology and Immunity*, 7th edn. Edward Arnold, London

3

The Culture of Specimens Normally Sterile

Any bacterium recovered from a body fluid which is normally sterile should be regarded as a potential pathogen. The aim of the cultures is to recover any known human pathogen. If, however, a microbe previously considered to be harmless is found, it must not lightly be dismissed as a contaminant (see Chapter 1).

All strains isolated are identified at least as far as the genus, and in most cases tests are carried further so that the species can be named. This is not unduly laborious because in many cases a single species only is found. Pleural and peritoneal fluids, however, commonly yield a mixed growth and anaerobes are often found in these sites. Mixed infection of the blood and cerebrospinal fluid does occasionally occur and it is important not to overlook it, since antibiotic therapy may fail if an unsuspected second invader is resistant to the drug chosen for treatment.

Blood

When blood is cultured for the diagnosis of bacteraemia, the number of viable organisms which may be circulating in it is usually small, often about one or two per millilitre, sometimes less. Among the species which may be found are several which are delicate and grow with comparative difficulty in culture media; for example, *Haemophilus influenzae, Neisseria meningitidis*, non-sporing anaerobes and the brucella group. Almost all known pathogens, and some organisms usually considered harmless, have been recovered from blood. It follows that a good technique is one in which a relatively large volume is cultured under conditions which favour, as far as possible, the growth of all known pathogens. The blood must not be allowed to clot since the few bacteria present may form colonies in the interior of the clot, making them inaccessible to examination. Finally the natural antibacterial power of the blood must be neutralized. Anticoagulants such as citrate and oxalate in the concentration necessary to prevent clotting are to some extent antibacterial; they may be dispensed with by adding blood to large volumes of nutrient medium so that clotting is prevented by dilution, or sodium polyanethol sulphonate (Liquoid) can be employed which is less inhibitory than other anticoagulants. Moreover, it neutralizes the bactericidal power of fresh blood and will withstand autoclaving; it is used at a final concentration of 0.03–0.05 g/dl (von

Haebler and Miles, 1938). (See page 313.) However, no single medium is ideal for all likely organisms; at least two different and complementary media should be employed (see below).

Selective and enrichment broths are not recommended for blood culture because selective agents are likely to inhibit slightly the bacteria selected. Enrichment is not necessary because a good quality broth must be employed and it is enriched by the presence of the blood. Even when *Mycoplasma hominis*, which is demonstrably inhibited by antibody, is the cause of bacteraemia it can be isolated from Liquoid blood broth without added enrichment (Stokes, 1955). The method described below is aimed at isolating bacteria from the blood of patients in Britain.

Method: media (see Chapter 10)

Diphasic medium incubated in air plus 5–10% CO_2

The two phases of this medium are 10 ml Liquoid broth and a nutrient agar slope. The bottle is incubated in the upright position and it can be subcultured daily without opening by tipping the blood broth over the agar slope, being careful not to wet the cap. It is particularly useful when large numbers of cultures have to be subcultured. A disadvantage is that the broth must be added after the slope has been made and therefore contamination during preparation is possible. (Commercially prepared medium containing air + CO_2 is available and recommended for use (see page 313).) Moreover, colonies on the slope must be inspected through the bottle glass and, when they are very small, or translucent and confluent, their presence may be missed. Colonies of rapidly growing organisms such as *Staphylococcus aureus* and *Salmonella typhi* can be easily seen and delay in reporting is minimal. Fungi and bacteria which tend to grow in clumps may be more quickly recognized because all the blood broth is tipped over the agar and therefore the chance that a few clumps will adhere to the slope and form visible colonies is greater than when a loopful only is subcultured. Incubation with added CO_2 is essential for the primary isolation of *Brucella abortus*. In our hands this medium has yielded growth of *Bruc. abortus* unexpectedly from the blood of an elderly patient with fever and arthritis, from a patient already treated with tetracycline as well as from febrile patients already diagnosed serologically; the addition of liver broth when brucellosis is suspected is not necessary. CO_2 is also required for the isolation of some streptococci causing endocarditis and, rarely, for other CO_2-dependent species. Its presence is not known to inhibit medically important aerobes. Liquoid is inhibitory to *Neisseria gonorrhoeae*. The addition of 1% gelatin to the medium is necessary to neutralize this effect if disseminated gonococcal infection is suspected (Staneck and Vincent, 1981).

Fastidious anaerobe broth (FAB)

Anaerobes are present in at least 10 per cent of positive blood cultures from patients in general hospitals. The only strict aerobes likely to be found are *Brucella* species and *Pseudomonas aeruginosa*. Enriched thioglycollate broths will support the growth of small inocula of both sporing and non-sporing anaerobes. These organisms may be inhibited by Liquoid. Clotting is prevented by diluting the blood sample in 75 ml of medium. Most pathogens will grow in this medium; however, the recovery of *Ps. aeruginosa* is unreliable. FAB (Ganguli *et al.*, 1982) is a thioglycollate-containing medium with resazurin as an indicator. The indicator turns blue if the anaerobiosis is inadequate, and the medium should not then be used.

Temperature of the medium

It is probably wise to warm the media before inoculation by leaving a few bottles ready for use in the incubator. Model and Peel (1973) cast doubt on the need for this provided the cultures can be incubated directly after venepuncture, but further evidence is needed before the practice can confidently be abandoned.

Time of sampling

The number of bacteria found in the blood varies from time to time in the same patient and it is clearly desirable to take the sample when many are present. When the pyrexia is intermittent, with rigors, sampling when the patient feels a rigor approaching is more likely to yield isolates than at other times. The time of maximum opportunity cannot often be predicted. Other febrile patients are not likely to have such extreme variation in the bacterial population of their blood and cultures may be taken at any time. When treatment is urgent, two cultures (4 bottles) can be taken within an hour so that treatment may proceed.

Obtaining the sample

To sample blood for culture is a sterile technique. It is no longer practicable for laboratory staff to obtain all specimens for blood cultures. Consequently, it is important to ensure that clinicians are aware of the need for care if contamination is to be avoided. Commensal organisms are frequently isolated from blood cultures. This can lead to confusion either due to more fastidious organisms being overgrown or in the interpretation of the significance of the isolate, particularly in the immunosuppressed patient. One advantage of laboratory staff obtaining the sample is that first-hand information on the patients' condition and previous antimicrobial chemotherapy can be obtained, which may affect the method of culture or interpretation of the results.

When blood is being withdrawn for multiple purposes, it is vital that blood culture media are inoculated first. This is particularly important when blood gas analysis is also comtemplated. Pseudobacteraemia may result from contamination of the syringe from the blood gas apparatus or from unsterile collection bottles.

The hands of the operator should be thoroughly washed and dried before the procedure. The wearing of a gown or mask is unnecessary. The proposed site for venepuncture should be prepared by cleaning the skin thoroughly without excessive friction. An isopropyl alcohol wipe should be used and the skin allowed to dry. Following disinfection, the venepuncture site should not be further palpated.

Commercially produced media are capped with perforated metal caps, covered with foil which is removed before inoculating the bottle. The penetrable part of the cap is sterile under the foil, and must not be touched or 'sterilized' before inserting the needle.

Venepuncture is performed in the usual way, 20 ml blood being withdrawn into a sterile syringe. The needle is then removed and replaced by a second sterile needle. Maintaining strict aseptic technique, 5 ml of blood is inoculated into each bottle. The remainder should be transferred to a plain sterile bottle and allowed to clot. The serum obtained from this bottle will be kept frozen for serological tests when required. Immunosuppressed patients are frequently on antimicrobial drugs during febrile episodes. High volume blood cultures (15–20 ml per bottle) will increase the yield of isolates in this group of patients. When only a small volume of blood can be obtained, it is better to inoculate a single bottle only, rather than distribute very small quantities among several bottles. For an adult, FAB is usually the best choice. In small children and infants, less than 20 ml is usually available. In general, all the blood should be cultured, none being saved for serology. If less than 5 ml is available, the diphasic medium should be used because the additional CO_2 is necessary for the isolation of some strains of *Str. pneumoniae*, *N. meningitidis* and *H. influenzae*. The possibility of anaerobic infection of neonates should be considered, and the FAB medium (which will support the growth of most coliforms also) should be inoculated unless *Ps. aeruginosa* is considered likely.

Number of samples

The idea that the more samples taken from each patient the greater the likelihood of a positive result is erroneous. A laboratory having to subculture innumerable blood broths, most of which are sterile, cannot be expected to give proper attention to those which really matter. It has been shown that when the first two samples are negative the chance of a positive result from further samples is remote (Crowley, 1970). More than one sample should, however, be taken before treatment is given because of the risk of contamination which may ruin a single sample. Two samples (4 bottles) are sufficient from patients suspected of acute generalized infection in whom treatment is urgent. Three samples (6 bottles) are recommended in other patients. It may sometimes be worthwhile to take another three samples when these prove to be negative but the microbiologist should be consulted before doing so.

Recognition of growth

All bottles should be checked daily for visible growth. Staphylococcal and coliform growth is easily seen; streptococci often form visible colonies on the surface of sedimented red cells when these are not lysed by streptococcal haemolysins. In addition to the presence of colonies on the solid phase of the diphasic medium, bottles that contain gas bubbles or are clouded after overnight incubation should be regarded as potentially containing organisms. It should not be assumed that when no growth is seen the blood broth is sterile. It is possible to obtain confluent growth when a loopful is subcultured from such a bottle. Moreover, bacteria such as non-sporing anaerobes which form small translucent colonies on blood agar may never produce visible opacity in blood broth. Growth in bottles is also very difficult to recognize when the red cells have degenerated and there is no longer clear supernatant fluid above them. White blood cells may aggregate on the surface of the sedimented red blood cells and give a false impression of bacterial colonies.

The thioglycollate bottle should be subcultured after 48 hours' incubation, unless evidence of growth is seen earlier, further subculturing to be done after 72 hours and 7 days of incubation. Unless growth is seen, it is unnecessary and unwise to subculture the diphasic medium until the seventh day. Most significant isolates will be obtained within 2–3 days of inoculation; prolonged incubation is necessary in only a few circumstances (e.g. infective endocarditis and brucellosis). All bottles for prolonged incubation should be subcultured weekly until discarded (usually after at least 3 weeks of incubation).

Subculturing is conveniently and economically carried out by spreading a loopful from each bottle over a sector of enriched agar, one-sixth of an 8.5 cm Petri dish. Two plates should be inoculated from each bottle. As growth of *Haemophilus* species may be unreliable on blood agar, a chocolate blood agar plate incubated in air plus CO_2 and a blood agar plate incubated anaerobically with 10% CO_2 should be used. The air-plus CO_2 plate should be examined after 24 hours' incubation, and reincubated for a further 24 hours if no growth is seen. When no growth is visible in the thioglycollate bottle, plates should be examined after 2 and 3 days' incubation. Delicate anaerobes are more likely to grow when they are not frequently exposed to air. The use of an anaerobic cabinet is recommended, but not essential provided that plates are returned to an anaerobic environment as soon as possible. A hand lens should be used to inspect all plate cultures; colonies of non-sporing anaerobes may be difficult to see. Plates prepared from day 7 subcultures should be incubated for 3 days before discard. Bottles should also be finally inspected at this time if they are to be discarded. Thus, routinely, blood cultures are kept for a total of 10 days.

When growth is seen or suspected in any bottle, both bottles should be examined further. Blood broth is inoculated onto whole chocolate and blood agar plates, for incubation as above. Growth on anaerobic plates from the thioglycollate bottle should be immediately subcultured to another blood agar plate and reincubated without delay. A further blood agar plate should be inoculated and incubated in air plus 10% CO_2, to check that the organism is an anaerobe. The addition of CO_2 for this purpose will prevent CO_2-dependent organisms from being misidentified as strict anaerobes. Discrete colonies seen in the broth media should be transferred by pipette into a sterile tube, taking with them as small a volume of fluid as possible so that Gram-stain, subculture and antibiotic sensitivity tests may be more easily performed. If facilities for gas-liquid chromatography (GLC) are available, analysis of the thioglycollate broth may assist identification of anaerobic organisms.

All organisms should be Gram-stained. The significance will be doubtful when the Gram-stains from each bottle are not identical. However, morphology may be affected by the broth medium; for example, streptococci (including *Str. pneumoniae*) are sometimes elongate and may be mistaken for diphtheroids. Typical streptococcal forms are usually visible, however, and on subculture the strain will revert to typical morphology. If there is any doubt, subculturing to Loeffler's medium will confirm the morphology.

Growth from each bottle must be identified. When a single isolate proves to be an unlikely contaminant, further blood cultures may be necessary to decide its significance. Contact with the clinical staff will be rewarding to gain further information on other risk factors, such as intravenous infusion lines, and immunological status. The disadvantage of using two bottles only is that growth from a single bottle may signify simply a preference of the microbe for these culture conditions; moreover, the sampling error is great. Any organism can be significant, and no isolate should be dismissed without further evidence to confirm that it is a contaminant. Growth deep in the thioglycollate bottle should be investigated without delay because Gram-stains of clostridia and anaerobic cocci can easily be mistaken for *Bacillus* species and micrococci.

Antibiotic sensitivity should be tested from each bottle when either *Staph. aureus* or coagulase-negative staphylococci are isolated. Major difference in senstitivity between strains casts doubt on the significance of the growth. With species of bacteria less commonly present on the skin this precaution can be omitted. Diphtheroid-like organisms should not be too easily dismissed. Streptococci can appear diphtheroid-like, as can *Listeria monocytogenes* which is an important cause of neonatal sepsis. Resistant diphtheroids of the J-K group cause septicaemia in immunosuppressed patients (see page 109).

Prevention of laboratory contamination

The use of a laminar-flow cabinet is not essential for subculture. The loop wire should be sufficiently long to sample the bottles without introducing the handle of the loop into them. When flaming, the bottle should be carried sideways to the flame, not scooped towards it, collecting air-borne contaminants *en route*.

When bottles are incubated in jars with plates they must be on top of the plates and either in racks made for the purpose or supported with clean paper to prevent them from falling over. Do not use cotton wool for this purpose; it is often contaminated with spores.

Penicillinase and other antimicrobial inhibitors

β-lactam antibiotics are the most likely treatment to have been given before blood culture is requested, and β-lactamase may be routinely incorporated in culture media but there are disadvantages in this. Because penicillinase is unstable it must be introduced after autoclaving, which may lead to contamination; moreover, it does not survive indefinitely, so large amounts have to be introduced if a sufficient quantity is to be guaranteed to neutralize penicillins at the time of culture. Since it is a biological product and is not normally tested for its effect on the growth of small numbers of a wide variety of pathogens, one cannot be sure that it does not also have slight antibacterial properties. For these reasons and because the culture of blood in the presence of antibiotics is to be discouraged, it is better to introduce an appropriate dose of penicillinase when it is required. This must be done by skilled laboratory staff because of the danger of contamination. There are a variety of β-lactamases, some of which inactivate penicillins but have little effect on cephalosporins, and others in which the position is reversed. A preparation which inactivates both groups of drugs can be obtained commercially and is best for routine use in blood cultures (Waterworth, 1973), (see page 14).

Para-aminobenzoic acid is an inhibitor of sulphonamides; it is also a growth factor for some species and will withstand autoclaving. It should be added routinely (50 mg/l) to blood culture broth. Resins are commercially available, designed to remove antimicrobial substances from the blood for culture. These resins are expensive and it is doubtful whether their routine use is justified. It is more important to try to obtain cultures before therapy is instigated, whenever possible.

Pour plates

These are of limited value though highly recommended by some. They are best made by transporting molten agar to the bedside and making the plates directly. Alternatively, 3 ml (i.e. 1 ml blood) can be withdrawn from one of the aerobic culture bottles to make a pour plate on return to the laboratory. There is no doubt that in some cases growth may be recognized earlier and, moreover, the number of colonies seen when coagulase-negative staphylococci are isolated may help to distinguish between true infection and contamination. However, laboratory contamination of these plates, especially when they are made by unskilled staff at night, makes interpretation difficult and diagnosis is usually rapid using the diphasic medium. When coagulase-negative staphylococcal bacteraemia is suspected, several blood cultures have usually been taken, and although a pour plate in addition would be helpful, this happens so rarely that it is not thought to be a sufficient reason for including it as a routine.

Glucose

The addition of glucose is not recommended although it may increase the rapidity of growth of some species. The bacteria having grown tend to die rapidly because of the changes in pH brought about by fermentation and it may prove impossible to subculture them successfully (Waterworth, 1972). Glucose is also used as a means of reducing Eh with the hope of culturing strict anaerobes but is totally inadequate for this purpose.

Cultures during antimicrobial treatment

If the laboratory is to give the best possible service it must be understood that to attempt culture in the presence of treatment should be done only in exceptional circumstances. Negative results for bacterial growth on such specimens are generally worthless. The idea that because the patient is not reponding to treatment the pathogen will grow is erroneous. An example is the *in vitro* sensitivity of *Salm. typhi* to tetracyclines which are useless in the treatment of typhoid fever. Blood cultures from undiagnosed typhoid patients treated with tetracycline will usually, therefore, be negative or growth will be delayed until the drug has degenerated and the bacilli have recovered sufficiently to grow.

It is usually possible, when treatment has been given, to stop it completely for 36 hours and then take cultures. A quicker result can be expected by stopping the drugs and sampling when the blood is free of them. A policy of culturing all blood sent regardless of the circumstances leads to an overwhelming number of cultures, none of which can be properly investigated through lack of laboratory time. The microbiologist should keep in close touch with clinicians to advise culture early, when appropriate, and to ensure that culture during antibiotic treatment is not undertaken unnecessarily.

When fever develops during treatment of bacteraemia the possibility of superadded infection due to resistant bacteria or fungi must be borne in mind, especially when antibiotics have been given intravenously. A more likely explanation is that the fever is a drug reaction. There are various ways in which this can be tested. Consultation between physician, pharmacologist and microbiologist is likely to solve the problem better than sending additional blood cultures which will usually be sterile.

When a sensitive organism is isolated and the patient fails to respond to appropriate treatment the possibility of a second unrecognized organism in the blood should be considered. This is most likely to happen when faecal organisms are found, the second invaders being non-sporing anaerobes which grow more slowly. Continued subculture from the anaerobic bottle on neomycin blood agar will usually reveal the additional pathogen.

Other methods

Over the past few years a number of automated methods for blood culture have become available. These involve techniques such as the radiometric or infra-red detection of carbon dioxide, measurement of changes in conductivity and lysis filtration/centrifugation. We have little personal experience of these techniques. The radiometric detection of carbon dioxide is the most reliable technique currently available and is widely employed. The method uses a relatively small volume of blood in a restricted choice of media. Caution is required in the disposal of radioactive waste, and the technique is comparatively expensive. A high standard of expertise and maintenance is required if contamination of cultures is to be minimized. Advantages centre mainly on labour saving and earlier detection of some isolates.

Bacteria found in febrile disease

Staph. aureus	*Str. pyogenes*
Coagulase-negative staphylococci	*Str. pneumoniae*
Coliforms and enteric group	Enterococci
Clostridia	*Streptococcus* spp.
Bacteroides spp.	*Haemophilus* spp.
Anaerobic cocci	*Campylobacter* spp.
Listeria monocytogenes	Corynebacteria
Neisseria spp.	Lactobacilli
	Mycoplasma hominis

It is possible to culture organisms, particularly of the salmonella group, from samples of clotted blood taken for agglutination tests, if the patient is not available for another blood sample or when antibiotics have been given after taking the clotted sample. The clot is broken by shaking with sterile beads in a screw-capped bottle and is then distributed into two tubes, one containing broth, the other bile broth or tetrathionate broth. Growth can be expected only if the blood was heavily infected; negative results are of little significance.

Marrow

In typhoid fever positive cultures are sometimes obtained from the marrow when blood culture is negative. In any undiagnosed general infection when the blood is sterile, the possibility of a positive result from marrow culture should be considered; if the marrow is to be examined microscopically it should also be cultured. The method is the same as for blood, but since the quantity of marrow withdrawn for culture is unlikely to exceed 2.5 ml it is best to place the whole of it in the diphasic bottle incubated in air plus 5–10% CO_2, because in Britain *Bruc. abortus*, a salmonella or other aerobe is most likely to be isolated. When only a very small amount is available, nutrient broth is added to the culture so that the proportion of marrow plus broth to Liquoid broth is approximately 1 : 2; otherwise the concentration of Liquoid may be too high and may inhibit the growth of delicate bacteria.

Cerebrospinal fluid

The fluid should arrive still warm and either be examined immediately or placed in the incubator for examination within an hour.

Macroscopic examination

Note the colour and the presence of turbidity, deposit or clot. When there is no clot, count the number of white cells per millilitre of fluid using a white blood cell counting chamber. When serial samples of fluid are obtained from a single lumbar puncture the last sample will contain the most representative cell count and distribution. Then transfer about 2 ml of the fluid to a sterile centrifuge tube and centrifuge at about 3000 r.p.m. for 5 minutes. Transfer the supernatant fluid to a separate clean container for chemical examination. Seed the deposit for culture, as described below, and make smears on three clean glass slides. If the specimen is clotted, transfer three small pieces of clot onto clean glass slides, tease them out and allow them to dry. Cells and bacteria, if present, are most likely to be found in the clot. Add some sterile beads to the remaining fluid and clot, and shake thoroughly to break it up before the fluid is centrifuged.

Microscopic examination

Stain one film with Gram's stain for bacteria, one with Leishman's stain for a differential cell count and leave the third for auramine or Ziehl–Neelsen stain for acid-fast bacilli, if required. Alternatively, the third slide can be stained for 30 seconds with methylene blue. This has the advantage that background debris stains poorly, allowing better contrast between organism and background, particularly with Gram-negative bacteria.

It is usually possibly to discover from the total and differential cell counts whether or not the patient has bacterial meningitis. When the fluid is turbid with white cells, mostly polymorphs, the causal organism is likely to be *N. meningitidis, Str. pneumoniae* or *H. influenzae.* The Gram-stain may show organisms resembling one of these. A positive result is a very valuable guide to treatment, which is urgent. No effort should therefore be spared in searching for bacteria. It is particularly important in tuberculosis because positive cultures cannot be observed quickly. Several drops of deposit should be placed on one spot on the slide, each being allowed to dry before the next is added; since there is little cell debris the acid-fast bacilli can be more easily seen when concentrated thus in a small area. A preliminary report may now be sent, but on no account should the investigation be allowed to stop at this stage; morphological appearances may be deceptive and a satisfactory diagnosis has not been made until the causal organism has been cultured and identified by appropriate tests. When the cell count shows only a few lymphocytes and when no abnormality is seen in fluid from a patient with meningism, an attempt to isolate virus is worthwhile. The fluid should either be dealt with by the virus laboratory forthwith or be frozen at a temperature not exceeding $-70°C$ until it can be received there. A sample of clotted blood, a throat swab in virus transport medium and a stool sample (not a rectal swab) should also be sent.

Culture

The deposit is seeded onto chocolate blood agar incubated in air plus 5–10% CO_2, a blood agar plate incubated anaerobically and into cooked meat broth. The anaerobic culture may be omitted if the fluid does not contain white blood cells. The remainder of the fluid which has not been centrifuged should be incubated overnight. When the primary cultures are sterile it is sometimes possible to recover the pathogen by repeating the cultures from the incubated fluid next day, or from subcultures from the cooked meat broth.

In most cases of meningitis if the fluid has been efficiently sampled before treatment, a pure growth of the pathogen will be obtained.

A co-agglutination slide test (Phadebact CSF Test) is available to detect capsular antigen to *H. influenzae* type b, *Str. pneumoniae*, *N. meningitidis* and *Str. agalactiae* (group B). The test is simple to perform on the original specimen, and is a useful additional test to the above. False negatives are not uncommon, whereas false positives are rare. Cross-reaction may occur between certain serotypes of *Str. pneumoniae* and *H. influenzae* type b, and between *N. meningitidis* type b and the Kl antigen of *Esch. coli*.

Bacteria found

ADULTS AND CHILDREN	NEONATES
N. meningitidis	Enterobacteriaceae
Str. pneumoniae	*Streprococcus* group B
H. influenzae	
Lis. monocytogenes	
Myco. tuberculosis	

The species listed are most commonly found in meningitis. The last two on the adult list are normally associated with lymphocytes rather than polymorphs in the infected fluid. Listeria resemble diphtheroids in the deposit and must not be disregarded. Almost all medically important bacteria have been isolated from the cerebrospinal fluid; moreover, if saprophytes find their way into the subdural space, either as a result of injury or when a needle is introduced, they may cause inflammation of the meninges, which are more vulnerable to attack than other tissues.

Serous fluids
(pleural, pericardial, ascitic, synovial, bursa, hydrocele)

Macroscopic and microscopic examination are made in the manner described for cerebrospinal fluid (page 34), omitting the total white cell count. When the fluid is purulent it is treated as pus (page 46).

Culture

The deposit is seeded on two blood agar plates and into cooked meat broth. One plate is incubated in air plus 5–10% CO_2, the other anaerobically plus about 10% CO_2.

When the plate cultures are sterile they are reincubated. The cooked meat culture is examined: when there is evidence of growth it is well mixed and seeded on two blood agar plates for incubation as above; when there is no evidence of growth it is reincubated and subcultured on the following day.

When growth is present on the original blood agar plates and all bacteria seen in the original Gram-stained smear have been accounted for the cooked meat broth may be discarded. It is used in the first place to encourage the growth of both anaerobes and aerobes when there are very few of them in the specimen. Even if large numbers of viable organisms were originally present they may have diminished very considerably by the time the fluid is cultured, particularly when it contains natural or therapeutic bactericides. The chance of recovering pathogens is increased by inoculation of a fluid medium with the whole of the deposit from a large volume of centrifuged fluid, but the significance of growth from a primary liquid culture is always difficult to assess, since one viable contaminating organism may yield abundant growth after overnight incubation.

Procedure

Examine the plate cultures, using a hand lens, and make a note of the amount of growth and the colonial morphology. Then pick a single colony of each type, Gram-stain and inoculate into suitable medium for identification. Colonial differences may be found to be due to variants of one species but such colonies must be assumed different until proved the same. Fluids from cavities which have opened either spontaneously (e.g. bronchopleural fistula) or at operation frequently become infected with several species; each must be identified.

Bacteria found

Str. pneumoniae
Str. pyogenes
Staph. aureus
Haemophilus spp.
Non-sporing anaerobic bacilli
Anaerobic streptococci
Myco. tuberculosis
Actinomyces

Secondary invaders

α-Haemolytic streptococci
Str. faecalis
Klebsiella spp.
Esch. coli
Ps. aeruginosa
Proteus spp.
Other coliforms
Diphtheroids

Urine

Urine is the only specimen normally sterile which need not be routinely cultured anaerobically. Anaerobic infection of the urinary tract is rare, but should be borne in mind if routine cultures are sterile in the presence of pus cells and symptoms. The normal human urethra is not sterile and even a carefully taken catheter specimen will usually contain a few organisms. For this reason, the use of broth cultures for urine is unsuitable unless the urine has been obtained direct from the bladder, either by aspiration at operation or through the abdominal wall. Small numbers of micro-organisms will flourish in broth culture and give misleading results.

Catheterization for the purpose of obtaining a urine specimen is seldom justifiable, owing to the risk of introducing infection. Carefully collected midstream urine should be obtained. In men the prepuce should be retracted if necessary, and the glans penis washed and dried. In women the labia should be parted, and the interlabial area washed and dried. The use of disinfectants to clean the perineum prior to obtaining the specimen is unnecessary, and may result in the inhibition of bacterial growth. Urine specimens should either be cultured within an hour of voiding or stored at 4°C immediately. No laboratory technique will give a reliable result on a poorly obtained specimen left for many hours at room temperature. There are a number of commercially prepared spoons or dip slides which, when dipped in freshly voided urine, will yield significant numbers of urinary pathogens after incubation. These are ideal for use in areas where rapid transport to the laboratory is difficult or refrigeration impracticable (e.g. from general practices). However, they are comparatively expensive and there is no advantage to be gained by using them in hospital. Further advice on the collection and transport of urine samples will be found in the PHLS Monograph No. 10 (1978).

Macroscopic and microscopic examination

Hospital laboratories receive very large numbers of urine samples daily, the majority of which are not infected. Macroscopic examination does not help to distinguish infected from sterile samples. Even clear urine may contain significant numbers of bacteria. Microscopic examination for the presence of pus cells was traditionally the indicator of infection but is unsatisfactory because in some infected samples the pus cells lyse. Screening culture identifies the samples worth investigating but does not exclude infection because samples from treated patients may be purulent, contain bacteria, but yield no growth. Moreover, the pathogen may be incapable of growth on the screening culture.

Microscopy is time consuming and is done only on request because to examine large numbers of negative samples is wasteful. The use of flat-bottomed microtitre trays and an inverted microscope will speed the processing of urine for microscopy.

Method

Using a pipette with disposable tips, add 60 μl of freshly mixed urine to the first well of the microtitre tray. Continue thus, discarding the tip between each specimen until all wells are filled. Allow the tray to stand for 5 minutes. Using a × 20 objective on the inverted microscope, scan each well briefly.

The cell count for one field multiplied by 4 approximates to the number of cells per millilitre of urine. Pus cell counts of > 200/ml are reported as numerous. For cells counts below this, the actual number is reported. For red blood cells and squamous cells, < 40/ml are reported as few, 40–200/ml as moderate and > 200/ml as numerous. The presence and type of casts when seen should be reported, although these are often insufficiently numerous to be seen without centrifugation. When examination for them is requested, 15 ml of urine should be centrifuged and the deposit examined in a wet preparation using an ordinary slide and coverslip. When requested to give total cell counts, the urine should be examined in a white blood cell counting chamber (but see above).

Culture methods

All urine samples are screened, further cultures being based on the results of the screening test. Since the common urinary pathogens are also likely contaminants from vagina, faeces or perineal skin, a culture method which distinguishes contamination from infection is required.

Urines are cultured on a well dried cystine–lysine–electrolyte-deficient (CLED) medium 8 cm plate. One-quarter of the plate is sufficient for each sample. Using a 1 μl disposable plastic loop, the urine is spread employing an inverted cone technique (Fig. 3.1).

The technique will usually yield single colonies, allowing assessment of

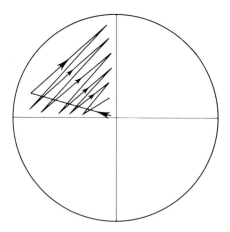

Fig. 3.1 Spreading using the inverted cone technique (initial streak from the centre to the outer edge, secondary spreading from the outer edge to the centre).

total count and enabling subculture to be performed without contamination. The urine will be sufficiently diluted over the surface of the agar to reduce the effect of any bacterial inhibitors present in the urine. Screening plates are incubated overnight in air. The urine samples are stored at 4°C.

After overnight incubation the majority of cultures will be sterile or show at most one or two colonies. Those which yield a heavy growth will be investigated further unless there is evidence of contamination, i.e. several colonial types on the CLED plate. CLED medium is well suited to this purpose because it prevents swarming as effectively as MacConkey agar but is less inhibitory, allowing contaminants to reveal their presence. The method of reporting screening culture results is given in Table 3.1.

Table 3.1   Examples of screening culture results

Culture	Report
Sterile	Screening culture negative.
Two or more colonial types	Specimen contaminated. Please repeat if required.
Apparently pure but scanty	Screening culture negative.
Apparently pure moderate or heavy growth	Screening culture under investigation.

Procedure

Significant growth is indicated by the presence of more than 100 colonies of a pure growth. This is equivalent to a total count in the original specimen of $> 10^5$ organisms per millilitre. Plate counts of between 10 and 100 colonies of a pure growth indicate total counts of 10^4–10^5. Ideally, a repeat specimen should be requested. However, frequently the patient will have commenced antibacterial therapy. Counts in this range should therefore be followed up, the organism identified and antibiotic sensitivities determined. The report should indicate that the count is of borderline significance. Occasionally, small numbers of a second colonial type will be found in the presence of a predominating organism. In this case, the predominant organism should be followed up and the report should state that there is evidence of contamination.

The count obtained by this method is adequate for routine use. Greater accuracy can be obtained with other methods, but there is little point unless the sampling technique can be relied upon. High counts due to contamination are not uncommon in urine sent from clinics and wards unless they have been refrigerated soon after voiding.

It is very important that the significance of growth should be carefully assessed in the laboratory and that the results of antibiotic sensitivity tests should not be reported unless the microbiologist is satisfied that the organisms tested are likely to be causing damage. *Esch. coli* and other common pathogens of the urinary tract are as likely as other harmless bacteria to contaminate specimens. Lack of judgement in the laboratory may lead to unnecessary treatment with antibiotics which are potentially harmful to the kidneys.

Usually infections are caused by a single species, but mixed infections are not unknown. When two species are constantly present in significant numbers in two or more specimens carefully taken, it is probable that both of them are infecting the urinary tract, but this is uncommon except in patients with a cystostomy when mixed infection is the rule.

Significant growth can usually be identified and tested for sensitivity directly from growth on the screening plate. Should this not prove possible, because of overcrowding and contamination, the original sample should be recultured using a whole CLED plate. A single colony is then picked off into peptone water, and this culture is used for further biochemical tests (e.g. API 10S, see page 111) and sensitivity testing.

Purulent specimens of urine yielding no growth by the above method on more than one occasion, in the absence of antimicrobial treatment, should be investigated as described for abacterial pyuria (see below). Prolonged incubation of the CLED plate may yield the presence of more fastidious organisms; for example, diphtheroids in significant numbers. Gram-stain of the urine deposit may prove useful. In addition to whole plate culture on CLED medium, a blood agar should be inoculated and incubated anaerobically plus 10% CO_2. Anaerobic infections will be revealed, although interpretation of growth must be made as described for aerobes, especially in women, since anaerobes or microaerophilic bacteria are likely contaminants from the vagina. Gram-stain smear of the urine in this circumstance will resemble smears from vaginal swabs.

Thymine-dependent variants of coliforms are not infrequently encountered in urinary tract infection. They will be unable to grow on sensitivity test medium which contains negligible quantities of thymine because of its inhibitory effect on sensitivity to sulphonamide and trimethoprim, but will usually grow normally on blood agar and other thymine-containing media.

'Abacterial pyuria' is a rare condition in which pus cells are found in the urine in a patient with symptoms of urinary tract infection but in the absence of bacterial growth by conventional techniques. *Myco. tuberculosis* should be excluded by culture (see page 150). The urinary deposit should be examined by both Gram and Ziehl–Neelsen (or auramine) stains and by phase-contrast or dark-ground illumination. The presence of acid-fast bacilli should be reported with caution, as they may be commensal mycobacteria. The presence of antibacterial substances in the urine should be excluded by testing it against the sensitive control *Staph. aureus* and *Esch. coli*.

When no organisms are seen in the deposit, *Mycoplasma hominis* may be the cause. Culture of the urine on a good quality defibrinated blood agar incubated anaerobically with additional CO_2 will reveal minute colonies of *Mycopl. hominis* after about 5 days. *Mycopl. hominis* may be recovered from the urine of normal people, but when present in significant numbers from uncentrifuged urine, and no other cause is found, it is reasonable to assume it is the infecting agent.

Further investigation should be based on fresh urine obtained by suprapubic aspiration. The deposit is cultured on blood agar (incubated aerobically, anaerobically plus CO_2) and in 50% human serum broth. Cultures should be examined daily for 7 days. If there is no visible growth after this time, the broth should be inoculated onto blood agar plates for anaerobic plus CO_2 and aerobic incubation before discard. Contamination of the liquid culture is inevitable unless aspirated specimens are cultured and very strict asepsis during sampling is observed.

Bacteria found (parentheses indicate exceptional finding)

Esch. coli	*Str. faecalis*	*Brucella* spp.
Klebsiella spp.	*Streptococcus* spp.	*Leptospira* spp.
Proteus spp.	*Staph. aureus*	*Bacteroides* spp.
Ps. aeruginosa	Coagulase-negative	*Mycoplasma* spp.
Salmonella spp.	staphylococci	*(Haemophilus* spp.)
(Shigella spp.)	*Corynebacterium* spp.	
Other coliforms		

Typhoid and salmonella carriers

When there are large numbers of these organisms in the urine the routine method will reveal them, but if a patient is an intermittent urinary carrier the organisms may be scanty and special methods will be necessary to recover them.

The whole of the deposit from about 30 ml of fresh clean urine is seeded into 10 ml of one or other of tetrathionate broth, selenite F or bile broth, and subcultured on MacConkey's medium after overnight incubation.

Leptospira interrogans (page 139)

Leptospira may be isolated from the urine in the second and subsequent weeks of Weil's disease. The urine should be made alkaline, when necessary, by giving the patient potassium citrate because the spirochaetes die rapidly in acid solutions.

Method

Centrifuge about 40 ml of fresh *warm* catheter urine and immediatley inoculate about 1 ml of deposit intraperitoneally into a guinea-pig. Make cultures in Fletcher's rabbit serum medium and examine the remainder under dark-ground illumination or by phase-contrast microscopy. The urine must be handled carefully since it may be highly infective. It is usually difficult to demonstrate the spirochaetes directly but they should be easily seen in the guinea-pig blood or peritoneal fluid if this is examined microscopically several times from the 4th to the 10th day after inoculation. The guinea-pig usually dies about the 10th to the 14th day, with typical postmortem findings (i.e. haemorrhages and jaundice). Samples of blood are obtained during life by heart puncture. Peritoneal fluid is most easily obtained by puncturing the abdomen with a sharp fine glass Pasteur pipette; the small quantity of fluid thus obtained is easier to handle than fluid taken with a syringe and needle. Peritoneal puncture is the method of choice.

Pathogenic viruses can be isolated from urine in various generalized infections but as far as is known they do not cause primary infection of the urinary tract in Britain. Most virus diseases are diagnosed more easily by other means. In cytomegalovirus infection in children, and in immuno-suppressed adults, examination of the urine is worthwhile. It may be possible to see inclusions in cells in the centrifuged deposit stained with Giemsa. Urine for culture should be sent fresh in an equal volume of virus transport medium. A throat swab or nasopharyngeal washings should also be sent preserved in virus transport medium at $-70°C$.

Tissue (biopsy and autopsy material)

Cultures of tissue removed at operation or post-mortem may sometimes reveal pathogens which have previously escaped isolation, either because the lesion was deep seated, beyond the reach of usual sampling methods, or because discharges from it were heavily infected with contaminating organisms. In the latter case cultures of tissues may prove successful because, unlike pus, it can first be washed free from contaminating organisms and then ground up so that the infecting bacteria within it are released into the surrounding medium.

The specimens are treated according to the nature of the investigation. Sometimes it may only be necessary to search for a known pathogen to confirm a diagnosis already made; for example, the culture of heart valves from a patient with endocarditis when the pathogen was isolated from the blood during life, or the culture of autopsy material from experimental animals infected with known strains. The method with uncontaminated specimens is to break up the tissue in a mechanical stomacher or to grind it in a sterile Griffith's tube (obtainable from Baird and Tatlock) (Fig. 3.2) or pestle and mortar, adding a little peptone water if necessary. The fluid from the grindings is seeded on solid and liquid media incubated in an atmosphere known to be suitable for the growth of the pathogen. Solid medium is used to enable identification to be made when a few organisms have contaminated the tissue during manipulation. Liquid medium usually gives a better chance of recovery if the number of the pathogen in the specimen is small, but a few contaminants will ruin the result.

Sometimes tissue, usually a lymph gland, is cultured when all other investigations have failed to establish the diagnosis in a patient with pro-longed pyrexia, when the infective nature of the pathological process is itself in doubt. In such a case it is necessary to provide conditions suitable for the growth of all known bacterial pathogens before a confident report can be made that there is no evidence of bacterial infection. This involves much labour and an extravagant use of medium but, as the result may be of vital importance, no effort should be spared. The following procedure is recommended.

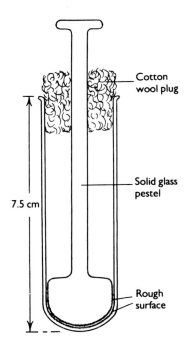

Cotton wool plug

Solid glass pestel

7.5 cm

Rough surface

Fig. 3.2   Griffith's tube.

The specimen is cut in half: one half for histological examination is placed in formal–saline; the other, in a dry sterile screw-capped container or in a sterile Petri dish, is sent to the laboratory for culture without delay. On arrival, a small piece is cut off and its inner surface is smeared on two clean glass slides for Leishman and Giemsa stains to show the presence of protozoa and inclusion bodies; the rest is ground as described above. Two smears are made for Gram and Ziehl–Neelsen's stains from the grindings and a little peptone water is added, if necessary, to make the volume of the remaining fluid sufficient for examination under dark-ground of phase-contrast microscopy (for motile spirochaetes) and to inoculate the following media:

Three blood agar plates and three glucose (0.5%) serum (10%) agar plates, for incubation in air, air plus 5–10% CO_2 and anaerobically plus CO_2.

Two 4% glycerol blood agar slopes and 4% glycerol blood broth, to be incubated in air plus 5–10% CO_2 for the diagnosis of glanders (page 121).

Two tubes of 30% human serum broth, two of glucose (0.5%) serum (10%) broth, to be incubated, one of each, in air plus CO_2 and the other anaerobically.

For aerobic incubation only, one tube of Robertson's cooked meat broth, and media for mycobacteria, see Chapter 6. The remainder of the fluid is inoculated intramuscularly into a guinea-pig and intraperitoneally into a guinea-pig and three mice.

The plate cultures and glycerol blood agar slopes are incubated for 7 days and examined after overnight incubation and then on alternate days. The liquid cultures are incubated for 4 weeks and subcultured every fourth day onto solid medium of similiar composition incubated in the same atmosphere. These secondary plates should be incubated for at least 4 days. They are seeded whether or not there is visible growth in the liquid cultures because, occasionally, growth which is insufficient to cause turbidity may be demonstrated by subculture on solid medium.

In recording the work done on this type of specimen is it helpful to label the original liquid cultures with large roman letters in addition to the specimen number so that subcultures can be easily distinguished. Thus the aerobic 30% serum broth culture of specimen No. 635 is 635A and all subcultures from it will be so labelled.

All the animals should be inspected daily. If the mice show signs of sickness, one of them is killed and an autopsy is performed with cultures of heart blood, spleen and peritoneal fluid (see Stokes and Ridgway, 1980). The others are left to see if the infection will prove fatal. If they die, autopsies are made. Should the guinea-pig which was inoculated intraperitoneally show signs of ill health, it is wise to take samples of its heart blood and peritoneal fluid for culture and microscopy, because if the animal survives there may be less chance later of recovering the pathogen. The fluids are examined by dark-ground illumination or phase-contrast microscopy and smears of them are stained by Gram and Ziehl–Neelsen's methods. If all the animals are alive and well after 6 weeks they are killed and examined for evidence of chronic infection; lesions found are cultured and examined histologically.

Tissue which is likely to be contaminated (i.e. all autopsy specimens collected more than 4 hours after death and tissue from superficial or 'open' lesions) must be washed free of contaminating bacteria before they are prepared for culture. A small piece of tissue showing macroscopic signs of recent infection is placed in a tube containing about 2 ml of peptone water and is then agitated thoroughly on a vortex shaker. The piece of tissue is then transferred with the aid of fine sterile forceps or a loop to another tube of peptone water and is shaken again. This is repeated until 6 tubes of peptone water have been used in washing. The piece of tissue is then ground with about 0.5 ml of sterile peptone water. It is better to use peptone water than saline or distilled water for washing because it can be relied on not to kill delicate organisms. The grindings are then treated in the manner described for uncontaminated specimens (page 43). The technique needs experience because if a rather friable specimen receives too much washing all the bacteria may be removed; on the other hand, if the washing is insufficient the surface contaminants will remain and spoil the cultures. The risk of losing all the bacteria can be avoided by seeding the washings on blood agar incubated aerobically and anaerobically plus CO_2. Contaminating organisms will be most plentiful in cultures from the first washings and will diminish in numbers in the

Primary anaerobic culture

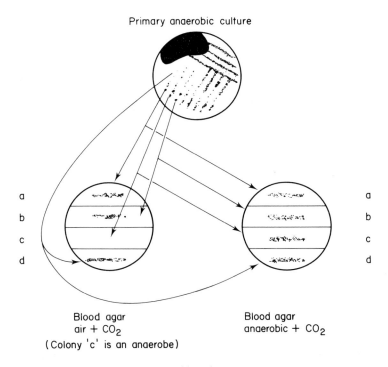

a
b
c
d

a
b
c
d

Blood agar
air + CO_2
(Colony 'c' is an anaerobe)

Blood agar
anaerobic + CO_2

Fig. 3.3   Procedure for primary anaerobic culture.

subsequent cultures. The last tube from which growth is obtained, and cultures of the ground tissue itself, should yield an almost pure growth of the pathogen.

Bacteria found

In subacute and chronic infections:
   Anaerobic streptococci
   Anaerobic non-sporing bacilli
   Erysipelothrix
   Listeria
Streptococci, staphylococci, coliforms, *Pasteurella* and other bacteria which
   more commonly give rise to acute infections.

Myco. tuberculosis, Actinomyces israeli and fungi often cause chronic lesions. Methods for their isolation are considered in Chapters 6 and 7. *Pseudomonas mallei, Myco. leprae*, amoebae and *Leishmania* are rare causes. Active syphilis and yaws can be excluded when serological tests are negative.

The somewhat laborious method described is intended for use on the rare occasions when it is necessary to exclude infection by any known pathogenic microbe, other than viruses. In an individual case the clinical findings may indicate infection by a member of a particular species, in which case selective media may be used *in addition* to those already recommended. If part of the routine is omitted the report is correspondingly modified. It is not reasonable to report 'cultures sterile' or 'no evidence of infection' until the whole investigation has been completed. As this takes 8 weeks (including cultures for *Myco. tuberculosis*) the microscopic findings are reported separately and a preliminary report on the cultures is sent at the end of the first week.

Pus

Although pus is usually sampled with a swab, it is more satisfactory whenever possible to take a liquid sample with a syringe or pipette. When the lesion is deep seated and opens through a sinus, the whole of the inner dressing should be sent in a sterile jar. Swabs should be placed in transport medium for the preservation of anaerobes and microbes sensitive to drying. There must be no delay in submitting swabs in transport medium because some species will grow in it at room temperature and may obliterate the true pathogens. When a small amount of liquid pus is sent, a swab of the pus in transport medium should also accompany it to protect any anaerobes from exposure to air.

Macroscopic and microscopic examination

Note the colour, consistency, odour and any peculiarity such as the presence of granules. The discharge may be coloured by bacterial pigments (e.g. pyocyanin) or by the breakdown of haemoglobin.

In all cases make a smear for Gram-stain; if the lesion is subacute or of long duration make another for Ziehl–Neelsen or auramine stain. The microscopic examination is very important and should never be omitted (see page 11). When a swab is examined the smears should be made first on sterile slides. One can then be sure that the bacteria seen have come from the lesion and cannot have been accidentally picked up from a minute contaminating colony on one of the culture plates. Gas-liquid chromatography may provide a rapid means of confirming the presence of anaerobes (Phillips *et al.*, 1976).

Culture

Seed the specimen on two blood agar plates (one incubated aerobically plus 5–10% CO_2, the other anaerobically plus 10% CO_2), on neomycin blood agar (incubated anaerobically plus CO_2) on MacConkey agar and in cooked meat broth. Refrigerate the remainder of the specimen. If there is any indication from the clinical condition of the patient or, when preliminary examination of the specimen incriminates a particular species, additional cultures may be made on selective media. For example, Wilkins–Chalgren supplemented for non-sporing anaerobes or Gram-negative anaerobes (see page 318) may be included for the selection of anaerobes in pus from abdominal and chest wounds and from all deep-seated abscesses. In some cases it may not be necessary to seed the pus on MacConkey agar, which is used mainly for rapid identification of bacteria is mixed cultures, but the routine of two blood agar plates and a cooked meat broth is followed in all cases.

When antibiotic sensitivity tests are required, seed the swab heavily and evenly on a separate sensitivity test blood agar plate (page 213) before immersing it in cooked meat broth.

Procedure

Examine the plate cultures with a hand lens in a good light. When they are sterile after overnight incubation, reincubate them. When growth is seen, describe each type of colony on all the plates, pick off single colonies of each type, Gram-stain them (for rapid method see page 85) and compare the appearance of the bacteria in the smears with those seen on the stained film of the specimen. There may be considerable discrepancy; if so, reincubate the cultures in the hope that those microbes seen in the original film which have failed to appear will grow after further incubation.

When the aerobic plate cultures reveal a pure growth of an organism resembling a common facultative anaerobe (e.g. *Staph. aureus*) and the anaerobic culture also shows only one type of colony, and, further, if the Gram-stain of both is identical, then it is reasonable to assume that they are the same and to continue identification from one plate culture only, disregarding corresponding growth on the other. If, however, there are several types of colony on each plate culture, it is impossible at this stage to be sure that they correspond, and even after Gram-staining it is not often possible to disregard one of the plates. They may apparently yield growth of the same species when an anaerobe is present in the following circumstances:

1. When a strict aerobe on the aerobic culture is similar microscopically to the anaerobe.

2. When a facultative aerobe with a colony variant is seen on the aerobic plate which fails to show the variant under anaerobic conditions. An anaerobe may then be mistaken for the variant.

It is necessary therefore to subculture all types of colony from a mixed anaerobic culture to an aerobic blood agar plate. If they grow, they can then be compared with the aerobes already under investigation and those which correspond can be discarded (see Fig. 3.3).

Further investigation for anaerobes

Fewer than 1 per cent of anaerobes encountered in pus in civilian practice are *Clostridia* and if the much commoner non-sporing anaerobes, which are found, for example, in about 30 per cent of samples of abdominal pus, are not to be missed it is necessary to reincubate the plates for a further day. Both plates should be reincubated, since when small colonies appear on the anaerobic plate on the second day they cannot be assumed to be anaerobes unless they have failed to appear after 48 hours' incubation aerobically. Routine reincubation of primary plates need not delay the

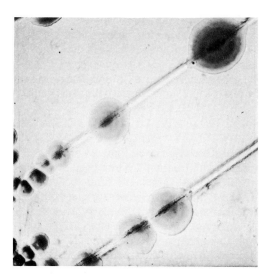

Fig. 3.4 Primary blood agar cultures of abdominal pus after 48 hours' incubation. Aerobic culture. *Esch. coli* colonies only.

final report because when growth is present on the first day identification almost always takes a further day, and when it is absent reincubation is needed in any case. Colonies are described and Gram-stained and when necessary retested for ability to grow in air plus CO_2. Unless the original sensitivity plate was cultured anaerobically, anaerobes must now be tested. Identification is desirable but our knowledge of the pathogenic role of various species of non-sporing anaerobes is at present rudimentary and full identification will not affect treatment, therefore they can be reported forthwith as *Bacteroides* spp. or anaerobic cocci. (See also Chapter 5.) *Clostridia* usually appear after overnight incubation and must be identified (see page 130). Sometimes colonies seen only on the anaerobic plate prove to be aerobes not found on the original aerobic culture, where they have been swamped by the growth of bacteria which are partly or completely inhibited by anaerobiosis. Haemolytic streptococci are sometimes isolated in this way when they would have been missed but for the anaerobic culture. Nalidixic acid blood agar (page 313) may be employed as a selective medium for isolating streptococci from pus.

When growth is present on the original plates, further procedure with the original cooked meat broth depends on the original Gram-film. When bacteria seen microscopically have not grown, the cooked meat culture must be investigated. After 2–3 days' incubation it is subcultured on neomycin blood agar incubated anaerobically plus CO_2. A parallel plate incubated in air plus CO_2 is also needed so that anaerobes can be recognized without further tests. Anaerobes will often be discovered in pus from deep wounds if the cooked meat broth is subcultured routinely, but isolation from the liquid culture only is hard to interpret. Inclusion of a selective anaerobic plate originally for such material is preferred; numbers of colonies grown then indicate numbers in the specimen not growth in the enrichment broth.

When numerous bacteria of apparently one kind are seen in the smear but growth is scanty (say, about 50 colonies per plate), further organisms should be sought because such a sample should yield a heavy growth. When the organisms seen are Gram-negative bacilli and only a scanty growth of coliforms has appeared overnight, *Bacteroides* may be present in much larger numbers (see Figs. 3.4 and 3.5). Similarly, anaerobic cocci may be accompanied by staphylococci from the skin which are of secondary importance.

When the original plates are sterile the cooked meat broth may bring to light the pathogen, aerobe or anaerobe, because it can be inoculated with a large volume of pus and therefore the chance of a positive result is greater. This often happens when the majority of organisms have been killed by an antibiotic. The significance of growth from liquid cultures, however, is often hard to assess. When cultures of pus on solid media are persistently sterile, analysis of the cooked meat broth after 5 days' incubation, by GLC, may prove useful (page 269).

Interpretation of results

Some bacteria are so often associated with pus that they are termed pyogenic, but this, like 'pathogenic', is not a precise term and organisms not usually called pyogenic are found in pus. If cultures yield a pure growth of an organism and no other type was seen in the stained smear of the specimen, it is usually, and often correctly, assumed to be the only

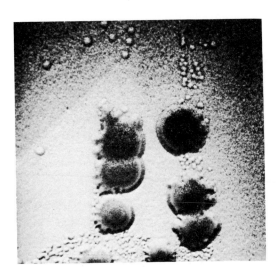

Fig. 3.5 Primary blood agar cultures of abdominal pus after 48 hours' incubation. Anaerobic culture. Numerous colonies of a *Bacteroides* species are also seen (they were not apparent after overnight incubation).

invading microbe; but a Gram-negative coliform bacillus in the smear may be any member of the coliform group, including *Proteus, Pseudomonas, Salmonella* and *Shigella*, it may be a parvobacterium or an anaerobe. The presence of an unsuspected second infecting organism may be revealed when the first is inhibited by antibiotics, either in the patient's tissues after therapy or during laboratory tests.

When pyogenic organisms are found, they are usually considered to be the primary cause of the infection and the rest to be secondary invaders or saprophytes. Sometimes disease caused by secondary invaders is more severe than the original infection; for example, gas gangrene caused by secondary invasion by Cl. *perfringens (welchii)* of a deep wound already infected with pyogenic cocci, and wound diphtheria in which the original infection may have been very mild.

Bacteria found

1. Open wounds and burns:

(a) *Staph. aureus*
Coagulase-negative staphylococci
Micrococcus spp.
Str. pyogenes
Esch. coli
Diphtheroids
Aerobic spore bearers

(b) *Proteus*
Ps. aeruginosa
Enterococci
Haemolytic streptococci
(other than group A)
α-Haemolytic streptococci
Anaerobic streptococci
Bacteroides spp.

(c) *Haemophilus* spp.
Pasteurella septica
Str. pneumoniae
Actinomyces spp.
C. diphtheriae

Cl. *perfringens (welchi)*
Cl. *tetani*
Cl. *novyi(oedematiens)*
Cl. *septicum*
Cl. *histolyticum*

This is a general frequency list which will vary with the age of the wound, its site and history. Pus from war wounds yields a higher proportion of anaerobes because of the extensive tissue damage and delay in surgical treatment which favours their growth.

2. Abscesses and other closed lesions:

The skin and environmental contaminants, coagulase-negative staphylococci, diphtheroids and spore bearers, are less frequent. All the rest listed above are found, and in addition:

Myco. tuberculosis
Brucella spp.
Salmonella spp.
N. gonorrhoeae
N. meningitidis

Ps. mallei
Erysipelothrix spp.
Bacillus anthracis
Mycoplasma spp.

Occasionally fungi and protozoa are encountered.

Of the bacteria listed, those usually called pyogenic are *Staph. aureus, Str. pyogenes, Str. pneumoniae, N. gonorrhoeae, N. meningitidis* and coliforms.

Specimens from neonates

When a newborn child is admitted for investigation, specimens must be taken immediately to diagnose or exclude infection. Clinical diagnosis of acute infection is often difficult but treatment cannot be delayed because the infant's life may depend on it. Since a normal infant gains its first contact with bacteria on its journey down the birth canal a pathogen is likely to be found superficially. It may also have been swallowed and may even multiply in the child's stomach, which is poorly protected against bacteria at this age. Often there is no indication of the site of infection; a routine procedure is therefore adopted, supplemented by blood culture (page 28) when necessary. Aspirate from the infant's stomach and swabs from the external auditory meatus, nose, umbilicus, pharynx and rectum are examined. Within 4 days of birth, growth from these sites should be very scanty. Microscopic examination of the gastric aspirate may reveal pus cells and numerous bacteria. Unsuspected gonorrhoea may be diagnosed by this means before the development of purulent ophthalmia, the infant having swallowed gonococcal pus during parturition. Specimens from the external ear, umbilicus and stomach are cultured as described for pus. Those from the nose, pharynx and rectum are cultured on blood agar and cetrimide agar to screen for hospital staphylococci and *Pseudomonas*. These aerobic cultures are repeated weekly while the infant is in the neonatal unit to give early warning of colonization by hospital pathogens (see page 282).

A cervical swab from the mother is also useful at this stage. The presence of a potential pathogen may indicate the need for prophylactic treatment of the baby.

References

Crowley, N. (1970). *Journal of Clinical Pathology* **23**, 166

Ganguli, L.A., Turton, L.T. and Tillotson, G.S. (1982) *Journal of Clinical Pathology* **35**, 458

Model, D.G, and Peel, R.N. (1973). *Journal of Clinical Pathology* **26**, 529

Phillips, K.D., Tearle, P.V. and Willis, A.T. (1976). *Journal of Clinical Pathology* **29**, 428

PHLS Monograph Series No. 10 (1978) *The Bacteriological Examination of Urine.* Ed. by P.D. Meers. HM Stationery Office, London

Staneck, J.L. and Vincent, S. (1981) *Journal of Clinical Microbiology* **13**, 463

Stokes, E.J. (1955). *Lancet* **i**, 276

Stokes, E.J. and Ridgway, G.L. (1980) *Clinical Bacteriology* 5th edn. Edward Arnold, London

von Haebler, T. and Miles, A.A. (1938). *Journal of Pathology and Bacteriology* **46**, 425

Waterworth, P.M. (1972). *Journal of Clinical Pathology* **25**, 227

Waterworth, P.M. (1973). *Journal of Clinical Pathology* **26**, 596

4

Specimens from Sites with a Normal Flora

The examination of these specimens presents the microbiologist with a dilemma. On one hand the clinician wants as quickly as possible, and within a few days at the latest, a detailed list of the microbes in the specimen; on the other hand the microbiologist knows that it is impossible in most cases to satisfy this demand in so short a time. Two courses are open to him. He may sacrifice the scientific integrity of his report by identifying perhaps one or two easily tested strains, guessing the rest by morphological appearances and his knowledge of the normal flora of the site from which the specimen was taken; or he may limit his investigation with a view to excluding known pathogens, making no attempt to identify the rest of the microbes found. The first method is unsatisfactory because the report is misleading. The clinician will assume that all the microbes have been equally well investigated and that their identity is certain, whereas in fact only one or two of the species mentioned have been identified and the chance that the guess-work applied to the rest is correct varies with the experience of the microbiologist but at best falls short of 100 per cent. Probably the individual patient will not suffer from this departure from the scientific method unless the microbiologists become overworked and overconfident and carry the guess-work a stage further so that the majority of bacteria are identified by colonial and microscopic morphology, or even colonial morphology alone. A more reasonable way of overcoming the difficulty is to explain it to the clinician and reach an agreement with him on the policy to be adopted. A convenient routine which reveals what he needs to know, quickly in most cases, without violating scientific principles, is to seek for known pathogens using appropriate selective media, and to report their presence or absence, taking no account of other bacteria which happen to grow on these media. This routine can be extended for a specific clinical situation after discussion between the clinician and the microbiologist. They will agree a suitable procedure of investigation, and keep full clinical and laboratory records which can be referred to later should similar cases be reported.

When the microbiologist examines the plate cultures he will note any change in the normal flora as judged by the appearance of the colonies, as well as searching for those resembling known pathogens. If further tests show that although no known pathogens are present the flora is unusual for the site from which the specimen was taken, suspicion of pathogenicity may be cast on bacteria previously thought to be harmless.

The amount of routine work which is done over and above the exclusion of pathogens will depend on the laboratory facilities. If the staff are hard pressed it may be just a note of the total amount of growth on the plate cultures, followed by a record of identification or exclusion of microbes resembling pathogens. If more time is available each type of colony can be described, Gram-stained and fully identified. In this case the work done will be recorded in the laboratory but will not be reported unless the microbiologist thinks it has some special significance. It is an excellent exercise for microbiologists in training, often brings to light interesting bacterial variants and may occasionally lead to the diagnosis of a rare infection which would otherwise have escaped notice.

It is better to use the laboratory for detailed investigation and full records of unusual cases than to squander time and effort on half-hearted attempts to identify all the bacteria in each culture. Hospital laboratories are seldom equipped to investigate satisfactorily the normal human flora as a part of the routine work. In many cases – for example, vaginal swab cultures – the colonies that appear overnight on blood agar give only the vaguest reflection of the total number and variety of species in the specimen. If it is seeded on several different enriched media, incubated in two or more different atmospheres and the cultures are examined frequently over a long period of incubation, a surprisingly large variety of bacteria can be isolated. Logically these are of as much importance as the ones of unproven pathogenicity which grow readily on blood agar, but it is clearly impossible to investigate them in every case.

To summarize: there are four types of investigation which can usefully be made in a hospital laboratory on specimens from sites with a normal flora:

1. Exclusion of known pathogens.
2. Exclusion of known pathogens plus partial investigation of normal flora.
3. Full microbiological investigation of clinically rare infections.
4. Full investigation of all the bacteria found in all specimens.

The first of these must be done as thoroughly as possible in all cases because on its reliability the well-being of the patient and all those exposed to the risk of infection from him depend. In well equipped laboratories it should be replaced by the second type. The extra work need not be reported unless it accompanies a request from the microbiologist to combine forces with the clinician in an effort to establish the cause of a rare infection.

The fourth type is not part of the routine work but is research which may suitably be undertaken in a hospital laboratory. The results are for scientific record, and perhaps publication, and may have little to do with the treatment of the individual patients from whom the specimens were taken.

Upper respiratory tract

Pathogens to be excluded

Group I	*Str. pyogenes* Haemolytic Streptococci (other than group A)	*C. diphtheriae*
Group II	*Str. pneumoniae* *Haemophilus* spp. *Klebsiella* spp. *Staph. aureus*	*N. meningitidis* Vincent's fusiform bacillus and spirilla *Candida albicans*

Other bacteria found

α-haemolytic streptococci
Branhamella catarrhalis
Coagulase-negative staphylococci
Micrococcus spp.
Non-haemolytic streptococci

Str. faecalis

Esch. coli and other coliforms
Yeasts and fungi
Other undifferentiated saprophytes
Diphtheroids
Aerobic and anaerobic spore bearers
Non-sporing anaerobic bacilli
Anaerobic streptococci

Throat swabs

Throat swabs from cases of acute tonsillitis are always examined for haemolytic streptococci and *C. diphtheriae*. In Britain by far the most common bacterial cause of upper respiratory infection is *Str. pyogenes*. Although diphtheria is becoming increasingly rare the consequences of overlooking the infection may be so serious, both to the patient and to those in contact with him, that is necessary to search for the organism in every case of febrile sore throat.

The pathogens in group II above are relatively benign and, provided the specimen has been properly taken, small numbers of them can be disregarded because they are often found in the upper respiratory tracts of healthy people. When one of them forms the major part of the growth it is generally, and probably correctly, assumed to be the cause of the infection because cultures from healthy people seldom yield these organisms in profusion.

Microscopic examination

In cases clinically suggestive of Vincent's angina and in all cases of tonsillitis with membrane or exudate, a film is made on a clean glass slide, stained with strong carbol fuchsin for 3 minutes without heating and examined for spirochaetes and fusiform bacilli. If a satisfactory specimen has been taken from a Vincent's infection they will be seen in large numbers. A few are often found in smears from normal mouths; there is no need therefore to search diligently for them as only large numbers are significant. Pseudomembranes are also seen in thrush caused by

C. albicans, which is a primary infection in infants but in adults is more often seen after prolonged antibiotic therapy. Masses of yeasts will be seen in the exudate. Stained films are useless for the diagnosis of infections other than these.

The morphology of the normal throat flora is extremely varied, streptococci can almost always be found and it is impossible to differentiate haemolytic streptococci from other streptococci by their microscopic morphology. Diphtheroids are very common and often resemble *C. diphtheriae*. Moreover, films from diphtheria membrane sometimes show nothing resembling a diphtheria bacillus. The stained film may therefore be omitted when it is not necessary to exclude Vincent's angina or thrush.

Exclusion of Str. pyogenes

The swab is seeded on a blood agar plate and incubated in an anaerobic jar plus 10% CO_2. The anaerobic atmosphere selects haemolytic streptococci from the rest of the throat flora. All strains grow well under these conditions; many yield larger colonies than they do on plates incubated in air. Moreover, larger zones of haemolysis are seen and it is not at all uncommon to find strains of *Str. pyogenes* (Lancefield's group A), which show very feeble haemolysis when incubated in air but clear zones on anaerobic plate cultures. Further, many throat commensals which flourish when grown in air yield minute colonies in this atmosphere. There is no doubt that in some cases anaerobic culture reveals the presence of *Str. pyogenes* which would otherwise be missed.

Anaerobiosis affects the other potentially pathogenic species listed as follows. Haemolytic streptococci (including varieties other than group A) and *Str. pneumoniae* grow well, many strains better than in air. *Haemophilus* species are not greatly affected; most strains show slightly smaller colonies under anaerobic conditions but the presence of CO_2 helps their growth. This is true only of culture on a highly nutrient defibrinated horse blood agar poured at least 3 mm deep; on some blood agar *Haemophilus* species grow poorly. The non-sporing anaerobes which are commonly found in the throat do not overcrowd the culture because they grow slowly and show, at most, very minute colonies after overnight incubation.

This method of selection is preferred for the following reasons: streptococcal growth is often actually stimulated and haemolysis improved; no special medium is required; all satisfactory swabs from the upper respiratory tract yield facultative anaerobes so that no further test of a satisfactory specimen by seeding on non-inhibitory medium is needed.

Procedure

1st day

Examine the plate culture with a hand lens by reflected light. If the specimen was satisfactory there should be confluent or almost confluent growth in the pool of inoculum. Now examine it by transmitted light and note the presence or absence of β-haemolytic colonies. If there is none the report can be sent 'No haemolytic streptococci isolated'. If β-haemolytic colonies are present, Gram-stain a single colony. If it is a streptococcus, the same colony should be subcultured onto blood agar and incubated. It is best to incubate this plate anaerobically, particularly if separation of the colony from other growth was difficult. The Lancefield group may then be determined (page 96).

Exclusion of *C. diphtheriae*

The swab is seeded on blood agar and blood tellurite agar. Tellurite selects corynebacteria from other throat flora very efficiently. It inhibits all growth to some extent, but the corynebacteria are much less affected than others. Even so, the plates should be incubated for 48 hours before discarding them as negative, because some strains fail to appear earlier. It also has the advantage of helping to differentiate typical strains of the three types of *C. diphtheriae*.* This, however, is of secondary importance in hospital work, because information about the type of infecting bacillus makes no difference to the treatment. The rapid identification of *C. diphtheriae* is all important; differentiation into gravis, mitis or intermedius strains follows later because it may have epidemiological significance. The blood agar culture is made for two reasons: first, because in all cases of sore throat suspected of diphtheria, haemolytic streptococci must also be sought – the two infections are often difficult to distinguish clinically and if the cultures are negative for diphtheria, *Str. pyogenes* is the most likely pathogen; second, because it is necessary to check that the specimen was satisfactory. Sterile cultures on tellurite medium may result either from the lack of organisms in the throat capable of growth on it or because the swab was unsatisfactory due to contamination with antiseptic or to some other fault in sampling or to antibiotic therapy.

When penicillin or other antibiotic has already been given, the microbiologist should warn the clinician that diphtheria cannot be excluded. *C. diphtheriae* is sensitive to all common antibiotics but antitoxin is the main requirement for treatment. There is no way in which infection by highly sensitive microbes can be excluded when swabs are sent from antibiotic-treated patients.

Procedure

Incubate the plates overnight – the tellurite culture in air, the blood agar anaerobically plus CO_2.

1st day

Examine the blood agar plate and make a note of the amount of growth. When it is very scanty the plates should be discarded and another specimen requested. If it is likely to be difficult to obtain another specimen,

---

*Of the numerous tellurite media available, Hoyle's blood tellurite agar has been found easy to prepare (page 314) and yields a good growth of most strains of *C. diphtheriae* after overnight incubation.

continue the investigation but make a note that a negative result is of no value. When haemolytic streptococci are found do not discard the tellurite culture; streptococcal carriers do sometimes become infected with diphtheria.

Make smears from isolated black colonies on the tellurite medium and stain with methylene blue. Although the bacilli do not show their classic morphology when grown on tellurite medium, they are recognizable as diphtheroids and strains of *C. diphtheriae* are usually highly pleomorphic compared with other species. As the colonies are picked, note their consistency. All three types emulsify easily; gravis colonies are friable, mitis colonies are butyrous. Although many strains of cocci are inhibited by Hoyle's tellurite blood agar (see page 314), some will grow and produce black colonies which may be mistaken for diphtheroids. They are easily distinguished when stained with methylene blue, but care must be taken not to mistake barred diphtheria bacilli for chains of cocci. Some strains of *Proteus* also yield black colonies on this medium but they are moist and brownish black and not likely to be mistaken for diphtheroids.

Table 4.1 lists descriptions of the various colonies commonly encountered on Hoyle's medium.

Corynebacterium ulcerans is a rare cause of diphtheria. The growth

Table 4.1

*Corynebacterium diphtheriae**			Diphtheroids	Cocci
			Hofmann and Xerosis group	Micrococci and Neisseria
Gravis	Mitis	Intermedius		
18–24 h ⎧ 0.5–0.8 mm grey-black matt ± haemolytic[†]	0.5–0.8 mm grey-black matt haemolytic[†]	Minute grey-black matt non-haemolytic[†]	0.1–0.8 mm grey matt non-haemolytic[†]	Minute deep black shiny or rugose surface
36–48 h 1.5–2 mm grey-black, matt, friable. Gently sloping edges with central eminence, occasionally typical 'daisyhead'	1.5–2 mm grey-black, dull or faintly glistening surface, butyrous. Shape of colony similar to gravis strain but no daisyhead	0.8–1 mm grey-black, matt colonies very flat. Resemble small drops of indian ink	0.5–2 mm grey-black, often with pale peripheral zone, sometimes shiny. Pool of inoculum often dense black with separate colonies paler	0.5–1.5 mm deep black, shiny or rugose surface, often difficult to emulsify

*Single colonies are as dark or darker in colour than those in crowded areas.
†Tested on blood agar.

resembles *C.diphtheriae* mitis but biochemical reactions may be mistaken for *C. diphtheriae* gravis. Haemolysis of horse blood agar is very rarely caused by harmless corynebacteria. This is a sign worth looking for by subculture from likely colonies on the tellurite plate to blood agar incubated in air. Sucrose-fermenting strains which show any degree of haemolysis (including that which is visible only when the colony has been removed) should be tested for toxigenicity (see page 108)

When an epidemic strain has been identified by biochemical tests and its behaviour on the tellurite medium is well known, it is reasonable, when examining subsequent specimens from the same patients and from contacts, to rely on the colonial morphology for a preliminary diagnosis and to test the strains later at leisure. But in routine hospital practice when single cases are investigated, fermentation reactions are essential for the identification of diphtheroids. Morphology is not sufficiently reliable for diagnosis and atypical strains are not infrequently encountered. An exception can perhaps safely be made when the appearance of the colonies suggests a diphtheroid and the stained film shows absolutely regular short diphtheroid bacilli with no long forms. Stains for metachromatic granules are not of much diagnostic value because young virulent gravis strains show no granules, and diphtheroids, particularly of the *C. xerosis* group, frequently show a large number of them.

Having established from colonial and microscopic appearances that diphtheroids are present, pick single colonies to a Loeffler slope and Hiss' serum water for fermentation, urea hydrolysis and virulence tests (see page 107) and also for further examination of microscopic morphology. The urease test should be incubated immediately, and examined preliminarily after 3 hours. Reincubate the tellurite culture.

Preliminary reports
When at this stage a culture from an infected throat shows a heavy growth of slightly haemolytic pleomorphic urease-negative diphtheroids and no other obvious pathogen, a preliminary positive report should be sent to initiate antitoxin therapy and isolation of the patient if these precautions have not already been taken. A heavy growth of diphtheroids is so common from nasal swabs that it is wiser to await the confirmation of the fermentation tests before giving an opinion unless the morphology is typical in every respect. It is usually impossible to give a preliminary report on swabs from carriers.

2nd day
Examine the reincubated tellurite culture. If it was negative on the first day but black colonies have now appeared, examine them as previously describe. If diphtheroids were found on the first day they will now show greater differentiation of colonial morphology, and when experience of the medium has been gained it is possible to guess fairly accurately whether they are *C. diphtheriae*. Stain a film from the Loeffler slope to see if the microscopic morphology bears out the diagnosis, and seed appropriate sugar media for final identification (page 107).

Other throat pathogens (group II, page 54)

These organisms are commonly found in moderate numbers in healthy throats; therefore only heavy predominant growth of them is significant.

1. Haemolytic streptococci other than group A will be differentiated by Lancefield grouping (pages 96–99).

2. *Str. pneumoniae* grows well anaerobically. It can therefore easily be identified if it is present on the anaerobic blood agar culture made for the recovery of *Str. pyogenes*. Atypical strains closely resemble other α-haemolytic streptococci; it is therefore necessary to subculture suspected colonies to blood agar for an Optochin sensitivity test (page 100).

3. *Haemophilus*. Haemolytic strains of *H. parainfluenzae* sometimes cause sore throats and their colonies are easily mistaken for haemolytic streptococci. Gram-stain reveals pleomorphic Gram-negative bacilli. Satellitism to other colonies may be seen on the original plate, but if there is no evidence of it a satellitism test is required for identification (see page 124). Most strains are slightly inhibited by anaerobiosis. Although the colonies are small, a heavy growth will not easily be overlooked on an anaerobic culture. Some strains of *Esch. coli* and *Bacillus* species are haemolytic when incubated anaerobically. They may be found in small numbers in throat swab cultures.

4. *Staph. aureus*. This is not a common throat pathogen and seldom causes simple sore throat. It sometimes causes quinsy and can be cultured from the pus when the abscess bursts. It is a facultative anaerobe and, although under strictly anaerobic conditions the colony size may be reduced tenfold, a predominant growth can be easily recognized after overnight incubation if the plate is carefully examined. Strains showing haemolysis aerobically are non-haemolytic on anaerobic plate cultures.

It is clear that, if throat swabs are seeded on blood agar to be incubated anaerobically and on tellurite blood agar, good results can be expected for the recovery of haemolytic streptococci, *C. diphtheriae* and *Str. pneumoniae*, but these two cultures alone are not ideal for the recovery of less common pathogens, some of which may need aerobic incubation. If numerous throat swabs have to be examined, routine seeding on three plates becomes very extravagant. This difficulty may be overcome by reincubating the anaerobic culture in air whenever no likely pathogen is found on the first day. It will not usually delay the result because in such cases the tellurite culture needs reincubation before a negative report can be sent. The method of choice for throat swabs depends on the prevalence of the various infections in the population investigated. In Britain *Str. pyogenes* is much the most important cause of tonsillitis. Diphtheria is now so rare that many general hospital laboratories encounter less than one case in a decade. The proportion of sore throats which can reasonably be attributed to the other pathogens listed is in our experience of the order of one for every twenty cases of streptococcal infection. Under these circumstances it is important to use a good selective method for *Str. pyogenes* and routine anaerobic culture is well worthwhile. If unlimited resources are available, aerobic blood agar cultures should also be made.

Sore throats associated with malaise and either low grade or no fever are usually viral in origin. A throat swab in virus transport medium frozen at $-70°C$ and a sample of clotted blood should be sent during the first 2 days of symptoms. The sooner the sample is taken the better the chance of isolation. A further sample of blood will be needed later to show a rise of antibody titre if virus is isolated. Glandular fever (page 266) is also a possible cause.

Nasal swabs

In all cases of rhinitis with a purulent nasal discharge three cultures are made. The swab is seeded on chocolate blood agar incubated in air plus 5-10% CO_2 for *N. meningitidis*, haemophilus and *Staph. aureus*; on blood agar incubated anaerobically for the selection of haemolytic streptococci and *Str. pneumoniae* and on blood tellurite medium for *C. diphtheriae*.

It is difficult to assess the significance of *Staph. aureus* isolated from nasal swabs. A heavy growth of this organism is common from apparently healthy noses but sometimes the formation of crusts on the nasal mucosa and nasal discharge may be caused by it. When no common pathogen is isolated from purulent discharge in a child, a foreign body in the nose is probably the cause.

Carriers

When nose and throat swabs are taken in a search for carriers, the full investigation can be modified. If *Str. pyogenes* be sought the swab is seeded on blood agar only, which is incubated anaerobically. Swabs from potential carriers of diphtheria are seeded first onto a small area of blood agar to test that the specimen is satisfactory (there is no need to spread the inoculum) and then onto tellurite blood agar.

Nasopharyngeal swabs and aspirates

Str. pneumoniae, N. meningitidis and members of the haemophilus group are more commonly found in the nasopharynx than in the nose or throat. Nasopharyngeal swabs are essential for the isolation of *N. meningitidis* from suspected carriers and for the recovery of *Bord. pertussis* from cases of whooping cough.

Meningococcal carriers are swabbed through the mouth, using a curved protected swab (West's swab) to prevent accidental contamination; alternatively, a laryngeal swab may be employed (see page 151). The swab is seeded immediately on warm blood agar or chocolated blood agar and incubated in air plus 10% CO_2. In children a pernasal swab may be preferred which must be seeded on selective medium for gonococci and meningococci (see page 314) to suppress the growth of nasal flora. The organism can be found in healthy people; carrier rates sometimes rise to 60 per cent in an apparently healthy population. The significance of a positive finding is therefore doubtful and swabbing of all contacts of patients with meningitis is not recommended. Spread within the family can be prevented by giving all members prophylactic treatment for one week. Three days after the end of treatment members of a family with children should be checked for clearance; nasopharyngeal swabs should be taken in the laboratory and cultured directly.

Examination of aspirated mucopus from the nasopharynx of patients with pneumonia, especially children, who have no sputum, sometimes enables a bacterial diagnosis to be achieved; the material obtained is comparatively free from contamination. A fine plastic catheter with a small collecting bottle attached can be obtained for the purpose. The catheter is gently introduced through the nose and suction is applied with a syringe attached at the distal end; the whole is sent in a plastic bag to the laboratory. Even a very small sample in the tubing only may give a useful result; it is removed by cutting the tubing. The specimen is treated as sputum; it is also suitable for virology and some of it can be extracted from the tubing and bottle and sent in an equal volume of virus transport medium frozen at $-70°C$. Smears of aspirated specimens from young children should also be sent for immunofluorescence of respiratory syncytial virus (see page 274).

Bord. pertussis

When there is no obstruction to the nasal passages, per nasal swabs are more satisfactory than nasopharyngeal swabs for the investigation of whooping cough. They are very small swabs made by wrapping cotton wool round thick loop wire instead of round the usual rigid metal or wooden applicator; they can be passed through the nose to the nasopharynx. Plates exposed in front of the mouth during coughing often yield a heavy growth of the pathogen in typical whooping cough and have the advantage that they do not distress the patient. They are not, however, as satisfactory as per nasal swabs for the investigation of early and atypical cases.

Special medium is essential for the isolation of *Bord. pertussis*. The classic Bordet–Gengou medium, screened with penicillin, gives good results when the commensals of the upper respiratory tract are penicillin sensitive; but, when pertussis has to be isolated from a swab contaminated with penicillin-resistant organisms, some additional selector is required. Cephalexin 40 mg/1 in charcoal blood agar is recommended. The medium at half strength, but containing the same concentration of cephalexin and blood, can be used for transport of swabs and for enrichment (Regan and Lowe, 1977) (see page 313). On arrival the swab in transport medium is seeded on the selective medium, replaced in the transport medium and incubated. After 48 hours the first culture is inspected and when negative the swab is again seeded on selective medium. Plates should be incubated in air in a moist atmosphere for 4 days, and inspected for typical pearly colonies (see page 126) using a hand lens, before they are discarded.

Bordetella pertussis does not withstand drying, and swabs must either be seeded at the bedside or be sent in transport medium which has a shelf-life at 4°C of 8 weeks. During an epidemic, medium will be constantly available but at other times the laboratory should be warned by telephone before specimens are taken.

Plates are seeded without spreading the inoculum, and are incubated in air in a moist atmosphere. They are examined on the third and fourth days for typical pearly colonies.

Laryngeal swabs

The larynx can be sampled under indirect vision using a laryngeal mirror, but the swabs are more often inserted 'blind'. The swab is made on a metal applicator which is bent to an angle of 120 degress 5 cm from its end, and is enclosed in a tube (18 cm × 3 cm) for sterilization. It is passed through the mouth over the back of the tongue, and when the long straight part of the applicator lies along the tongue the swab should be in the larynx. The patient will be stimulated to cough and material from the trachea as well as from the larynx itself will be deposited on the swab. For a more detailed account of the method, see page 151.

It is essential to swab the larynx in cases of suspected laryngeal diphtheria because tonsillar swabs may be negative when the patient has an extensive laryngeal membrane. This is a rare condition and the larynx is more often swabbed for the diagnosis of pulmonary tuberculosis in patients with no sputum. Laryngeal swabs are also of use for the diagnosis of acute lung infections in children when a nasopharyngeal aspirate is unobtainable. The specimen is cultured on media employed for sputum.

Epiglottitis

Haemophilus influenzae type b causes acute epiglottitis in young children and may be recovered from the blood and from the upper respiratory tract in this dangerous condition. A clinical diagnosis must be made and treatment given immediately. Results of culture will confirm the diagnosis but by the time this is known the child will be either dead or well on the way to recovery.

Mouth swabs

Ulcers of the mouth are sometimes caused by bacteria. The commonest infection is Vincent's angina, which is diagnosed by finding numerous spirochaetes and fusiform bacilli in a stained film of the exudate (see 'Throat swabs'). Ulceration due to *Str. pyogenes* and *Staph. aureus* is uncommon but may be severe and lead to cancrum oris. If swabs are taken carefully from dental abscesses they should be relatively uncontaminated with mouth flora and are treated as pus (see page 46). Thrush, caused by the yeast *Candida albicans*, is common in children. Stained films of the exudate show numerous yeasts which can be identified by culture (page 164).

When the stained film reveals no yeasts or Vincent's organisms, the swab is seeded onto a blood agar plate for anaerobic incubation, and examined next day for haemolytic streptococci and *Staph. aureus* or for a heavy growth of any other organism not commonly found in profusion in the mouth. Aphthous ulcers are not, as far as is known, caused by bacterial infection; it may occasionally be necessary to take cultures from them to exclude the infections previously mentioned. Syphilis and tuberculosis must also be borne in mind as possible causes of mouth ulcers.

Herpes simplex virus sometimes causes painful ulcers inside the mouth, particularly in immunosuppressed patients. Mouth lesions may also be seen in herpangina or in hand, foot and mouth disease caused by members of the Coxsackie A group of viruses. A swab in virus transport medium frozen at $-70°C$ should be sent with a sample of clotted blood. Isolation and a rise in antibody titre to the virus isolated will confirm the diagnosis.

Antrum wash-out fluid

Pus aspirated from the antrum is treated as described in Chapter 3 but it is worthwhile in addition to set up a primary Optochin sensitivity test for the rapid indentification or exclusion of *Str. pneumoniae*. Primary tests of sputum can be made on the same plate (for method, see page 100). Common pathogens found are *Str. pneumoniae, Str. pyogenes, Staph. aureus* and *H. influenzae*. Non-sporing anaerobes, particularly cocci, may also be seen in almost pure growth. Examination of pus by gas-liquid chromatography (GLC) is useful to identify anaerobic infection.

Saline washings from patients with chronic antrum infections are always contaminated with the upper respiratory tract commensals, and detailed investigation of them is of doubtful value. Moreover, the saline may kill delicate organisms within an hour or two, so predominance of growth of different species in cultures is more than usually unreliable as an indication of their predominance in the material sampled. Usually the main purpose of the investigation is to find which, if any, of the available antibiotics or chemotherapeutic agents is likely to be successful in treatment. Antimicrobial agents should not be recommended when there is no clear indication of a bacterial pathogen.

Procedure

As soon as possible after the fluid has been collected, make a stained film and seed on three blood agar plates for aerobic and anaerobic incubation and for antibiotic sensitivity tests by the paper disc method described in Chapter 9. Common pathogens encountered are *Str. pneumoniae* and *Haemophilus* (for their identification, see Chapter 5). Often a very scanty growth of several different species is found, which do not resemble known pathogens. This may be reported forthwith: 'Cultures yield no significant growth'.

Sputum

Examination for *Myco. tuberculosis* will be considered in Chapter 6 and for fungal infection in Chapter 7. Other primary pathogens which must be excluded in respiratory infections are: *Str. pneumoniae, Str. pyogenes, Staph. aureus, H. influenzae, Legionella pneumophila*, occasionally *Branhamella catarrhalis* and, rarely, Friedlander's bacillus.

General considerations*

In acute bacterial pneumonia the pathogen is seen in smears and recovered almost pure from all the cultures. With the exception of tubercle bacilli, all the common lung pathogens can be recovered from the upper respiratory tract of apparently healthy people. Their recovery in small numbers from sputum is not therefore sufficient evidence that they are the cause of a particular infection. Often when sputum is examined from an acutely ill patient the cultures yield a scanty mixed growth of mouth and upper respiratory tract commensals, mainly streptococci. A few colonies of *Str. pneumoniae, H. influenzae*, diphtheroids, neisseria, yeasts, coliforms and haemolytic streptococci (often Lancefield's group C) may also be found. The proportion of each type of colony on the different cultures often varies and this cannot be accounted for by the different atmospheres in which the plates were incubated. Moreover, if different portions of purulent material are cultured from the same specimen, different organisms may be found. The cause of many acute respiratory infections is still largely a matter for speculation; if they are fully investigated a proportion prove to be virus or mycoplasma pneumonias, rickettsial infections or Legionnaire's disease, but in a large number of cases the patient recovers and no satisfactory laboratory diagnosis is made. Some of these are not true infections but are due to aspiration of secretions followed by blockage of small bronchi and collapse of the lung distally. Physiotherapy will do more to help the patient than antibiotic treatment aimed at the commensals isolated. Most of the remainder are probably caused by viruses but proof must await more effective diagnostic virological methods. From the physician's point of view, two questions are asked: first, 'Is the patient suffering from an acute bacterial respiratory infection?'; second, 'Is treatment with specific chemotherapeutic agents likely to be beneficial?' Routine examination of sputum is therefore aimed at answering them.

Sputum samples should be collected early in the morning. To avoid misleading results, samples more than 24 hours old should not be processed. Because of overgrowth by organisms of doubtful pathogenicity, the routine culture of sputum from patients receiving antimicrobial agents should be discouraged.

Interpretation of sputum cultures is facilitated by liquefaction and dilution of the specimen (Dixon and Miller, 1965). Pneumococci and haemophilus normally present in the nasopharynx may contaminate the specimen; dilution will prevent their appearance in the cultures. A true pathogen will be present in sufficient numbers to appear in almost pure culture from the diluted specimen. Untreated sputum is very difficult to

*See also page 52.

sample for culture, and liquefaction avoids the risk of accidentally choosing a non-purulent part of the specimen.

Liquefaction must be rapid and preferably carried out at room temperature to prevent overgrowth in the specimen of contaminating staphylococci and coliforms. A solution of N-acetyl-L-cysteine will liquefy sputum in 30 minutes at room temperature (18°C) if it is constantly shaken (Mead and Woodhams, 1964). The solution must be freshly made; for convenience, bottles containing each of the three reagents (see below) are prepared ready for use. The procedure should be carried out in a safety cabinet and the bottles should be shaken upright to avoid wetting the caps.

Procedure
Choose a purulent part of the specimen; tease two small pieces of it on two slides to make films for Gram and acid-fast stains. Streak the remainder across a blood agar plate for direct Optochin sensitivity. This is most easily done with a short sterile swab as used for antibiotic sensitivity tests (see Chapter 9); at least 6 samples of sputum can be tested on one plate (page 100). This often saves time because it enables pneumococci to be differentiated from other α-haemolytic streptococci after overnight incubation. Samples of antral pus can be tested on the same plate. An additional advantage is that this pre-liquefaction culture checks that the specimen was satisfactory and that lack of growth on the dilution cultures means few organisms were present.

Dilution method (Dixon and Miller (1965) modified)
Material

> N-acetyl-L-cysteine 2 g in sterile screw-capped bottles.
> 80 ml phosphate buffer (sterile) containing 0.15 ml universal indicator; the solution should be pale green pH 7.
> 13 ml sterile 4% NaOH.
> 10 ml ¼ strength Ringer solution (sterile) in a sterile screw-capped bottle.

Method*
Add the cysteine to the buffer and mix well; the solution will turn pink. Add the sodium hydroxide and mix well. Add an equal volume of this fresh green solution to sputum and shake for 30 minutes at room temperature, being careful not to wet the cap of the sputum pot.

Using an automatic pipette transfer 0.1 ml homogenate to the Ringer solution and mix well. With a sterile disposable loop, transfer 0.01 ml of the dilution to blood agar and incubate in air plus 5–10% CO_2 because some strains of *Str. pneumoniae* and *H. influenzae* fail to grow on first isolation without it. Chocolate blood agar can be used but good quality defibrinated horse-blood agar is satisfactory and there is no need to use a special medium.

Presumptive identification of *H. influenzae* may be facilitated by

---

*Note. All sputum specimens should be handled with care and processed in a safety cabinet.

inhibiting coccal growth with a bacitracin disc, leaving *Haemophilus* species, which are resistant, to grow within the zone of inhibition. Although the colonies are small on blood agar, they are easily seen with a hand lens. Satellitism around colonies of commensals is often visible. Similarly, an Optochin disc may give presumptive evidence of *Str. pneumoniae*. In both situations the discs are a guide, and further tests are necessary to confirm the presence of the organisms (see pages 99, 123).

Sputum from acute respiratory infection

Microscopy

A clinical diagnosis of acute bacterial pneumonia can often be strengthened by examining a Gram-stained film of a mucopurulent part of the sputum, when the pathogen will be seen in areas full of pus cells, uncontaminated by other bacteria. Because the relation of the bacteria to pus cells is important in assessing their significance, the film must be made before liquefaction.

Culture

Examine the cultures, using a hand lens, and record a description of the colonies seen; Gram-stain them. If any resemble the important lung pathogens, inoculate single colonies into suitable media for identification. Colonies of *Str. pneumoniae* and other α-haemolytic streptococci frequently resemble each other morphologically. An Optochin sensitivity test (described on page 100) is always required if cultures yield a moderate or heavy growth of small α-haemolytic colonies which are Gram-positive cocci.

Significance of culture results: reports

When *Str. pneumoniae* is recovered in almost pure culture from sputum, it is considered to be the primary pathogen. Staphylococcal pneumonia may occur as part of a generalized septicaemia but *Staph. aureus* is also found as a secondary invader in acute influenza virus pneumonia. When it is found in pure culture in sputum from acute primary pneumonia and there is no evidence of recent staphylococcal infection elsewhere, a virus infection should be suspected. In such a case the infection may fail to respond to rigorous antibiotic therapy. *H. influenzae* is well known as a secondary invader in influenzal pneumonia and is probably incapable of causing acute infection of a healthy normal lung, although it may do so postoperatively and in the elderly. *Branhamella catarrhalis* (see page 106) is occasionally implicated as a secondary invader in lower respiratory tract infection (Slevin *et al.*, 1984). The organism is often β-lactamase producing, which may result in therapeutic failure.

When the predominant organism has been identified the report may read thus:

'Smear: Numerous pus cells and Gram-positive capsulated diplococci; no acid-fast bacilli seen.

'Cultures yield a mixed growth, mainly *Str. pneumoniae* which is sensitive to pencillin.'

When cultures yield a scanty mixed growth, or when an organism, not one of the known pathogens, is predominant on one plate culture and absent on the others, no attempt is made to identify all the species found. The report might then read:

'Smear: Numerous pus cells, small numbers of various organisms; no acid-fast bacilli seen.
'Cultures yield a scanty mixed growth of doubtful significance.'

The result of antibiotic sensitivity tests should not be reported unless the microbiologist is satisfied that the organisms tested are likely pathogens. It is foolish to expect that treatment with a drug which is active against commensals will necessarily benefit the patient. In treated patients such reports may be a positive danger. Resistant commensals appear within a day or two of the onset of treatment, and physicians have been known to change the antibiotic in spite of a good clinical response because the laboratory reported that organisms in the sputum were resistant.

This is particularly likely when patients have received ampicillin-like antibiotics and cultures yield antibiotic-resistant Enterobacteriaceae or *Pseudomonas*. Since their colonies are large the quantity of growth, and hence its significance, tends to be overestimated. The dilution procedure recommended avoids this pitfall because when they are contaminants they will not appear on the dilution culture. When an almost pure growth of them is seen it is important to check that a fresh specimen has been received and that large numbers cannot be due to growth in the sample after collection. Serious and even fatal infection is sometimes caused by them, especially as a complication of immunosuppression. The difficulty of assessment is similar to the problem of contaminated urine samples.

The bacillus responsible for Legionnaire's disease, which usually presents as an atypical pneumonia, cannot easily be isolated from sputum but may be seen. It is a pleomorphic coccobacillus which stains irregularly or Gram-negative and can be identified by immunofluorescence. Strong carbol fuchsin (as used for the Ziehl–Neelsen stain) unheated is likely to reveal its presence in specimens better than the Gram stain (Porschen, 1979). The organism may be cultured on supplemented buffered charcoal yeast extract agar (see page 314). Cultures are incubated at $35°C$ in a moist atmosphere, for up to 14 days. Grey-blue or purple colonies indicate presumptive legionellae. Contaminating organisms may be suppressed by heating the specimen to $50°C$ for 30 minutes before inoculating the plate; *L. pneumophila* will withstand this treatment, other species may not. Culture is unlikely to be successful unless large numbers of the organism are present in the specimen.

Samples of serum should also be obtained to be examined for specific antibody (page 260). When the patient is seriously ill and not responding to treatment, a trial of erythromycin, or this drug combined with rifampicin, is indicated since, at present, a firm diagnosis is likely to be too much delayed to be useful as a guide to treatment.

Chronic bronchitis; emphysema; asthma

It is doubtful whether routine blood agar cultures of sputum from such cases are of any value as an aid to diagnosis or treatment.

Acute exacerbations in chronically infected patients are usually caused by pneumococci, *H. influenzae* or, occasionally, *B. catarrhalis*. As these species are at present usually sensitive to antibiotics, it is reasonable and quicker to make a clinical therapeutic trial, particularly as there can be no guarantee that the pathogen will be isolated from the first sample of sputum examined. Cultures should be made when an exacerbation is sufficiently severe for admission to hospital, as guidance may be needed if treatment fails and the chance of a useful result is greater in these circumstances.

Bronchiectasis

In this condition the bronchi are abnormally susceptible to acute infection. During an attack the sputum is investigated as already described for acute pneumonia. Cultures may be requested of sputum from a patient with localized chronic disease, to test the antibiotic sensitivity of the organisms before operation. Numular sputum from bronchiectatic cavities yields a very varied growth of any or all of the organisms previously mentioned. An extra blood agar culture incubated anaerobically plus 10% CO_2 should be made from a purulent part of the untreated specimen because non-sporing anaerobes may predominate; they are unlikely to survive the prolonged exposure to air which is inevitable during liquefaction.

Lung abscess and bronchoscopy specimens

These specimens are treated as pus (see page 46).

Gastric aspiration and vomit

Samples aspirated from the stomach of newborn infants suspected of infection are examined for pus cells and bacteria. Likely pathogens are *N. gonorrhoeae* and *Str. agalactiae* (group B). Gonococci may be seen associated with pus cells in their typical form, pus from the mother's cervix having been swallowed during labour. When pus cells or bacteria are seen in a Gram-stained smear of the specimen, it is cultured as described for pus (page 46), with an additional plate for selection of *N. gonorrhoeae* (page 314). Gastric aspiration from a healthy newborn infant yields very scanty or no growth.

Gastric aspiration from adults may be sent from patients with ulcers suspected of *Campylobacter pylori* infection. They are examined for the presence of urease (Owen *et al.*, 1985) and cultured (see page 73).

Vomit is occasionally submitted for culture from patients with food poisoning. Culture methods are as described for faeces. Microscopy may show Gram-positive bacilli when *Bac. cereus* or *Cl. perfringens* has been swallowed. Filtrate of vomit may contain bacterial toxins and should be sent to a reference laboratory for examination when symptoms suggest botulism.

Botulism

In many cases only the toxin is ingested, the organisms having multiplied, formed their toxin and died before the food was eaten. When *Cl. botulinum* is still viable it will isolated more easily from the remains of food than from the patient's excreta.

Faeces

The majority of faecal specimens examined come from patients with acute intestinal symptoms. The most important organisms to be considered are the salmonellae, shigellae and *Campylobacter* species. Selective methods are required for the reliable isolation of these organisms, and numerous media have been described for the purpose. All have advantages and limitations. Selective media in general act by inhibition of normal commensal organisms. However, to a lesser extent they may also inhibit the pathogens themselves. The success of a selective medium for a particular pathogen therefore depends on the absence of harmless organisms in the faecal flora able to grow well on it. *Proteus, Ps. aeruginosa* and other non-lactose-fermenting organisms are commonly found in loose stools from any cause, and may outgrow the pathogen. No enrichment medium will inhibit *Proteus* and *Ps. aeruginosa* and yet guarantee to yield a good growth of *Salmonella* and *Shigella* after overnight incubation. During the acute stage of infection, pathogens are present in large numbers, and may be readily isolated. However, the variable nature of the faecal flora will account for the difficulty in recovering pathogens late in the infection, and from suspected carriers.

Selection of *Campylobacter* species is achieved by using medium screened with antibiotics (page 73). The need for a microaerophilic atmosphere and an increased incubation temperature also inhibits overgrowth by commensal organisms. The ability to isolate *Camp. jejuni* from faeces is essential for the diagnostic laboratory because it is one of the commonest causes of acute diarrhoea (Wilson *et al.*, 1983). Cholera and other pathogenic vibrios are uncommon, but when a history of possible exposure is given a suitable medium must be inoculated (see page 74). *Yersinia enterocolitica*, and occasionally *Y. pseudotuberculosis*, may be recovered from the faeces of symptomatic patients (see page 127).

For examination of specimens from an outbreak of food poisoning see page 291.

Macroscopic and microscopic examination

Note colour, consistency and any abnormality such as pus, blood and excess mucus.

Microscopy of faecal specimens is required when requested and when diarrhoea persists in the absence of a bacterial diagnosis. Fresh stool samples should be processed as described in Chapter 8.

Culture

Isolation of *Salmonella* and *Shigella*

When the stool is liquid it can be seeded without preparation. When it is solid take a piece about the size of a small pea on the end of a swab or stout wire loop and make a thick emulsion in peptone water. Seed the specimen or emulsion on MacConkey agar, XLD agar and desoxycholate citrate agar (DCA) and inoculate about 1 ml of it into selenite broth;* incubate the plates and the broth culture at 37°C.

1st day

(*a*) When lactose fermenters only are found on the MacConkey agar, make a note of the growth. (It should be very heavy if the specimen is satisfactory, unless the patient has received antibiotics by mouth.) Cultures from infants and young children must be examined for the serological types of *Esch. coli* known to cause infantile enteritis (see page 110). This may also be required occasionally in outbreaks of diarrhoea in adults since particular types of *Esch. coli* foreign to the country of origin of the patient may cause travellers' diarrhoea (Rowe *et al.*, 1970). There are two main categories which cause disease in adults: enterotoxic *Esch. coli* are rare in Britain but may be seen in travellers from the East; enteroinvasive *Esch. coli* are non-lactose-fermenting and resemble *Shigella*. Sera for their identification are not generally available at present; therefore, when an outbreak of infection by one of them is suspected, strains must be sent to a reference laboratory for typing. The MacConkey agar plate is incubated at room temperature for a further 24 hours. When the specimen is loose and the patient has undiagnosed diarrhoea, test lactose-fermenting colonies for oxidase production, *Aeromonas* is a possible cause (see below).

The desoxycholate citrate culture usually shows much less growth of lactose-fermenters and may be sterile, when no non-lactose-fermenting colonies are found reincubate it. Subculture a large loopful of the selenite broth onto XLD agar incubated at 37°C. XLD agar (xylose lysine desoxycholate) medium (Taylor, 1965) was originally formulated for the isolation of shigellae from faeces. McCarthy (1966) demonstrated its suitability for the presumptive identification of both salmonellae and shigellae. Commensal organisms ferment xylose and will appear as yellow colonies on the medium. When yellow colonies only are present, the plate should be reincubated.

(*b*) Non-lactose-fermenting colonies seen on the MacConkey or desoxycholate citrate agar will require further investigation. Shigellae do not ferment xylose and will appear as red colonies on the XLD agar. Salmonellae do ferment xylose but in addition will decarboxylate lysine

---

*Faeces from a suspected typhoid carrier should, addition, be cultivated on Wilson and Blair's bismuth sulphite medium.

(except *Salm. paratypi* A), maintaining the pH of the medium alkaline, and then mimicking colonies of *Shigella* species. In addition, salmonellae will produce hydrogen sulphide and appear as red colonies with black centres. Commensal hydrogen-sulphide-producing organisms do not decarboxylate lysine and generally produce black pigment only after reincubation.

Potential enteric pathogens (one of each kind from each plate) are subcultured to peptone water and a urea slope. The remains of each colony is Gram-stained. It is essential that *single* colonies only should be picked. It is false economy in time and materials to risk contaminating a culture which is to be used for fermentation tests. Contamination may not be recognized and may lead to delay in identification or a wrong diagnosis. Consequently, if there is the slightest possibility that a colony may be contaminated by other close colonies, it should be seeded first onto MacConkey agar and picked off as a single colony on the next day.

Non-lactose-fermenting colonies are easily overlooked, particularly on desoxycholate citrate agar, because they are translucent and the same colour as the medium. *Sh. sonnei* is a late lactose fermenter, but may be mistaken for a poorly fermenting strain of *Esch. coli* after overnight culture owing to the development of a pale pink colour. Occasional strains of lactose-fermenting salmonellae occur but will be distinguishable on the XLD medium. If MacConkey plates have been poured rather deeper than usual or are heavily coloured with neutral red, non-lactose-fermenting colonies may appear pink because the colour is transmitted through them from the medium, translucency is a better guide than colour. All translucent colonies should be regarded as non-lactose fermenters until proved otherwise.

After 2–4 hours' incubation the urea slope may appear pink. This is due to the growth of a urease producer and is evidence that the colony seeded on it is not a *Salmonella* or *Shigella*; the peptone water culture may therefore be discarded. When there is no evidence of urease production, inoculate each peptone water culture to MacConkey agar for purity and into a series of media for biochemical tests. Examination of a hanging drop preparation from the peptone water culture may obviate the need for further investigation when *Shigella* only is of interest (e.g. in specimens from a dysentery epidemic or in a search for carriers) because highly motile strains are not *Shigella*. The hanging drop method is the most rapid and reliable way of estimating motility, which is one of the essential tests for preliminary identification, but in unskilled hands it is hazardous. When there is no urgency, motility can be demonstrated in an overnight culture by stab-inoculating a semi-solid, clear, nutrient medium in a tube. Motile organisms will grow out from the stab to give cloudiness throughout the medium and non-motile growth will be confined to the stab, the surrounding medium remaining clear: this is the safer and therefore the preferred method for routine use.

When larger numbers of stools and rectal swabs are examined a short range of tests including sucrose and Kligler's composite medium saves time and materials (Kligler, 1918; Bailey and Lacey, 1927). In laboratories where most Enterobacteriaceae come from urine or wound cultures and

Table 4.2

| Probable identity | Motility | Indole | Sucrose* | Kligler's medium | | | |
				Butt	Slope	Gas	Blackening
Salm. typhi	+(−)	−	−	Yellow	Pink	−	+
Salmonella spp.	+(−)	−	−	Yellow	Pink	+	+
Shigella spp.	−	+−	−	Yellow	Pink	−	−

* Sh. sonnei may show very weak fermentation after overnight incubation.

therefore need full identification, it may be economical to put non-lactose-fermenters which fail to split urea through the full range of tests rather than to prepare an extra composite medium. Commercially produced miniaturized biochemical tests for screening (API 10S) can be employed but are costly (see page 111). Laboratories processing a large number of faecal specimens can screen cultures economically (see Table 4.2), leaving the API system for final identification of presumed positive strains.

2nd day
Examine the subcultures from the selenite broths and proceed with them in the manner described for the original plate cultures. Reincubated DCA plates are also examined, and if non-fermenters have not appeared they may be discarded. Small colonies seen on the MacConkey agar after 48 hours may indicate *Yersinia* infection (see page 127).

Examine the tubes inoculated from the peptone water cultures of non-lactose-fermenters. The media inoculated for biochemical tests are chosen for their usefulness in excluding as rapidly as possible non-lactose-fermenters which are not members of the *Salmonella* or *Shigella* groups. No attempt is made to identify these organisms and they are not mentioned in the report. The following is a list of media for first-line tests on non-lactose-fermenters, with notes on the value of each of them.

Peptone water
Examined after 2–4 hours' growth for motility, if it is actively motile, *Shigella* is excluded. After overnight incubation test for indole; if it is present, the organism is not a *Salmonella* (see Chapter 5).

Fermentation of carbohydrates
   Glucose and mannite: All salmonellae ferment these sugars, with the formation of acid and gas, except *Salm. typhi* which ferments them without gas production. Many shigellae ferment them both, forming acid but no gas.
   Sucrose: Not fermented by *Salmonella*. Salicin can also be employed for the exclusion of *Salmonella* and *Shigella*, which do not ferment it.
   Lactose: Confirms that the bacterium under investigation is a non-lactose-fermenter. Note that *Sh. sonnei* ferments lactose late.
   Dulcite: Fermented by almost all salmonellae except *Salm. typhi* which may not ferment it. Not fermented by *Shigella*.

Urea slope
Proteus and other organisms produce urease which changes urea to ammonium carbonate and ammonia. The intestinal pathogens do not give this reaction.

Agar slope
Pigmented growth or colour diffusing into the agar excludes *Salmonella* and *Shigella*. The culture will be used for agglutination tests when necessary. After overnight incubation, refer to Table 5.6 (page 113) which indicates possible identity of strains. Cultures giving positive reactions alien to *Salmonella* and *Shigella* may be discarded.

When Kligler's medium and sucrose only have been inoculated, strains giving reactions seen in Table 4.2 after overnight incubation need further investigation; others can be discarded.

Growth on the Kligler slope can be used for slide agglutination. When this confirms the probable identification, the physician can be telephoned. Weak positive slide agglutination should be ignored and the strain fully identified before a report is sent. Final identification must await a full set of biochemical reactions and further agglutination tests (see Chapter 5). *Aeromonas hydrophila* and *Plesiomonas shigelloides* may be occasional causes of diarrhoea (Sawle *et al.*, 1984; Mandal *et al.*, 1982). There is still some controversy as to the significance of these organisms, but identification of them by field laboratories will help to elucidate their pathogenesis and epidemiology. *Plesiomonas* may be presumptively identified by using the procedures for salmonellae and shigellae, and *Aeromonas* by testing lactose-fermenting colonies for oxidase production (see above). Table 4.3 summarizes the relevant results, including *Pseudomonas* species for comparison. Identification of *Aeromonas hydrophila* and *Plesiomonas shigelloides* is confirmed by API 20E (see page 111). Presumptive *Pseudomonas* species are discarded as not significant. For the possible role of *Edwardsiella tarda*, see page 119.

Table 4.3   Scheme for presumptive identification of *Aeromonas* and *Plesiomonas* species

	Aeromonas	*Plesiomonas*	*Pseudomonas*
Indole	+	+	−
Urea	−	−	−
Sucrose	V	−	−
Glucose	A(G)	A	−
Lactose	+	−	−
H$_2$S	−	−	−
Oxidase	+	+	+

A = acid G = gas; V = variable; () = some strains negative.

Isolation of *Campylobacter* species (from Skirrow, 1977)
Using blood agar containing polymyxin, vancomycin and trimethoprim (for preparation, see page 314), seed the liquid or emulsified faeces in the

usual way. Two specimens or even four can be inoculated per 8-cm plate because selection is very efficient and the medium is costly. However, the organism tends to spread to some extent and specimens must not, therefore, be inoculated very close to each other. Place the plates in an anaerobic jar without a catalyst, evacuate to minus 50 mmHg and run in hydrogen or hydrogen–nitrogen mixture, containing 10% CO_2. Incubate the jars at 42°C.

Examine the cultures after 48 hours' incubation. The colonies are about 0.5 mm in diameter, grey and moist. Moist grey confluent growth spreading from the area of inoculation may be seen; it has a well defined edge unlike spreading *Proteus*. Gram stain will reveal small s-shaped or spiral Gram-negative bacilli typical in appearance. When a suspension is made in peptone water for examination in a hanging drop, typical tumbling motility is seen and some of the organisms make a short spurt in one direction and then go rapidly into reverse. At this stage a preliminary diagnosis is possible but subcultures in parallel should be made to blood agar incubated at 37°C in air and to blood agar incubated microaerophilically, as described above, at 42°C to confirm that the organism will grow only in conditions suitable for *Campylobacter*.

Isolation of vibrios

Although cholera has not been endemic in Britain for more than a century, it may be necessary to exclude it in patients with diarrhoea who have visited endemic areas within the previous 2 weeks; special medium will be required.

Procedure (from Furniss and Donovan, 1974)
Inoculate 20 ml alkaline peptone water, pH 8, with 2 ml liquid faeces or the same quantity of emulsified faeces from a suspected carrier.

Seed heavily on thiosulphate–citrate–bile–salt–sucrose agar (TCBS) medium.

After 5 hours' incubation, inoculate another TCBS plate from the top of the peptone water culture and also another alkaline peptone water from this first tube. Incubate for a further 5 hours or overnight and inoculate a third TCBS plate from the second alkaline peptone water.

Vibrio cholerae forms 2 mm yellow colonies on TCBS. It is Gram-negative but not necessarily curved and vibrio-like. Slide agglutination with polyvalent serum will confirm a tentative diagnosis. When it is negative it should be repeated from growth on nutrient agar. When it is positive the nearest reference laboratory should be telephoned forthwith so that final identification can be made and the appropriate public health measures instituted without delay.

Patients arriving by air from the Far East may suffer from infection by *Vibrio parahaemolyticus*, which can also be isolated on TCBS. It does not ferment sucrose and the colonies will therefore appear green.

These methods are also described in PHLS Monograph No.11 (1978).

Pseudomembranous colitis

This potentially fatal disease is now recognized to be an important cause of diarrhoea following antibiotic treatment, especially in patients undergoing abdominal surgery.

The diagnosis is made by sigmoidoscopy, when plaques of necrotic epithelium can be seen. The most common cause is toxin produced by *Cl. difficile*, which can be neutralized by *Cl. sordelli* antitoxin; it can be demonstrated in high titre in the stools (Larson *et al.*, 1978). *Cl. difficile*, which is uncommon in normal adult faeces, can be isolated from the faeces of those affected. It is often resistant to lincomycin and clindamycin but sensitive to metronidazole and vancomycin. The disease needs urgent treatment and therefore vancomycin (Tedesco *et al.*, 1978) is given by mouth and all other antimicrobials are stopped. Unlike vancomycin, metronidazole is rapidly absorbed and is unlikely to be present in the lumen of the colon in sufficient quantity to inhibit toxin production when given orally.

The introduction of selective media for *Cl. difficile* (see page 316) has considerably simplified isolation. However, toxin, either in the specimen or produced by the strain in culture, must be demonstrated before isolation can be considered significant (see page 132). Laboratory findings must be interpreted in the light of the patient's clinical condition. Cases of pseudomembranous colitis responding to vancomycin therapy in the absence of organisms or demonstrable toxin are well documented (Phillips *et al.*, 1981). Both organism and toxin, in low titre, have been demonstrated in the faeces of normal infants (Larson *et al.*, 1978).

Method

Prepare tenfold dilutions of faeces (10^{-1} to 10^{-5}) by emulsifying a pea-sized portion of faeces in 9 ml of saline. Inoculate a whole plate of *Cl. difficile* selective agar from the 10^{-1} dilution and half-plates with the remaining dilutions. Incubate plates anaerobically for 48 hours at 37°C. In addition, inoculate a Robertson's cooked meat medium for incubation at 37°C for 5 days. Examine culture plates under ultra-violet light (Wood's lamp) for fluorescing yellow/green colonies (George *et al.*, 1979). If suspected colonies are Gram-positive bacilli, inoculate them into a Robertson's cooked meat medium for a further 48 hours' incubation. (Products of metabolism may be identified using gas-liquid chromatography when available.) Subculture the 5-day cooked meat medium onto *Cl. difficile* selective medium or nalidixic blood agar (see page 313) for anaerobic incubation. If colonies resembling *Cl. difficile* are isolated at any stage, test the cooked meat cultures for the presence of toxin (see page 132). The original sample of faeces may also be tested similarly for the presence of toxin.

Viral enteritis

Intestinal symptoms are commonly associated with virus infections, especially in children, but it is not often possible to culture virus causing enteritis from faeces. Direct electron microscopy reveals large numbers of virions in faeces of infected patients which cannot be grown. Antigen-detection kits for the diagnosis of rotavirus infection are now available (see page 275). Electron microscopy remains the method of choice for infections caused by adenoviruses, astroviruses and caliciviruses. Specimens of faeces from patients with suspected viral diarrhoea should be sent to a virus laboratory with full facilities. They do not require freezing or special transport media.

Necrotizing enterocolitis

This is a disease of neonates, usually premature, in neonatal units. Its cause is unknown and although symptoms are caused by escape of microbes from the gut into tissues it is unlikely to be primarily infective (Kliegman and Fanaroff, 1984). An attempt at microbial diagnosis is not likely to be helpful once known causes of infection have been excluded.

Genital specimens

The bacteriological diagnosis of genital infections is comparatively straightforward in acute venereal disease, but many non-specific acute infections are encountered in which even prolonged and detailed investigation fails to reveal sufficient evidence to incriminate a particular species as pathogen. Examination of these specimens from women is particularly difficult because they are often contaminated by the normal vaginal flora which is largely composed of slow-growing organisms, many of which are microaerophilic or anaerobic and which show very poor colonial differentiation for the first 2 or 3 days of incubation. The lactobacilli, diphtheroids, anaerobic non-sporing bacilli, anaerobic Gram-positive cocci, Gram-variable coccobacilli and *Listeria* isolated from the vagina have been studied by many microbiologists, but so far these groups of organisms are not satisfactorily classified, and, although there is no doubt that some of them can under suitable conditions assume a pathogenic role, in individual cases it is often impossible to assign it to a particular species. Unless the suspected organism is a well established pathogen, its presence in large numbers in the cultures is not by itself sufficient evidence of pathogenicity. (For evidence required to establish a strain as pathogen, see Chapter 1.)

It is convenient to consider specimens according to the clinical state of the patient from whom they are taken.

Acute infections

Puerperal sepsis, septic abortion and pelvic inflammatory disease

Bacteria found

RECOGNIZED PATHOGENS	OTHER BACTERIA
Str. pyogenes	*Corynebacterium* spp.
Cl. perfringens	*Lactobacillus* spp.
Anaerobic streptococci	*Staphylococcus* spp.

Staph. aureus
Streptoccoccus group B
Str. faecalis
Esch. coli
Neisseria gonorrhoeae
Listeria monocytogenes
Mycoplasma hominis
Bacteroides spp.
Chlamydia trachomatis

Streptococcus spp.
Actinomyces israeli
Anaerobic Gram-positive cocci
Anaerobic Gram-negative cocci
Any of the bacteria, particularly
anaerobes, which invade wounds (see
Chapter 3)

Since puerperal fever may be rapidly fatal if untreated, the usual practice when pyrexia is discovered is to swab the cervix and begin treatment without waiting for the results of culture. Fortunately, many common uterine pathogens are penicillin sensitive and the patient is often convalescent by the time the report reaches the ward. Nevertheless, these infections should be thoroughly investigated. When Str. pyogenes or antibiotic-resistant 'hospital' Staph. aureus are found in puerperal infection it is a sign that the aseptic surgical technique may have failed, and it is important to discover how this has occurred so that future accidents may be avoided. Infection by the other pathogens listed above indicates that bacteria from the patient's own vagina or perineum have invaded the uterus, and epidemic spread of the infection is extremely unlikely. Stuart's transport medium is recommended for cervical or high vaginal swabs because anaerobes survive well in it and microbes such as Mycoplasma hominis which will not stand drying are preserved. For Chlamydia trachomatis investigations see pages 259 and 270.

Procedure
Make a smear for Gram-stain. Seed the swab on two blood agar plates and a neomycin blood agar plate for incubation in air plus CO_2 and anaerobically. In addition, MacConkey's bile salt agar, a mycoplasma agar (incubated anaerobically plus CO_2) and a gonococcal selective (GC) agar (incubated in air plus CO_2), should be inoculated. For economy, a quarter of a GC agar plate may be used.

1st day. Examine the cultures carefully for colonies resembling the species in the first list above. When any of them are present in profusion they are considered to be the cause of the infection because they have been proved pathogenic on numerous previous occasions. Str. pyogenes is so rarely found in a healthy vagina that even a few colonies signify the possibility of infection. When, however, a satisfactory specimen yields only a few colonies of Cl. perfringens, Esch. coli, Str. faecalis, Staph. aureus or anaerobic streptococci, it may well be that they are harmless and the pyrexia may be caused by infection with a slow growing species which has not yet appeared, or by infection elsewhere, perhaps in the urinary tract or chest. Single colonies of all types resembling bacteria in the first list above are Gram-stained and subcultured into suitable medium for identification tests. At this stage a preliminary report may be sent. Reincubate aerobic and anaerobic blood agar and neomycin agar plates and note further growth the next day. Non-sporing anaerobes, particularly anaerobic streptoccocci, often need at least 48 hours' incubation before colonies are visible. The GC agar should be examined at 48 hours for typical colonies, which are picked off and identified (see page 103). The mycoplasma medium is examined after 72 hours' incubation (see page 137). The application of a penicillin-impregnated disc to the plate after initial inoculation will aid recognition of suspect colonies because the mycoplasmas are resistant to it.

When in the Gram-stained smear of the specimen pus cells are few or absent, and on the second day none of the recognized pathogens listed above has appeared, a report can be sent worded to show that complete identification of all species has not been attempted (see page 5). When the smear shows evidence of infection as judged by numerous pus cells, few squamous cells and lack of the normal varied vaginal flora, the specimen is treated as pus. Prolonged incubation may lead to the implication of non-sporing anaerobes, *Mycoplasma, Listeria monocytogenes* or some other slow-growing microbe as the cause of a particular infection.

For the investigation of actinomycosis in patients with an intrauterine device (IUD) (Traynor *et al.*, 1981), the device is smeared onto two blood agar plates, using sterile forceps. The IUD is then placed into fastidious anaerobic broth (FAB) (see page 26). Plates are incubated, one in air plus 5-10% CO_2 and the other anaerobically for 5 days. After 5 days the FAB is subcultured onto two further blood agar plates, for aerobic plus CO_2 and anaerobic incubation as above. The presence of whitish granules growing below the surface of the broth is suggestive of actinomyces. On the anaerobic blood agar, colonies are cream coloured, opaque and crumb-like (see page 156). No comparable growth is seen on the aerobic culture.

Acute cervicitis in non-pueperal women; acute urethritis; vulvovaginitis in children

Bacteria found

N. gonorrhoeae	*Chlamydia trachomatis*
Str. pyogenes	
Any of the bacteria listed under the previous section.	

Specially prepared swabs and transport medium* are required for gonococci; they are also satisfactory for other bacteria. A smear from material taken with an ordinary swab sent separately is desirable for two reasons. The transport medium swab is impregnated with charcoal which neutralizes inhibitors sometimes present in the medium and particles of it will spoil the appearance of the smear. Best results for the isolation of *N. gonorrhoeae* are achieved when patients attend a clinic where trained staff culture directly to warm selective medium. A small, sterile disposable loop introduced into cervix or urethra collects a much better sample for direct culture than a swab, which is usually too large to reach the site of infection. Culture plates are incubated immediately in the clinic and at the

*For preparations, see page 311.

end of the session are taken without delay for incubation in the laboratory in air plus 5–10% CO_2. Alternatively, laboratory staff should prepare smears and inoculate culture media at the bedside. Rectal and urethral swabs, in addition to the cervical specimen, should be taken from all women suspected of gonorrhoea. Swabbing the pharynx of both men and women, and the rectum of men, will occasionally be indicated for the diagnosis of gonorrhoea. Swabs should be cultured on the selective medium as described above. Direct examination of a Gram-stained preparation from these sites serves little purpose and may be misleading.

Where facilities for the isolation of *Chlam. trachomatis* are available, specimen collection is of extreme importance if a useful yield is to be obtained. A suitable transport medium is required (see page 311) and facilities for either deep freezing ($-70°C$) or rapid transport to the laboratory are necessary. Collection of specimens from the male urethra should be made by the insertion of a *small* wire-mounted cotton-wool-tipped swab 4–5 cm into the urethra; the swab is rotated before withdrawal. To obtain satisfactory specimens from the cervix the patient should be examined in the lithotomy position. The cervix is visualized using a bivalve speculum and wiped with sterile gauze held on sponge forceps. An ordinary wood-mounted swab is then inserted into the cervical canal and rotated. Swabs obtained in the above manner are squeezed out into the transport medium. Swabs should *not* be left in the medium. Recently, highly specific monoclonal and polyclonal antibodies have become commercially available for the detection of chlamydial antigen in ocular and genital specimens (see page 270).

Procedure*
Gram-stain the smear. Seed the swab from transport medium onto two blood agar plates and selective medium (see page 314). Incubate one blood agar and the selective medium in air plus 5–10% CO_2 and the other blood agar anaerobically plus 10% CO_2. Occasional strains of *N.gonorrhoeae* are inhibited by the selective medium. Therefore, for maximum success, plain blood agar or chocolate blood agar should also be included; this is very extravagant when a large clinic is served. An alternative is to use the selective medium alone, which will succeed for almost all actively infected patients, and repeat cultures on two media when a negative result is obtained from purulent material.

1st day
Gram-stain any colonies resembling *N. gonorrhoeae*. If none is found, reincubate the culture because many strains need 48 hours' incubation before growth is visible on first isolation. Do not allow the culture to stand on the bench until it is cold. Examine it quickly and reincubate it.

---

*This is equally applicable to the examination of discharges of *N. meningitidis*; the colonies closely resemble *N. gonorrhoeae*.

2nd day
After 48 hours' incubation, colonies of *N. gonorrhoeae* are typically
0.5–1.5 mm in diameter, moist, domed, with entire edge, translucent and
easily emulsifiable. They are never matt, rugose, heavily pigmented or
absolutely opaque. All colonies which resemble them are Gram-stained.
Any which prove to be Gram-negative cocci are identified by a coagglutination test (page 105). Alternatively, they may be subcultured to blood
agar for further tests.

Fluorescence microscopy
   Fluorescent antibody techniques can be applied to smears of pus from
suspected gonorrhoea. In positive cases the cocci fluoresce but
occasionally non-specific positives are seen. Therefore, culture followed
by rapid identification of the Gram-negative cocci by fluorescence
microscopy or coagglutination (see page 105) is recommended. A reliable
report 1–2 days later is preferable to risking an early false positive report.
N. gonorrhoeae and *N. meningitidis* have antigens in common and the
immunofluorescence test will be positive with either. Fermentation tests
will confirm the presumptive diagnosis of gonococcal infection (see page
104).

Acute microbial vaginitis and vaginosis
   There are three common microbial infections of the vagina. The fungus
Candida albicans and the protozoan *Trichomonas vaginalis* are readily
identifiable (Chapters 7 and 8). The third condition, previously termed
non-specific vaginitis, has been the subject of discussion and controversy
for many years. The association of *Gardnerella vaginalis* with the condition has long been recognized. More recently, various anaerobic non-
sporing bacteria and vibrios have also been implicated. However, their
role as primary pathogens remains unclear. The term 'bacterial vaginosis',
implying infection without overt inflammation, is preferable to the older
'non-specific vaginitis'. The diagnosis is essentially clinical, based on the
criteria described on page 137. The routine culture of specimens for
G. vaginalis is unnecessary, but when specific requests are received the
procedure described on page 137 is recommended.
   Gonorrhoea in adults is a disease of cervix and urethra not of the
vagina. Vaginal swabs are therefore not suitable for the diagnosis of
gonorrhoea except in childhood. Nevertheless, vaginal swabs sent from
general practitioners, who may find it impracticable always to take
cervical swabs, are worth examining; gonococci can be isolated from them
in acute infection.

Chronic infections

Leucorrhoea
   A large number of gynaecological patients complain of chronic vaginal
discharge. The causes of this symptom are manifold and in only relatively
few cases can leucorrhoea be attributed primarily to infection. In Britain

there are two important pathogens which need to be excluded: *Trichomonas vaginalis* and *Candida albicans*. There are almost certainly other infective causes of chronic vaginitis, but in most hospital laboratories it is impossible to make a full investigation of specimens from every case of vaginal discharge. The cultures yield a profuse growth of micro-aerophilic and anaerobic bacteria which need many days' incubation before pure cultures can be obtained for identification. Moreover, to establish any one of them as pathogen would need prolonged investigation and a search for more patients similarly infected. A compromise must therefore be made and the following routine has been found satisfactory both to clinician and microbiologist.

Procedure
Examine microscopically a wet preparation and Gram-stained film of all specimens. When numerous pus cells, yeasts or Gram-negative diplococci are seen, the preliminary diagnosis must be confirmed by culture. When there are very few pus cells the condition is most unlikely to be infective and cultures are not made. When chronic gonorrhoea is suspected, take *cervical*, urethral and rectal swabs in transport medium and use the method already described for acute cervicitis. When a patient shows any unusual sign, such as ulceration of the vaginal wall, and cultures may be expected to yield valuable information, a special note is sent with the swab explaining the need for culture in the first instance and the specimen is treated as pus.

Syphilis
Clean around the site of the suspected chancre with sterile gauze and saline. Induce bleeding by rubbing with a dry sterile swab or scarifier. Allow the clot to retract before collecting the serum onto a glass slide. Examine under dark-ground illumination or phase-contrast microscopy as soon as possible. Stained films of the fluid are much less satisfactory. Spirochaetes other than *Treponema pallidum* are often found in fluid from chronic ulcers; consequently, serological tests are mandatory, including the absorbed fluorescent treponemal antibody test.

Skin and conjunctiva

Bacteria found

Staph.aureus	Enterobacteriaceae
Coagulase-negative staphylococci	*Pseudomonas* spp.
Str. pyogenes	*Myco. tuberculosis*
Streptococcus spp.	*Mycobacterium* spp.
Anaerobic streptococci	*Erysipelothrix* spp.
Diphtheroids (some anaerobic or	*Actinomyces* spp.
microaerophilic)	*Nocardia* spp.
C. diphtheriae (rarely)	*Ps. mallei* and *B. anthracis* (very rarely)

Staph. aureus is the only pathogen which commonly inhabits the normal skin. Carrier rates vary from 10 to 20 per cent in apparently healthy adults, and the organism may remain in the skin for months or even years. Skin carriers are almost always nasal carriers and the skin population is probably maintained by reinoculation from the nose. Coagulase-negative staphylococci, micrococci and diphtheroids are often found on normal skin but they are usually harmless. The other microbes listed are present either as casual superficial contaminants, which are quickly removed by the antibacterial action of the skin secretions and by washing, or they are found in discharges from skin lesions.

Acute infections

Examine swabs from inflamed areas, impetigo, superficial wounds, burns, etc., by the method described for pus (see page 46). Bacteria found are *Str. pyogenes* and *Staph. aureus* very commonly, *C. diphtheriae* rarely. The skin of the buttocks, lower abdomen and thighs is often contaminated with coliforms and *Str. faecalis*; these may be found in other areas, especially after antibiotic therapy when they replace the antibiotic-sensitive pyogenic cocci.

Fluid from blisters is difficult to sample without accidental contamination. The following procedure is usually successful.

Select an intact bulla with as firm a layer of skin over it as possible. Clean the skin with liquid soap and spirit. It is very important that it should be dry before sampling. Pierce the skin of the bulla with the broken end of a sterile glass capillary tube (the fluid tends to be lost in a needle and syringe), and suck out the fluid. Place drops of it immediately onto two blood agar plates and into cooked meat broth. Incubate the plates in air and anaerobically. The fluid is often found to be sterile when broken blisters are heavily infected with pyogenic cocci.

Virus in vesicle fluid can be seen by electron microscopy. The fluid should be sent in a capillary tube sealed at each end. When herpes simplex is suspected and there is no possibility of smallpox, a small drop of fluid can be sent dried on a glass slide but this will not be suitable for culture and is potentially infective. It should be covered with another clean slide to avoid contamination of the container. A swab in virus transport medium frozen at $-70°C$, should be sent for culture in all cases when examination for virus cannot immediately be performed.

Chronic ulcers*

It is usually impossible to determine the cause of a chronic spreading ulcer by taking swabs from the weeping surface except when acid-fast bacilli are seen (see page 150). Secondary invaders (e.g. *Proteus, Ps. aeruginosa* and the pyogenic cocci) may sometimes be avoided by sampling in the following manner. Clean the healthy skin just beyond the edge of the ulcer with spirit, allow it to dry and then pierce the skin with a sterile hypodermic

*It is assumed that before these investigations are begun syphilis has been excluded by negative serological tests.

needle so that its point travels near the edge of the ulcer but below the surface; gently press the indurated tissue around the needle, withdraw it and, using a sterile syringe, squirt any tissue fluid which may be in it onto two glass slides, two blood agar plates, into cooked meat broth and 0.2% glucose broth for *Erysipelothrix*. When the quantity of fluid is insufficient, deliver one small drop onto blood agar and another onto a glass slide. The plate culture is best incubated anaerobically, as obligate aerobes are much less common than anaerobes.

When a biopsy is performed, take a small piece of the tissue in a sterile tube, wash it free of contaminants, grind it in a sterile tube or stomacher and make cultures as described for culture of tissue (page 42).

Bacteria found

Str. pyogenes
Streptococcus spp.
Anaerobic streptoccocci
Staph. aureus
C. diphtheriae (rarely)

Mycobacterium spp.
Actinomyces spp.
Norcardia spp.
Pseudomonas mallei
Erysipelothrix spp.

Bear in mind also the possibility of fungal infections, and, when necessary, stain smears for Leishman–Donovan bodies (see Chapter 8).

Conjunctival swabs

When the conjunctiva is acutely inflamed, the discharge is treated by the method described for pus.

The discharge is best cultured at the bedside (outpatients can attend the laboratory) because lysozyme in tears will kill some bacteria during transit. When direct culture cannot be made, a swab in transport medium should be sent. The anaerobic culture sometimes enables *Str. pneumoniae* or *Str. pyogenes* to be more easily recognized but anaerobic infection of this superficial site is very unlikely. Carbon dioxide, 5–10%, should be added for aerobic culture for the isolation of CO_2-dependent strains of *Haemophilus, Neisseria* and *Str. pneumoniae*. Additional primary culture on a Leoffler serum slope will aid recognition of *Moraxella*.

Conjunctivitis is also caused by adenoviruses and *Chlamydia trachomatis*. A swab in virus transport medium frozen at $-70°C$ should be sent when adenovirus culture is required. Chlamydial inclusions may be seen in a smear of the discharge stained by Giemsa or Lugol's iodine, but infection in Britain is seldom sufficiently florid to be able to diagnose the condition thus. The use of an indirect immunofluorescence test (see page 270) is particularly useful for the rapid diagnosis of ocular chlamydial infection. For culture a swab in chlamydial transport medium should be sent direct to the laboratory (see page 271). For the diagnosis of trachoma, conjunctival scrapings from the upper lid are required, whilst from cases of ophthalmia neonatorum, a dry swab rubbed across the lower conjunctival surface (after wiping away any pus) is preferred. When delay is unavoidable, specimens may be held at $4°C$, but for delay beyond 24 hours, specimens must be stored at $-70°C$.

Bacteria found

ADULTS AND CHILDREN
Haemophilus spp.
Str. pneumoniae
Staph. aureus
Haemolytic streptococci
Neisseria
Moraxella
Enterobacteriaceae
Pseudomonas
Chlam. trachomatis
Corynebacterium spp.
Coagulase-negative staphylococci (as commensals)

INFANTS
Stap. aureus
Coagulase-negative staphylococci
Enterobacteriaceae
Pseudomonas
Neisseria
Chlam. trachomatis
Rarely, other bacteria listed under adults

References

Bailey, S.F. and Lacey, G.R. (1927) *Journal of Bacteriology* **13**, 182

Dixon, J.M.S. and Miller, D.C. (1965) *Lancet* **ii**, 1046

Furniss, A.L. and Donovan, T.J. (1974) *Journal of Clinical Pathology* **27**, 764

George, W.L., Sutter, V.L., Citron, D. and Finegold, S.M. (1979) *Journal of Clinical Microbiology* **9**, 214

Kliegman, R.M. and Fanaroff, A.A. (1984) *New England Journal of Medicine* **310**, 1093

Kligler, I.J. (1918) *Journal of Experimental Medicine* **28**, 319

Larson, H.E., Price, A.B., Honour, P. and Borriello, S.P. (1978) *Lancet* **i**, 1063

McCarthy, M.D. (1966) *New Zealand Journal of Medical Laboratory Technology* **20**, 127

Mandal, B.K., What, K. and Morson, B.C. (1982) *British Medical Journal* **285**, 1539

Mead, G.R. and Woodhams, A.W. (1964) *Tubercle* **45**, 370

Owen, R.J., Martin, S.R. and Borman, P. (1985) *Lancet* **i**, 111

Phillips, R.K.S., Glazer, G. and Borriello, S.P. (1981) *British Medical Journal* **283**, 823

Porschen, R.K. (1979) *New England Journal of Medicine* **300**, 369

Public Health Laboratory Service Monograph No. 11 (1978) *Vibrios*, Furniss, A.L., Lee, J.V. and Donovan, T.J. HM Stationery Office London

Regan, J. and Lowe, F. (1977) *Journal of Clinical Microbiology* **6**, 303

Rowe, B., Taylor, J. and Bettelheim, K.A. (1970) *Lancet* **i**, 1

Sawle, G.V., Das, B.C., Acland, P.R. and Heath, D.A. (1984) *British Medical Journal* **292**, 526

Skirrow, M.B. (1977) *British Medical Journal* **ii**, 9

Slevin, N.J., Aitken, J. and Thornley, P.E. (1984) *Lancet* **i**, 782

Taylor, W.I. (1965) *American Journal of Clinical Pathology* **44**, 471

Tedesco, F., Gurwith, M., Markham, R., Christie, D. and Bartlett, J.G. (1978) *Lancet* **ii**, 226

Traynor, R.M., Parratt, D., Duguid, H. and Duncan, I.D. (1981) *Journal of Clinical Pathology* **34**, 914

Wilson, G.S. Miles, A.A. and Parker, M.T. (Eds.) (1983) In *Topley and Wilson's Principles of Bacteriology, Immunology and Virology*, 7th edn, Vol. 3, page 469. Edward Arnold, London

5

Identification of Bacteria

Introduction

Given cultures of infected material, a textbook of systematic bacteriology and a knowledge of bacteriological technique, it should be possible in theory to identify any bacteria found; in practice, however, the road to identification is full of pitfalls. This chapter is a guide to the inexperienced traveller. It is not an abbreviated system of bacteriology but deals with the special problem of rapid identification in a hospital laboratory. It should be used in conjunction with, not as a substitute for, the standard textbooks. We have followed the nomenclature of internationally approved names in *Topley and Wilson's Principles of Bacteriology, Virology and Immunity*, 7th edition (Wilson *et al.*, 1983).

It is often possible after examination of the primary overnight plate cultures to gain a fairly accurate idea of the nature of the organisms present. It is, however, extremely important to approach identification with an open mind and not to be too much influenced by colonial appearance, by the clinical symptoms and by a knowledge of the bacteria commonly found at the site of sampling. Previous experience indicates in which order tests are to be made but none must be omitted on the grounds that the presence of a particular species is improbable (see Chapter 1).

In every case the first step is to examine isolated colonies carefully with a hand lens by reflected and by transmitted light, then pick a single colony of each type, Gram-stain smears of them and examine them under the microscope.

Rapid Gram-stain

Smears of specimens are normally stained mechanically, but mechanization is not practical for examining smears of colonies for identification. The need is for a rapid stain which is immediately available for examination while the appearance of the colonies is still in mind. Written descriptions of Gram-staining do not fulfill the need. It is possible, however, to Gram-stain very quickly and reliably. Having wasted much time and effort on false identification trails because of omission of this simple test, we think it worthwhile to include this description.

Example of Gram-stain from a wound swab culture

It is assumed that there are three colony types on the aerobic and three on the anaerobic plate cultures.

85

1. Using a diamond marker, write the culture number on each of two glass slides, one for each plate culture, and number positions for the smears.

2. Take a loop, *not more than 2 mm external diameter* and place 3 loopfuls of water on the first slide to receive each of the colonies to be examined.

3. Pick each colony in turn, starting with the largest, and make a narrow band of smeared bacteria.

4. Repeat this procedure for the second culture plate.

5. The smears on the first slide will now be dry and ready to fix by flaming. After fixing, mark the undersurface of the slide with a grease pencil between each band (to aid examination) and flood the slide with gentian violet.

6. The second slide will now be ready for fixing, marking and flooding with gentian violet.

7. Wash the first slide under a running tap, shake off excess water and flood with double-strength Gram's iodine. Repeat for slide two.

8. Wash the iodine off the first slide under the tap and, while the tap is till running and the slide in your hand, allow acetone to run over the surface of the slide; wash it off immediately. Counter-stain with carbol fuchsin. Repeat for the second slide.

9. Wash the carbol fuchsin off the first slide and blot it dry. Repeat for second slide.

Note. Gram-positive and Gram-negative bacteria may not always be found on the same slide; therefore, until experience is gained it is wise to include smears of a known positive and a known negative bacterium on each slide, making five smears per slide in the example as a check of the technique.

The result of the Gram-stain can only be expected to indicate to which family the microbe belongs and which identification tests are likely to be helpful. In all cases the next step is to seed the remains of the colony, or another exactly like it, into a medium which is likely to yield prolific growth. This pure culture is then used for identification tests. When the original plating technique has failed to yield well isolated colonies, it is imperative to replate for purity. Failure to identify correctly is probably more often due to testing impure cultures than to any other cause.

Tests for specific antigens can be done directly from colonies on over-crowded plate cultures (e.g. rapid identification of *N. gonorrhoeae*). A preliminary Gram-stain is essential because the specific antigen test is valid only when used on Gram-negative diplococci. Little is known about the test when applied to other bacteria and antigenic cross-reactions are common. Even when identification is to be achieved by this means, a subculture for purity should be made; further tests may be required.

Table 5.1 indicates to which genus a bacterium may belong as judged by its colonial appearance on blood agar, result of Gram-stain and ability to grow on MacConkey agar after overnight incubation. In addition to this, the results of primary antimicrobial sensitivity tests are also a useful guide

Table 5.1   Colonial appearance on primary blood agar cultures

Blood agar (aerobic) after overnight incubation	Blood agar (anaerobic + 10% CO_2) after overnight incubation, no equivalent growth on aerobic culture
1. *Colonies 1 mm or more in diameter* *	1. *Colonies about 1 mm diameter or spreading*
Gram-positive cocci Staphylococci Micrococci (Streptococci)	Clostridium
Gram-negative cocci *Neisseria*	
Gram-positive bacilli *Corynebactrium* *Bacillus*	
Gram-negative bacilli	
(a) Growth on MacConkey's medium Enterobacteriaceae *Pseudomonas* (*Brucella, Yersinia*)	
(b) No growth on MacConkey's medium (*Pasteurella*)	
2. *Colonies less than 1 mm in diameter*	2. *Colonies less than 0.5 mm diameter*[†]
Gram-positive cocci in pairs or short chains	Gram-positive cocci Anaerobic streptococci Anaerobic cocci
	Gram-negative cocci *Veillonella*
(a) Growth on MacConkey's medium *Str. faecalis* (group D) Streptococci of groups B, C, G	Gram-positive bacilli *Lactobacillus* spp. *Actinomyces* *Corynebacterium* spp.
(b) No growth on MacConkey's medium *Str. pyogenes* (group A) Streptococci of groups other than group D *Str. pneumoniae* *Str. viridans*	Gram-negative bacilli *Bacteroides* *Fusiformia* (a few are Gram +)
Gram-positive cocci in clumps (Staphylococci) Micrococci	
Gram-negative cocci *Neisseria*	
Gram-positive bacilli *Cornyebacterium* *Actinomyces* *Listeria* *Erysipelothrix*	
Gram-negative bacilli Parvobacteria	

*Species listed within parentheses are those which may yield smaller colonies.
†These small colonies may fail to appear for several days. Some may prove to be micro-aerophilic, not true anaerobes.

to identity. For example, a Gram-positive coccus having a colony slightly less than 1 mm diameter which is fully sensitive to gentamicin is most unlikely to be a streptococcus. A slow-growing variant of a staphylococcus or micrococcus is much more likely since streptococci are not naturally fully sensitive to this drug. In general, sensitivity is a better guide to identification than resistance because acquired resistance is common. When checking reports it is important to relate identification to antibiotic sensitivity. Unexpected results should lead to repeat identification and sensitivity tests; a laboratory error may then be brought to light before the final report is sent.

Essential tests for the identification of each medically important species will now be described, starting with the colonial appearance after overnight incubation on the media recommended in Chapters 3 and 4 (see Table 5.1). When in a particular investigation the results are equivocal, the reader is advised to turn to a textbook of systematic bacteriology where he will find descriptions of further tests appropriate to the problem.

Note. Colonial morphology is so variable that description is useful only when the preparation and constituents of the medium are defined as precisely as possible. The species of blood in blood agar will obviously make a difference to the appearance of haemolytic organisms but colonies will also vary with the presence of anticoagulant and its nature, with the method of extraction of the meat broth base, the peptone, the thickness of the medium in the plates and the concentration of agar. Some medium sold as MacConkey agar contains bile salt which commonly inhibits species which are normally described as capable of growth on it; Difco MacConkey agar yields colonies as described here. The description of colonies on blood agar applies to Oxoid No. 2 nutrient agar base in layered plates, the top layer containing the base plus 10 per cent defibrinated horse blood. The total depth of medium is about 4 mm (2 mm for each layer); this is equivalent to 5 per cent blood in unlayered plates. Thin plates will not yield satisfactory growth of fastidious organisms.

Procedure when tests fail to identify

When a bacterium gives reactions which fail to fit the description of any known species it may in fact be a new species, but one of the following possibilities is more likely.

1. *The culture may be contaminated*. To reveal contamination, subculture on a blood agar plate so that numerous well isolated colonies are obtained. Even if no contaminants are visible after overnight incubation, pick a single colony and repeat the subculture in the same manner twice consecutively. A single colony from the third blood agar plate is assumed to be pure and a culture from it is retested. Identification tests may be repeated from a single, well isolated, colony on the first subculture to save time, but it is useless to repeat the tests without any attempt at purification.

2. *The strain may have lost its true staining properties or colonial morphology with the result that the wrong tests have been made*. To reveal lost staining properties and colonial variation, subculture to a Loeffler serum slope because growth on this medium usually yields typical microscopic morphology. After overnight incubation, Gram-stain very carefully including a known positive and negative control on the same

slide. When there is no change in morphology, subculture from the Loeffler slope to a blood agar plate and examine the colonies carefully next day for any sign of reversion to a different colonial form. (Common variants are described with typical members of their species later.)

3. *It may be a microbe which lies outside the field of medical bacteriology but would be familiar to veterinary or plant pathologists.* Make three comparable cultures, on blood agar, on nutrient agar incubated at 37°C and on nutrient agar incubated at room temperature in the dark. Also, since growth may be inhibited by broth, test in peptone water at 37°C and at room temperature, and in broth and peptone water at 50–56°C. Medically important bacteria grow at least as well on blood agar as on nutrient agar and usually better at 37°C than at other temperatures.

Appropriate tests for the identification of members of each medically important genus will be found under separate headings in this chapter.

Staphylococci

Gram-stained smear of infected discharge

The cocci appear rather large, mainly in pairs, a few single. They may be intra- or extracellular. Dead cocci stain poorly and can easily be mistaken for *Neisseria*.

Culture (18–24 hours)

1. *Blood agar aerobic.* Smooth, slightly domed colonies with entire edge 1 to 2 mm diameter; sometimes beta-haemolytic, opaque or translucent. Pigmentation variable but usually not marked in a young culture.

2. *Blood agar anaerobic* (plus about 10% CO_2). Opaque domed colonies 0.1–0.5 mm diameter. Strains which are beta-haemolytic on the aerobic culture show no haemolysis. No pigment formed.

3. *MacConkey's bile salt agar.* Colonies 0.1–0.5 mm; opaque. Pigment often marked which may mask the pink colour of lactose-fermenting strains. See Note, page 88.

4. *Microscopic examination.* Gram-positive cocci in clusters regular in size; some strains stain poorly and show a mixture of positive and negative cocci.

Staph. aureus is the most important pathogen. It can be identified by its power to form human plasma-coagulating substances, coagulases, which are possessed by no other Gram-positive coccus. Some animal pathogens previously called *Staph. aureus* which normally coagulate rabbit plasma occasionally coagulate human plasma also. They are now categorized as *Staph. intermedius*.

Although human blood transfusion blood is screened for hepatitis and HIV viruses, the possibility of the presence of other pathogenic viruses cannot be excluded. The use of human plasma as a routine diagnostic reagent has therefore been abandoned. Rabbit plasma can be substituted but will not distinguish between *Staph. aureus* and *Staph. intermedius*.

For routine purposes a rapid latex agglutination test has replaced the slide coagulase test.

Human plasma-coated latex particles will agglutinate in the presence of clumping factor (responsible for positive slide coagulation) or staphylococcal protein A. This is the basis of the Staphaurex (Wellcome Diagnostics) test. Almost all *Staph. aureus* will react when tested with Staphaurex.

Provided the test is done carefully with Gram-positive staphylococci from an overnight blood agar culture, false negative reactions are rare. The latex reagent must be in fine suspension without visible particles and the staphylococcal suspension must also be uniformly opaque. When mixed, agglutination will be seen within 20 seconds, easily visible to the naked eye. Stringy and very fine agglutination, visible only with a lens, is disregarded. The reagent is supplied in dropping bottles with sticks and cards with which to make the test. A laboratory performing many tests will find it more economical to use a loop in place of the dropper; care must be taken not to contaminate the reagent. A positive and negative control should be tested daily.

Micrococci sometimes give false positive results with Staphaurex and the test should not be performed without a Gram-stain showing typical staphylococci. Staphaurex-positive strains isolated from serious or generalized infection need to be checked by a coagulase test. The tube test described below is recommended. Coagulase-negative strains isolated from sites normally sterile in circumstances which indicate pathogenicity (see Chapter 3) should be investigated further. Table 5.2 lists reactions of the pathogenic species. Biochemical tests are difficult to perform reliably and such strains are best examined by experts in a reference laboratory where phage typing can also be carried out when appropriate.

Table 5.2 Staphylococci pathogenic to man

	Staph. aureus	*Staph. epidermidis*	*Staph. saprophyticus*
Coagulase	+	−	−
DNAase	+	−	−
Phosphatase	+	+	−
Novobiocin 2 mg/l (normal strain)	S	S	R
Acid from mannitol (anaerobic)	+	−	+

R = resistant; S − sensitive.

Coagulase test

Tube culture method

Inoculate 5 ml broth with a single colony of the staphylococcus. Add ten drops of rabbit plasma and incubate for 18 hours. (The proportion of plasma to broth is important.) Control positive and negative tests should be set up each time.

False positives
Provided the test is made as described, these do not occur. Heavy granular growth may be mistaken for clot but it will disintegrate on shaking, whereas a clot will contract but will remain solid.

False negatives
If the culture is incubated longer than 20 hours the clot may lyse. Contaminated cultures will give negative results when fibrinolysin-producing organisms, such as streptococci, are present.

DNAase production

The demonstration of DNAase production is useful for identification when coagulase tests are equivocal or when plasma is not available. Colonies are spot-inoculated on agar medium containing deoxyribonucleic acid; a positive control, *Staph. aureus*, and a negative control, *Esch. coli*, should be included. After overnight incubation the plate is flooded with normal hydrochloric acid which causes precipitation with the nucleic acid, making the medium cloudy. Spots of heavy growth of DNAase-producing bacteria are surrounded by a clear zone where the nucleic acid has been hydrolysed by the enzyme they have formed (Blair *et al.*, 1967). Weak reactions must be disregarded because they can be caused by other staphylococci which form a heat-labile enzyme. *Staph. intermedius*, an animal pathogen, is DNAase positive but, unlike *Staph. aureus*, it fails to ferment mannite and will not normally coagulate human plasma. However, occasional strains are Staphaurex positive.

Pigmentation

The name 'aureus' is misleading because pigmentation is variable and cannot be relied on for identification. If after overnight incubation the culture is allowed to stand on the bench for 24 hours, pigmentation may become more marked and colonies, which were apparently identical immediately after incubation, may now show a difference in colour. Difference in pigmentation is often well marked on MacConkey's bile salt agar which, if it is included in the primary culture media, may show two varieties of staphylococcus when the colonies on blood agar are apparently all of one kind. It must be stressed that there are many harmless yellow-pigmented Gram-positive cocci and that the differentiation is only of value in demonstrating two types of colony *both* needing a coagulase test. It may well be that the pigmented coccus is harmless and the pale one a strain of *Staph. aureus* incapable of forming much pigment. Different strains of *Staph. aureus* may appear golden, buff coloured, yellow, creamy, white or even greyish in colour.

Variants

Other variants are also encountered. One is very common: a pure growth of *Staph aureus* shows on the aerobic blood agar plate two types of colony – one large and typical, the other small, about 0.5 mm in diameter. Both are found to be coagulase positive; the large one on subculture usually gives rise to large colonies only, the small one to a mixture of the two types. A less common variant is one which on the primary aerobic blood agar culture shows very minute colonies. They are so small as to be barely visible to the naked eye after overnight incubation. The variant needs CO_2 for maximum growth, and if the culture is incubated in air plus 5–10% CO_2 all the colonies become large and typical. The small colony looks normal microscopically and is coagulase positive even without added CO_2. If cultures are made as recommended on blood agar incubated in air and incubated anaerobically plus CO_2, these strains will be easily identified, even though the aerobic culture is unrecognizable at first sight because, since there is CO_2 in the anerobic jar, they grow like a normal strain under these conditions. This variant is not harmless; it has been isolated in pure culture from clinically typical staphylococcal lesions (Hale, 1951).

Staph. aureus causing endocarditis which has received prolonged treatment with bacteriosatic drugs may temporarily lose its power to produce coagulase and the cocci may resemble micrococci. When subcultured or stored in antibiotic-free medium it reverts to the typical form and becomes coagulase positive (Clinicopathological Conference, 1966).

Small colony variants can be distinguished from streptococci by a catalase test (see page 101).

Enterotoxin-producing strains of Staph. aureus may be isolated from vomit, faeces and food in outbreaks of food poisoning. Bacteriophage typing is employed in epidemiological investigations of staphylococcal infection. Almost all enterotoxic strains belong to phage groups III and IV, but not all strains in these groups are enterotoxic (Williams et al., 1953). Reference laboratories now have antisera to two toxins, A and B, and strains can be tested for toxin production in vitro. Moreover, a tentative diagnosis can sometimes be confirmed by demonstrating toxin in the food when the staphylococci have been killed in cooking.

Selective media for Staph. aureus

Isolation of Staph. aureus from faeces or food in an outbreak of food poisoning cannot be expected to succeed without selective media. The symptoms are caused by heat-stable toxin and the bacteria may be few or absent. Small numbers of Staph. aureus can be recovered from heavily contaminated material by enrichment in Robertson's cooked meat broth containing 10% sodium chloride. After overnight incubation it should be subcultured on nutrient agar containing 3 g/l nalidixic acid. This is preferred to selection with polymyxin B because Proteus is more often a contaminant than Pseudomonas.

When carriers and the environment are being investigated to find the source of an outbreak of Staph. aureus wound infection, direct plating on phenolphthalein phosphate agar (page 315) is recommended because staphylococci are likely to be present in large numbers and differentiation between the epidemic strain and other staphylococci is the main problem. Epidemic strains are usually resistant to a number of antibiotics and selection can be achieved by placing a strip of blotting paper impregnated with the appropriate (differentiating) antibiotic at right angles to the areas of heavy inoculation in the manner described for the Optochin sensitivity test (page 100). We find that four inoculation areas per 8 cm culture plate is the maximum practicable for this method.

Coagulase-negative staphylococci

These have been divided into numerous biotypes (Baird-Parker, 1974). Those of medical importance are *Staph. epidermidis* biotype 1, which may cause severe infection in immunoincompetent patients, and *Staph. saprophyticus* biotype 3, which causes cystitis in young women. *Staph. epidermidis* is a common commensal; its identity should be confirmed when isolated in significant numbers from a site normally sterile. The term '*Staph. albus*', although it can no longer be considered a final identification, may usefully be retained for coagulase-negative staphylococci, which, being skin commensals, often appear in small numbers in wound swabs. Full identification serves no useful purpose and the clinician understands this term. '*Staphylococcus* species' is unsatisfactory because it is not clear that *Staph. aureus* has been excluded; 'coagulase-negative staphylococcus' is correct but cumbersome, and it is better to retain the old name than to report *Staph. epidermidis* without confirmatory tests.

Antibiotic sensitivity patterns

Penicillin-sensitive (β-lactamase negative) strains are uncommon in populations exposed to antibiotics. Resistance of *Staph. aureus* to methicillin and other staphylococcal β-lactamase-resistant penicillins is increasing, and serious outbreaks of wound infection in some hospitals have been caused by these strains. Most of them are resistant to a number of antibiotics, a few to all therapeutic antimicrobials except glycopeptides (eg. vancomycin and teicoplanin). Methicillin-resistant strains are resistant, completely or partially, to cephalosporins (see page 219). Penicillin-sensitive strains are sensitive to cephalosporins but may be resistant to chemically unrelated antimicrobials. Methicillin-resistant, penicillin-sensitive strains are very rare.

Staphylococci acquire resistance by transduction. Bacteriophages carrying plasmids from resistant *Staph. aureus* infect sensitive strains with them, sometimes conferring resistance to a number of chemically unrelated antimicrobials at a time. *Staph. epidermidis* is also often resistant to a number of drugs and can confer resistance by transduction *in vitro* to *Staph. aureus*. When exposure to antimicrobials is prevented, no biological advantage is gained and strains tend to lose their resistance-conferring plasmids within weeks or months and revert to sensitivity. When the recipient strain was originally a β-lactamase producer it retains the ability to form this enzyme and remains penicillin resistant.

Staphylococci are naturally resistant to polymyxin B and nalidixic acid; *Staph. saprophyticus* is naturally more resistant than other staphylococci to novobiocin (see Table 5.2) but they may also become resistant when exposed to it.

Micrococci

These coagulase-negative, catalase-positive, Gram-positive cocci tend to be larger than staphylococci, less regular in size and to occur in packets of four or eight. They are widespread in nature and often encountered as commensals. Strains resembling staphylococci are coagulase tested. Those forming comparatively small colonies may be mistaken for streptococci; they can be differentiated by the catalase test (page 101).

Streptococci

Gram-stained smear of infected discharge

The stained smear may show Gram-positive cocci in short or long chains or in pairs. Slightly elongated cocci have their long axis in line, not in parallel like staphylococci and neisseria. They may be intra- or extra-cellular. Capsules are sometimes seen.

When streptococci and pus cells are seen in the original smear of the specimen, especially a uterine or vaginal swab, notification to the clinician in charge of the patient is urgent. *Str. pyogenes* can kill a previously healthy young patient within hours, and penicillin treatment may save her.

Culture (18–24 hours)

1. *Blood agar aerobic.* Colonies are 0.1–1.0 mm in diameter and variable in appearance. They may be non-haemolytic, β-haemolytic, α-haemolytic or show α'-haemolysis (Fig. 5.1). They may be smooth, domed, entire and translucent, mucoid, or tough, opaque and triangular with a rolled edge. Their surface may be matt or glossy.

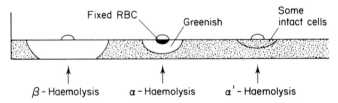

Fig. 5.1   Section of colonies on blood agar.

2. *Blood agar anaerobic plus 10% CO_2.* All streptococci grow well anaerobically. The growth is similar to that on the aerobic culture but the colonies tend to be a little larger and haemolysis more marked. Strains of *Str. pyogenes* showing α'-haemolysis aerobically and β-haemolysis anaerobically are not at all uncommon; occasionally the aerobic culture shows α-haemolysis or is non-haemolytic.

3. *MacConkey's bile salt agar* (see *Note*, page 88). Primary culture of wound or uterine swabs on this medium is helpful because *Str. pyogenes*, the most dangerous pathogen, is incapable of growth on it. *Str. faecalis* appears as a lactose-fermenter about 1 mm in diameter and some strains

of *Str. agalactiae* (group B) yield similar growth and may or may not ferment lactose. Group C and G strains may grow on it but may fail to appear.

Beta-haemolytic streptococci

It is possible to prepare 'blood agar' culture plates, each apparently acceptable, and show that a single virulent strain of *Str. pyogenes* can be β-haemolytic, non-haemolytic or show α'-haemolysis according to the medium and the conditions of growth. Blood agar mentioned throughout this text contains 5% defibrinated horse blood (see page 312). Anaerobic culture selects all streptococci from common commensals, many of which grow less well under these conditions. Haemolysis of *Str. pyogenes* is improved, the O (oxygen-labile) haemolysin effect being added to that of streptolysin S. Table 5.3 lists the results expected of typical strains grown under conditions suitable for the production of haemolysins. Lancefield grouping is essential for identification. All β-haemolytic streptococci should be grouped and also all streptococci, whether haemolytic or not, which are isolated in pure culture from a site normally sterile. Lancefield grouping is the best indicator we have of the pathogenic potential of streptococci. Even when isolated from a site showing no sign of infection, grouping is important because *Str. pyogenes* in a carrier may infect others and its presence must be reported.

Table 5.3   Streptococci pathogenic to man

	Group	Haemolysis	Need for CO_2	Primary growth on MacConkey's agar *
Pyogenic streptococci:				
pyogenes	A	β	−	−
equisimilis	C	β	−	−(+)
sp.	G	β	−	−(+)
agalactiae	B	β (N, α)	−	+(−)
milleri	(A, C, G, F)	N (α, β)	+	−
Enterococci:				
faecalis	D	N (β)	−	+
bovis	D	N (α)	−	+
Str. pneumoniae	−	α	+(−)	−
Other streptococci:				
salivarius	− (K)	N	−	−
sanguis	− (H)	α (N, β)	−	−
mitior (mitis)	− (O, K, M)	α (N, β)	−	−
mutans	− (E)	N	+	−

N = non-haemolytic. () = less common alternatives.
*See page 88.

Lancefield grouping

Extraction of group antigens A, B, C, D, F and G by which medically important, mainly β-haemolytic, streptococci can be identified has been greatly simplified by the commercial preparation, in freeze-dried form, of the proteolytic fraction of the *Streptomyces griseus* enzyme, described for this purpose by Maxted in 1948. After extraction the antigen can be recognized by agglutination of latex particles coated with appropriate antiserum. This is the basis of the Streptex latex streptococcal grouping kit (Wellcome Diagnostics) which is now the method of choice in most British laboratories. The method is very sensitive and can even be used to detect *Str. pyogenes* on a skin or wound swab before culture if present in sufficient quantity (Petts, 1984). Although grouping can be done direct from throat swabs, in practice this is seldom advantageous and has the theoretical disadvantage of the possibility of cross-reactions with unkown bacterial antigens in the specimen. A much more practical advantage is grouping from colonies on the original blood agar culture without the need for subculture and rapid grouping of streptococci when they are first seen in a blood culture (Wellstood, 1982). The commercially prepared enzyme is more efficient than the original preparation and extracts the group D antigen, a protein, enabling enterococci to be recognized by this means.

Method

The method described by the manufacturers can safely be modified to save cost by using loops instead of the droppers provided (Castle *et al.*, 1982), the number of tests possible from one pack being increased from 40 to up to 200. The latex suspensions are ready for use and are stored upright between 2 and 8°C; they must not be frozen. In addition to separate antigens A, B, C, D, F and G, a polyvalent positive control is provided which reacts with any of these antigens. The extraction enzyme is reconstituted by adding 10 ml sterile distilled water. This is also stable at 2–8°C for up to 3 months or it can be frozen in convenient aliquots and stored at −20°C when it will remain stable for at least 6 months. If part of an aliquot remains, it must not be refrozen.

Preparation of extract

Deliver 0.2 ml reconstituted enzyme into a small tube for each strain to be tested. Label one of the tubes and pick 7 or 8 colonies *exactly similar* from the original blood agar plate. The possibility that there are two different strains of β-haemolytic streptococci in the culture must be borne in mind; if two colonial forms are seen, both should be tested. Suspend the colonies in the enzyme and incubate for 1 hour in a waterbath at 37°C. A smooth suspension is not necessary, and slight contamination when colonies are not well separated does not matter.

Remove the broth from a positive blood culture (avoiding red cells) and centrifuge. Resuspend the pellet in enzyme and proceed as above.

When identification of streptococci in skin or wound swabs is urgent, the swab should be sent in transport medium without charcoal (page 311).

After primary culture, place the swab in enzyme and vortex to aid penetration. Incubate with the swab *in situ*. Remove the swab and centrifuge briefly to remove visible particles before testing.

Test

Take a clean glass slide and mark it into seven divisions, one for each group to be tested plus the positive control. The minimum for a satisfactory test is four – groups A, C and G and the control – because cross-reactions cannot be recognized and investigated if the test is performed against only one group antibody. Moreover, lack of reaction with one suspension is needed as a negative control. Group G strains may require further investigation (see below). Shake the latex suspension gently to ensure a smooth suspension. Using 10 μl loops, place drops of equal volume side by side in each marked area: one of the extract, the other of the latex suspension. The extract will contain living streptococci and care must be taken to prevent splashing by removing the loop edgewise; bubbles must not be allowed to form. The loop must be flamed between each latex suspension to prevent contamination. When all drops are in position, take a straight wire and mix each pair of drops together. Flaming between pairs of drops is not necessary because carry-over is insignificant. Rock the slide to and fro for up to 1 minute. A strong extract will produce a positive agglutination within seconds, but with a weak extract, when colonies are small or comparatively few, the reaction will be slower and the agglutinating particles smaller. After recording the result, discard the slide into disinfectant.

Interpretation of results

Most β-haemolytic streptococci isolated in circumstances where they appear to be the main pathogen give an unequivocal strong reaction with one of the test latex suspensions. Sometimes additional weak cross-reactions are seen; these should be ignored.

When a single weak reaction is seen the result is probably valid, the poor reaction being caused by insufficient antigen from too few or too small colonies. The test should be repeated from a pure culture. The addition of 0.5–1% glucose to the subculture medium will enhance antigen production.

Occasionally more than one fairly strong reaction is seen. It is then worth retesting the extract diluted 1 : 2; the difference between the reactions may become obvious and the identity of the strain no longer in doubt. Some β-haemolytic *Str. faecalis* produce both D and G antigens and have characteristic antibiotic resistance patterns (Birch *et al.*, 1984). When testing against A, C and G antisera only, the possibility that a group G strain may be *Str. faecalis* must be considered.

Negative results indicate either that the strain does not belong to any of these groups or that antigen production is insufficient. The latter is most likely to be the case with group D strains.

Additional tests
The presence of group D antigen is not sufficient for final identification of enterococci because other strains, some harmless to man, possess this antigen. All group D strains, and group G strains which have not been tested for group D antigen, should be tested for hydrolysis of aesculin and ability to grow on 40% bile medium (page 101).

The most likely difficulties in identification are: (1) that the culture is a mixture of two β-haemolytic streptococci; (2) that it is contaminated; (3) that the haemolytic colony is not in fact a streptococcus. All these possibilities must be checked before proceeding further: (3) by repeat Gram-stain and a catalase test (page 101) and (2) by subculture incubated in air. If anaerobiosis was originally used to select streptococci, an aerobic contaminant may have been suppressed; (1) is checked by subculture to blood agar from several of the original colonies, or the pool of inoculum when this is mainly streptococcal. This may show more than one colonial type when inoculated in a manner to yield as many isolated colonies as possible. Subculture to MacConkey agar may also help because group B, C, D or G strains contaminating a culture of *Str. pyogenes* will probably grow on this medium, unlike *Str. pyogenes* itself.

When the culture has been purified and the faults listed above eliminated, biochemical tests are indicated. These tests are seldom needed and the cost of an API 20STREP identification test kit is worth the speed and reliability of these 20 commercially prepared biochemical reagents. The microtubes of the test kit are inoculated with a dense suspension of the pure streptococcal culture which rehydrates the substrates. Instructions for the procedure and interpretation of the results are supplied by the manufacturer.

The significance of streptococci of various groups isolated from clinical specimens is as follows.

Group A
Str. pyogenes is one of the most dangerous of all bacterial pathogens. Its continued sensitivity to penicillin, which is the drug of choice, and its potential for causing epidemics make rapid identification and reporting imperative.

Group B
Str. agalactiae has replaced *Str. pyogenes* as the main streptococcal cause of neonatal death and postpartum morbidity. Unlike *Str. pyogenes*, it is a normal commensal in the healthy vagina and in faeces and so cannot be excluded from obstetric wards (see page 281). Colonies on blood agar tend to be large, at least 1 mm diameter, and either non-haemolytic or show a small zone of β-haemolysis. On columbia blood agar, colonies can be recognized by orange pigmentation. Enrichment broth containing 15 mg/l nalidixic acid can be employed for the recovery of small numbers from contaminated specimens. Strains causing bovine mastitis are a different biotype of this species.

Group C

Str. equisimilis is antigenically related to *Str. pyogenes* but is much less pathogenic. It is found as a commensal in throat swabs and faeces, and is an uncommon cause of tonsillitis and systemic infection.

Group D

All enterococci produce this antigen in common with other streptococci harmless to man. The two important human pathogens are *Str. faecalis* and *Str. bovis*. It is important to distinguish between them in endocarditis because *Str. faecalis* is naturally more resistant to antibiotics than *Str. bovis*. API 20STREP can be employed. Some strains of *Str. faecalis* also produce group G antigen.

Group F

Str. milleri may produce this antigen; it is the only important human pathogen to do so. It may produce other group antigens (see Table 5.3). It is usually CO_2 dependent. In a study of streptococci isolated from internal abscesses in man, *Str. milleri* was the commonest isolate (Parker and Ball, 1976) and this has been confirmed by other workers (Leading Article, 1985). Those adding CO_2 to anaerobic, but not to aerobic, cultures may misidentify *Str. milleri* as an anaerobic streptococcus. Unfortunately, there is as yet no international agreement about nomenclature. *Str. angiosus*, *Str. intermedius* and *Str. constellatus* in the USA would usually be identified as *Str. milleri* in Britian. It is found as a commensal in the human mouth, vagina and faeces. It is normally highly sensitive to penicillin but sufficient penetration into abscesses may be hard to achieve. When isolated from blood a primary pyogenic site should be sought.

Group G

These strains usually produce rather large smooth colonies and wide zones of β-haemolysis. They occasionally cause severe infection (e.g. endo-carditis) but relatively benign tonsillitis is more usual. Urinary tract infection is sometimes seen. They are antigenically related to *Str. pyogenes*.

Alpha-haemolytic streptococci

Str. pneumoniae, the pneumococcus, is by far the most pathogenic α-haemolysin producer. It is a common cause of meningitis, the only cause of lobar pneumonia and the commonest cause of all adult pneumonia in Britain (Report 1987). It also causes otitis media, sinusitis, suppurative arthritis and peritonitis.

In Gram-stained smears of specimens, pneumococci usually appear associated with pus cells in their typical encapsulated, lanceolate, diplo-coccal form. However, they may not be seen when the patient has already received penicillin which is still the drug of choice. *Str. pneumoniae* has remained penicillin sensitive and although some strains have become suffi-ciently resistant to require very high dosage, or alternative antibiotic treatment, they are uncommon. Lack of response to penicillin in patients suffering from pneumonia is, in our experience, more often due to inadequate dosage than to the wrong choice of drug. Fortunately, a laboratory diagnosis can be achieved even in treated patients, by recognizing pneumococcal antigens in specimens (see Chapter 10).

Descriptions of typical colonies can be found in any textbook of systematic bacteriology but, unfortunately, variants are common. Like other streptococci, *Str. pneumoniae* grows well anaerobically with added CO_2, some strains are CO_2 dependent. Encapsulated strains yield mucoid colonies. Variants are non-mucoid and resemble other α-haemolytic streptococci, Gram-stain shows no capsules and they may appear in short chains. Sometimes elongated forms resemble diphtheroids (but α-haemolysis by diphtheroids is very rare). They are incapable of growth on MacConkey's medium and colonies are soluble in bile salt. Spontaneous autolysis occurs with prolonged incubation and sometimes within 24 hours. It produces further haemolysis, the pneumococcus appearing β-haemolytic.

Str. pneumoniae is identified by sensitivity to Optochin but encapsulated strains may be rapidly identified using type-specific antisera which cause swelling of the capsules of homologous strains which can be observed microscopically – the Quellung reaction.

Optochin sensitivity test

Optochin (ethyl hydrocuprein hydrochloride) inhibits the growth of pneumococci much more than that of other streptococci. Strips of blotting paper about 8 mm wide are soaked in 1 in 4000 Optochin in distilled water, blotted and then dried in the incubator; they can be obtained commercially. Colonies resembling pneumococci are picked from the original plate cultures and streaked across a blood agar plate. A known pneumococcus is included as a control and the strip is laid on the culture at right angles to the streaks immediately before incubation. About 12 colonies can be tested on one plate. Pneumococci show a zone of inhibition about 7 mm wide; other streptococci grow up to the strip except for occasional strains which show very slight inhibition. The test may also be employed for rapid identification on original cultures. The control is best maintained by daily subculture on blood agar.

Alpha-haemolytic streptococci other than *Str. pneumoniae* were given the descriptive name 'streptococcus viridans' because their properties and pathogenicity had not been differentiated. Streptococcus viridans is not a streptococcal species. Some streptococci, possessing Lancefield group antigens, appear as α-haemolytic variants (see Table 5.3); they have been described above.

Streptococci isolated from blood culture, or any other site normally sterile, should be fully identified. As can be seen from the Table, haemolysis, even of typical strains, is variable; it is not necessarily related to pathogenicity.

Other streptococci

Streptococci listed in Table 5.3 are commonly isolated as commensals in throat swabs and sputum. They are identified and reported only when isolated from blood culture or other sites normally sterile. They may also be found in small numbers in wound swabs contaminated by upper respiratory, vaginal or faecal flora. Those which grow on the original MacConkey agar culture can be identified as enterococci by the aesculin–bile test. When, as judged by the Gram-stained smear of the specimen, they are playing no pathogenic role, they can be reported as *Streptococcus* species. Those with larger than usual colonies and equivocal Gram-stain can be differentiated from staphylococci, micrococci and neisseria by the catalase test.

Aesculin–bile test for enterococci

Enterococci, unlike other streptococci, grow on medium containing 40% bile; they also hydrolyse aesculin. Single colonies of streptococci are streaked across agar medium containing these two ingredients (page 317). Those which hydrolyse aesculin blacken it after overnight incubation, sometimes within a few hours.

Catalase test

Differentiation between streptococci, staphylococci, micrococci and neisseria by their morphology is not always possible. In such cases a test for catalase production is of value, since staphylococci, micrococci and neisseria produce catalase whereas streptococci do not.

Seed a single colony on a nutrient agar slope. After overnight incubation pour several drops of a 10-volume solution of hydrogen peroxide down the slope. When catalase is present, bubbles of gas will be seen. Colonies which can be easily picked from the plate without scraping off medium with them can be tested rapidly by emulsifying them in small loopful of water on a glass slide. The addition of a large loopful of hydrogen peroxide will cause very vigorous bubbling when the strain is catalase positive. The slide should be placed in a covered Petri dish to avoid the risk of contaminating the bench. Some bubbling is caused by catalase in blood from the medium, and a doubtful result must be disregarded and the strain retested by the overnight method.

Anaerobic streptococci

The anaerobic streptococci and other anaerobic cocci grow more slowly and form smaller colonies than the aerobic cocci. Some are strict anaerobes, others are capable of growth in a microaerophilic atmosphere. Microscopically they are Gram-positive and may show long or short chains. The cocci may be large, elongated or very small. On blood agar incubated anaerobically plus about 10% CO_2, growth is sometimes visible after overnight incubation, but more often 48–72 hours' incubation is required before it appears as minute, shiny, smooth, non-haemolytic colonies. Some strains show slight greenish discoloration of the medium after prolonged incubation but true haemolysis of horse blood is rare. They can be isolated from the mouth, vagina and faeces of healthy people. Some strains produce gas and some have a foul odour. Some of the strict anaerobes are very sensitive to oxygen and die after a few hours' exposure on the bench. For this reason cervical and uterine swabs are taken with specially prepared swabs and plunged in transport medium which prevents exposure to oxygen (see page 311).

This group of cocci is not well differentiated but some are undoubted human pathogens and cause severe puerperal sepsis with invasion of the blood stream. Gas-forming strains sometimes give rise to pseudogas-gangrene when they invade wounds. They are also commonly found in association with other anaerobes in chronic infection of the mouth and they can be recovered from pus in chronic empyema, from lung abscesses, abdominal abscesses and from pilonidal sinuses and umbilical sepsis. They are also found in tissue at the edge of chronic ulcers of the skin and in infected sebaceous cysts.

If these delicate microbes are not to be missed in routine work the following procedure must be followed. When Gram-positive cocci are seen in the stained film of the original material and do not appear on the plate cultures within 48 hours' incubation, reincubate for 2 more days. The cocci will probably appear on the anaerobic plate. When cultures of purulent material, in which no acid-fast bacilli have been seen, are sterile after 48 hours' incubation, continue incubation for a week if necessary. Subculture the original cooked meat broth culture, after 48 hours, on blood agar and incubate the plate anaerobically for at least 48 hours. The gas-forming strains show obvious signs of growth in cooked meat medium but non-gas producers may show none for several days. The cooked meat broth should therefore be subcultured on the fourth day whether there is evidence of growth by this time or not.

Strains which form chains and fail to grow in air plus 5% CO_2 are reported as anaerobic streptococci. Strains which fail to form chains, even in liquid media, are called anaerobic Gram-positive cocci. Further tests of identification are not made routinely because they throw no further light on pathogenicity. Those wishing to identify these cocci should turn to *Anaerobic Laboratory Manual* (Holdeman and Moore, 1977). There are three genera: *Peptococcus* does not form chains and does not ferment carbohydrates actively; *Peptostreptococcus* forms chains and attacks carbohydrates more vigorously. The name *Sarcina* is reserved for anaerobic cocci which form packets and are catalase positive; the aerobic cocci which have a similar microscopic appearance are now included in the genus *Micrococcus*. We think the proper names of these genera are best reserved for strains which have been fully identified because the differentiation between *Peptococcus* and *Peptostreptococcus* is not straightforward; chain formation depends on the constituents of medium (Thomas and Hare, 1954). Sarcinae are more easily identified but of less importance clinically.

Antibiotic sensitivity patterns

Str. pyogenes is at present always sensitive to penicillin but resistance to sulphonamide and tetracycline is now fairly common. Resistance to erythromycin and other drugs has been reported but is rare. Multiple acquired resistance, i.e. to at least three drugs belonging to different categories, has not been seen. This species is comparatively resistant to the aminoglycosides, especially kanamycin, to fusidic acid and to trimethoprim. Like other Gram-positive cocci, it is sensitive to vancomyin and resistant to polymyxin (colistin) and nalidixic acid. It is more sensitive to bacitracin than other species. This property has been used in identification, but the test must be well controlled and the concentration of bacitracin is critical.

Str. pneumoniae is now occasionally partly resistant to penicillin, but no resistance due to penicillinase production has so far been reported and increased dosage may succeed in treatment. Resistance to tetracycline is fairly common in Britain (Report, 1977). Multiple resistance has been reported from South Africa (Leading Article, 1977) and elsewhere but at present shows no sign of becoming widespread. In other respects *Str. pneumoniae* behaves like other streptococci.

Other streptococci have normally the same sensitivity pattern as *Str. pneumoniae* but comparative resistance to penicillin was reported earlier and in general resistance to a single drug is more common. Multiple resistance is rare.

Enterococci, with the exception of *Str. bovis* which is sensitive, are about 100-fold more resistant to penicillin than other streptococci, having a minimal inhibitory concentration to penicillin and ampicillin of about 2 mg/l. The belief that ampicillin is significantly more active is due to testing with a high content ampicillin and a low content penicillin disc. Enterococci are also comparatively resistant to cephalosporins and trimethoprim. *Str. faecalis* is invariably resistant to sulphonamides in our experience although other enterococci may be sensitive.

All streptococci are comparatively resistant to aminoglycosides, especially kanamycin, and to fusidic acid. They are resistant to polymyxin (colistin) and nalidixic acid; they are sensitive to vancomycin.

Neisseria, Branhamella and *Moraxella*

The potential human pathogens of these genera (Table 5.4) are all Gram-negative, oxidase and catalase positive and normally sensitive to penicillin. In Gram-stains of pus they are indistinguishable, except for *Moraxella lacunata* which is a short, fat bacillus but may appear coccoid.

Neisseria

The only members of this genus of widespread medical importance are the pathogens *N. meningitidis* and *N. gonorrhoeae*. They are Gram-negative diplococci, catalase and oxidase positive, which need enriched medium for

Table 5.4 *Neisseria, Branhamella* and *Moraxella* Pathogenic for Man

	Acid from				
	Glucose	Maltose	Sucrose	Pigment	Growth at 22°C
N. gonorrhoeae	+	−	−	−	−
N. meningitidis	+	+	−	−	−
N. flavescens	−	−	−	+	+
B. catarrhalis	−	−	−	−	+
M. lacunata	−	−	−	−	s

s = scanty.

growth (neither grows on MacConkey's medium). They are closely related to each other antigenically. *N. meningitidis* is the most important cause of bacterial meningitis and *N. gonorrhoeae* causes widespread genital infection and neonatal ophthalmia. Both are responsible for epidemics, but *N. meningitidis* is more difficult to control because it can spread by droplet infection from the nasopharynx. *N. flavescens* is a rare cause of meningitis; it resembles *N. meningitidis* but is antigenically distinct.

Gram-stained films of infected discharge

These show Gram-negative, oval, bean-shaped diplococci with the long axis of the cocci parallel; many of them can be seen within pus cells. It should be borne in mind that dead staphylococci will be Gram-negative and may be mistaken for *Neisseria*.

Culture (18–24 hours)

1. *Blood agar aerobic plus 5–10% CO_2.* 0.2–1 mm colonies smooth, shiny, grey or colourless with entire edge, opaque, usually no haemolysis. *N. meningitidis* tends to produce larger colonies than *N. gonorrhoeae*. Because the gonococcus most commonly infects the urethra and cervix it will be seen on selective medium used for its recovery from these sites (page 314).

2. *Blood agar anaerobic plus 10% CO_2.* Colonies very small. Some strains are strict aerobes.

3. *Microscopic examination.* Large Gram-negative cocci, many of them round and single, unlike the bean-shaped diplococci seen in the original material. The cocci are fragile and some disintegrating ones are almost always seen; they are particularly numerous in films of gonococcal cultures.

Some strains of *N. meningitidis* and *N. gonorrhoeae* are difficult to maintain in culture and are sensitive to cold. Therefore the cultures should be kept in the incubator except during actual examination, and subcultured on alternate days, while tests are being made, to keep the strain alive. For primary isolation the blood agar must be fresh and moist. An open test tube containing water and a blotting paper 'wick' will help to keep the atmosphere moist in a CO_2 jar. 'Chocolate' blood agar is often recommended for *Neisseria* and *Haemophilus* and it supports their growth well. It is not, however, much superior to a highly nutrient defibrinated horse blood agar, which will yield as many colonies from a small inoculum although they will not be quite so large. The advantage in diagnostic work of relying on blood agar is that growth of fastidious organisms will be obtained even when it was not anticipated. Logically one must either include 'chocolate' blood agar for all primary cultures or have a blood agar medium sufficiently good to make it unnecessary.

It is likely that isolates from the urogenital tract are *N. gonorrhoeae* and those from cerebrospinal fluid are *N. meningitidis* but this is by no means certain. Isolates from other sites (e.g. throat and rectum) need rapid precise identification. *N. meningitidis* and *N. gonorrhoeae* are very similar but murine monoclonal antibodies prepared against two antigenic components of the gonococcal cell wall will react specifically with gonococci. This test has been developed in Sweden as the Phadebact Monoclonal GC Test (obtainable from Pharmacia Ltd). It is a coagglutination test; each monoclonal antibody is attached to protein A of nonviable staphylococci which agglutinate in the presence of gonococci carrying the homologous antigen. Gonococci having the specific protein 1A in their cell membrane are classified to sero group WI, those carrying the specific protein 1B belong to sero group WII/III. The kit comprises two reagents, WI and WII/III. To make agglutination more easily visible, methylene blue has been added to the specific staphylococcal suspensions. They are stored at between 2 and 8°C ready for use and must not be frozen. Dropping pipettes for reagents and cards on which to do the test are provided. Colonies from primary plates can be tested provided that growth is sufficient.

Method

Emulsify colonies of Gram-negative, oxidase-positive cocci in 0.25 ml saline to give visible turbidity. Heat the emulsion in a boiling waterbath or, more conveniently, in a metal block at 100°C for 5 minutes. After cooling, mix a drop of the emulsion with a drop of each of the antibody suspensions, as described by the manufacturer. Gonococci will agglutinate one or other of the suspensions within 30 seconds to 1 minute.

Interpretation

Agglutination with both suspensions may occasionally be seen. This is possible when two different strains of gonococci are present, or it may be a non-specific reaction possibly caused by contamination. The culture must be re-examined, purified and retested. The Phadebact test is more than 95 per cent specific but on first isolation from a newly infected patient the result should be confirmed by sugar reactions (Table 5.4). *Neisseria* grow poorly in liquid culture; sugar reactions are therefore tested on highly nutrient sugar slopes obtainable from Difco (page 325). The slopes are seeded heavily from a pure culture and incubated upright with the caps loosened in air plus 10% CO. The medium must be fresh and sufficiently moist but not wet. Good growth and fermentation can be expected from 1 to 4 days' incubation.

Monoclonal antibody is also available for the identification of *N. meningitidis* but is too costly for routine use. It is differentiated from *N. gonorrhoeae* by fermentation of maltose (Table 5.4). Strains can be classified by agglutination tests into four groups, A, B, C and D. In Britain group B strains are most often isolated; they are antigenically the least homogeneous. Recognition of meningococcal antigens in cerebrospinal fluid or urine is valuable for rapid diagnosis, particularly in treated patients when there is little hope of isolating the pathogen (see page 35). It is more often successful with group A and C strains than with group B.

Branhamella

These are also Gram-negative diplococci resembling *Neisseria*. Only one species, *B. catarrhalis* (previously *N. catarrhalis*), can cause human infection. *Branhamella* are less fastidious than *Neisseria*, grow on nutrient agar and are capable of growth at room temperature. *B. catarrhalis* is a common commensal of the upper respiratory tract and an occasional cause of respiratory infection, both in children and in adults; it can also infect the middle ear (Leinonen *et al.*, 1981). It is frequently a β-lactamase producer (McLeod *et al.*, 1986) and, when present in mixed infection, may interfere with penicillin treatment.

Moraxella

Although these are short fat bacilli which, when seen in Gram-stained smears of pus, resemble *Klebsiella*, in other respects they resemble much more closely *Neisseria* and *Branhamella* and are therefore included here. Their morphology is variable and they can easily be mistaken for cocci unless a careful search is made for long forms which are never seen in the other two genera.

Moraxella lacunata (the Morax–Axenfeld bacillus) causes conjunctivitis and occasionally other purulent infections. It resembles *Neisseria* in being fastidious, oxidase and catalase positive and normally sensitive to penicillin. It grows better on Loeffler serum or Dorset egg medium than on blood agar. On serum slopes, pitting and liquefaction of the medium will be seen after 1 or more days' incubation. These features are sufficient for identification.

Antibiotic sensitivity patterns

Unlike other Gram-negative bacteria, *Neisseria, Branhamella* and *Moraxella* are normally highly sensitive to penicillins and sensitive to most other antibiotics. They are resistant to lincomycin and polymyxin. Many strains of *Neisseria* have acquired resistance to sulphonamide and moderate resistance to penicillin. Some strains of *N. gonorrhoeae* are highly resistant β-lactamase producers. (For recognition of β-lactamase production, see page 310). *Neisseria* resemble other Gram-negative species in their sensitivity to nalidixic acid.

Gram-negative anaerobic cocci

There is one genus, *Veillonella*, and they are probably harmless. They are normal commensals of the upper respiratory tract, mouth and intestine. They are often isolated, with other non-sporing anaerobes, from chronic infective discharges. The colonies are minute, moist, non-haemolytic and usually take at least 48 hours' anaerobic incubation to make their appearance. The cocci are small and round, unlike *Neisseria*, and tend to stick together to form quite large groups. They are easily recognizable and no further identification, other than checking that they are indeed anaerobes (page 47), is normally required.

Corynebacteria

Corynebacteria are Gram-positive, pleomorphic bacilli, often showing club-shaped ends and irregular staining. Some species form metachromatic granules and occasional branching is seen. The genus comprises the toxin-producing pathogen *C. diphtheriae* (of which there are three subspecies), *C. ulcerans* and numerous commensals, diphtheroids, common on skin and mucous surfaces in man and animals. In clinical bacteriology the main problem is to distinguish as quickly as possible *C. diphtheriae* from other members of the genus. The main points of difference after overnight culture may be tabulated thus:

C. diphtheriae	Other species
Bacilli very pleomorphic with many long slender forms	Bacilli fairly regular, often short
Many metachromatic granules	Few granules
Typical grey-black colonies on tellurite medium	Pale grey or lampblack colonies on tellurite medium
Some strains haemolytic	Haemolysis very rare

None of these findings is significant when taken singly, but consideration of all of them usually makes it possible to send a preliminary report.

The preliminary stages of identification have already been described in

Table 5.5 Screening for *Corynebacterium* species

Species	Urea	Acid produced from				Haem	Toxin
		Gluc	Suc	Malt	Starch		
C. diphtheriae gravis	−	+	−	+	+	+(−)	+
C. diphtheriae mitis	−	+	−	+	−	+	+(−)
C. diphtheriae intermedius	−	+	−	+	−	+(−)	+
C. ulcerans	+	+	−	+	+	−	[+]
C. xerosis	−	+	+	+	−	−	−
C. hofmanni	+	−	−	−	−	−	−
Other species	−+	+−	−+	+−	−+	−	−

Haem = haemolysis of horse blood agar; () = less frequent result; [] = clinically less effect.

Chapter 4. The preliminary screening test for urea hydrolysis distinguishes between *C. diphtheriae*, and *C. ulcerans* plus many of the harmless commensals (Table 5.5). Urea-positive strains need no further investigation unless they have been isolated from a throat swab in tonsillitis or from a site normally sterile. *C. ulcerans* is a variant of *C. diphtheriae* which resembles animal pathogens. It is a rare cause of tonsillitis and skin infection, and, although it produces toxin, toxaemia in man is not seen and epidemics do not occur. Urea-negative strains are investigated biochemically and for toxin production.

Although corynebacteria grow on nutrient agar, they will not yield sufficient growth in peptone water without added serum. Liquid serum sugars are difficult to maintain in good condition and it is better to add serum by inoculating about 5 drops per tube of Hiss serum water culture. Starch hydrolyses easily in solution and should not be stored in this condition for more than a few days. Suitable media for biochemical tests are obtainable from Southern Group Laboratories (page 326).

Toxin production test

   C. diphtheriae gravis and intermedius strains are almost always toxigenic, and confirmation of toxigenicity is not essential when they are isolated from a throat swab in clinical diphtheria, but mitis strains are sometimes non-toxigenic and need testing. The *in vitro*, Elek, test for toxin production is not difficult; the basic medium can be obtained commercially. However, like most laboratory tests, if it is performed infrequently, reliability is difficult to maintain (see page 23). We therefore recommend that all urease-negative Corynebacteria should be tested as described below. This will ensure that rare sucrose-fermenting strains of *C. diphtheriae* will be recognized. Alternatively, toxigenicity should be tested in a reference laboratory. Guinea-pig inoculation is required when the *in vitro* test is equivocal or positive, or when the patient shows no clinical signs of diphtheria. For technique and evaluation, see previous editions of this book (Stokes and Ridgway, 1980).

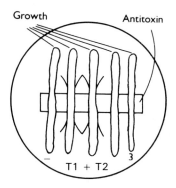

Fig. 5.2   Elek's test for toxogenicity. T = test strains.

Elek's plate virulence test for _C. diphtheriae_ (Elek, 1949, modified)
Method
Melt 15 ml Elek agar base (Southern Group Laboratory) in the steamer and cool to 56°C. Add 3 ml good quality sterile horse serum. Pour into a Petri dish and, when set, dry at 37°C.

Soak a strip of Whatman No. 1 filter paper in 750 units/ml Berna antitoxin, drain and place on the surface of the agar. Inoculate the strain to be tested heavily at right angles to the strip. Include a positive and a negative control inoculated one on either side of the test strain (Fig. 5.2). If lines of precipitation are not seen after overnight incubation, reincubate for a further 24 hours (see PHLS Monograph No. 5, 1974).

Interpretation
False negative and false positive results are sometimes seen (Bickham and Jones, 1972). Even lines of identity with the control may occasionally be due to non-specific substances. Public Health measures should not be instituted on the evidence of a diffusion test alone in the absence of clinical diphtheria.

In populations where the carrier rate is high, especially in hot climates, toxigenic strains may be isolated from wounds or ulcers.

Antibiotic sensitivity
Corynebacteria are normally sensitive to penicillin and the macrolides. Since antitoxin dominates treatment, sensitivity to antibiotics has been studied less for this than for other genera. Resistance can develop and sensitivity patterns are not helpful in identification of toxigenic strains.

In 1970 Johnson and Kaye reviewed 52 published cases of serious infections by antibiotic-resistant diphtheroids. Since then their presence in opportunistic infection has been increasingly reported and they are known as JK diphtheroids. All are resistant to penicillin and sensitive to vancomycin, but, although they are all mutiply resistant, the resistance pattern to other antimicrobials varies. They grow slowly on columbia agar. After 48 hours' incubation the colonies of some species are of normal size, but the more resistant and typical JK strains have very small colonies. They are aerobes and resemble _C. genitalium_. They do not infect previously healthy people. For selective methods of culture and identification, see Bayston and Higgins (1986).

Coliforms

'Coliform' is a convenient term which needs clarification. Here it means a bacterium resembling _Esch. coli_ on primary culture, i.e. any aerobic non-sporing Gram-negative bacillus capable of forming colonies about 1–2 mm in diameter on nutrient agar without enrichment. Most of the coliforms as here defined are Enterobacteriaceae, but _Pseudomonas_ and _Aeromonas_ are also coliforms. Although _Yersinia_ are now classified as Enterobacteriaceae, they do not resemble _Esch. coli_ morphologically and so are included under Parvobacteria (page 127).

Coliforms are found in normal and abnormal human and animal faeces, from whence they contaminate other sites, especially the urinary tract and wounds, causing infection which may be severe or even fatal. Biochemical and serological tests are usually needed for identification because there are many atypical strains of pathogenic species and entero-pathogens sometimes possess antigens in common with those of faecal commensals. Identification of atypical strains may necessitate numerous biochemical tests and typing methods outside the scope of this book; *Identification of Medical Bacteria* by Cowan and Steel, and volume 2 of *Topley and Wilson's Principles of Bacteriology, Virology and Immunity* (Wilson *et al.*, 1983) are recommended as further guides.

Since lactose fermentation after overnight incubation on lactose-containing agar media is the first biochemical reaction to be noted, it is convenient to consider identification of lactose and non-lactose ferm-enters separately.

1. Lactose-fermenting coliforms isolated from faeces

In faeces from individual adults investigated because of enteritis these can normally be disregarded, but in infants up to the age of 3 years some strains of *Esch. coli* cause acute diarrhoea. These enteropathogenic strains are agglutinated by specific antisera; there is as yet no satisfactory selective medium. Traveller's diarrhoea may be caused by unfamiliar types of *Esch. coli* (Rowe *et al.*, 1970) but investigation of *Esch. coli* isolated from individual patients is unrewarding. When an outbreak has occurred and no other cause can be found, *Esch. coli* strains should be sent to a reference laboratory for typing.

Method (Taylor and Charter, 1952)
Using a polyvalent serum, pick at least five colonies including all morphological types and test each for slide agglutination (see page 114). Test also the confluent growth if these are negative. When the confluent growth but no single colony is positive, replate from the agglutinated particles.

When slide agglutination is positive with the polyvalent serum, test further with specific O sera to discover to which serotype the strain belongs.

Slide agglutination must always be checked by tube agglutination. Inoculate broth with a single colony and incubate overnight. Heat the culture in a boiling water bath for half an hour, adjust the opacity with saline to about 250×10^6 organisms per ml and test as described for Salmonella (page 140).

Aeromonas hydrophila is an ocasional cause of diarrhoea in man. It is a lactose fermenter but, unlike Enterobacteriaceae, it is oxidase positive and produces DNAase. It is usually β-haemolytic on blood sugar, the growth becoming dark green on further incubation. Colonies suspected of being *Aer. hydrophila* can be screened with API 10S and followed up with API 20E when necessary (see below and page 73).

2. Lactose-fermenting coliforms isolated from specimens normally sterile

Identification must be precise when it is necessary to follow up episodes in repeated urinary tract infection and also for coliforms isolated from blood, from cerebrospinal fluid and under other circumstances where infection is judged to be potentially lethal. The API 20E system of commercially produced miniaturized biochemical tests is worth its comparatively high cost and has been widely adopted. Results have been compared with conventional tests on strains held at the National Collection of Type Cultures (NCTC) (Holmes *et al.,* 1977) and are satisfactory.

The API identification system (Appareils et Procedes d'Identification)

API manufactures identification systems for staphylococci, streptococci, Enterobacteriaceae, anaerobes, non-fermenting Gram-negative bacteria and yeasts. Of these, the API 10S system backed up by the more comprehensive 20E system are particularly useful for the identification of Enterobacteriaceae and some non-fermenting Gram-negative bacteria.

The test system consists of a plastic chamber containing a plastic strip of cupules. These contain a variety of substrates and indicator chemicals. The addition of a standard inoculum of the test organism to each cupule results, after incubation, in a series of colour changes. The pattern of colour change will identify the organism either directly or by converting the pattern to a numerical profile allowing identification using a manual derived from an extensive computer database.

Pitfalls with the system must be avoided. It is imperative that the manufacturer's instructions be followed. The organism should be either recently isolated or, if from stock, passaged at least three times. Emulsification to the standard concentration in the correct carrier medium is necessary. Before incubation, certain cupules need to be overlain with sterile mineral oil to prevent interaction between the constituents. The plastic incubation chamber should contain the recommended quantity of water to maintain high humidity. A purity plate must be inoculated with each strip, as mixed cultures may otherwise go undetected and lead to false identification.

Because the majority of test systems rely on pH change to produce the colour reaction, strips should not be incubated in a CO_2-enriched atmosphere. Incubation time may also affect the final results and has proved the most common cause of error (Holmes and Dawson, 1985). Most organisms will produce reliable results after 18–24 hours' incubation in API 10S or API 20E. The manufacturer recommends that when three or more cupules show definite colour change the strip is ready for interpretation. This may require up to 48 hours' incubation for slow growers.

Beyond 48 hours' incubation, results are unreliable because some substrates deteriorate.

Interpretation is an exercise in probabilities. The numerical profile will lead to a series of options for identification, expressed in the manual as a percentage probability. The nearer to 100 per cent the result, the more likely the correct identification. The decision to accept the profile result rests with the user. However, the skill of the microbiologist will be required to avoid obvious errors of identification. There is much to be said for basing identification on knowledge of biochemical reactions of commonly encountered bacteria plus the morphology and growth requirements of the test strain, reserving the use of numerical profile and computer-generated database for the more obscure results. Further assistance can be obtained by telephoning the API laboratories with the test results, and using an enlarged database.

Esch. coli is the most frequently encountered species in sites normally sterile but *Citrobacter*, *Enterobacter* and *Klebsiella* will also be isolated. Their clinical importance in acute urinary infection is similar to *Esch. coli* but *Klebsiella* and *Enterobacter* are naturally more resistant to antibiotics (see page 122). They tend to cause epidemics of hospital infection after acquiring multiple resistance (page 283). In tracing epidemics precise identification, including serological or bacteriocine typing, is required and is best done in a reference laboratory.

Klebs. pneumoniae differs from other coliforms in pathogenicity because it occasionally causes primary pneumonia. Respiratory pathogens are similar to other strains biochemically and serologically but are much more pathogenic to mice. Death follows intraperitoneal injection of a 10^{-5} dilution of a peptone water culture. *Klebsiella* are non-motile and usually show mucoid colonies caused by capsules or free slime. Non-mucoid strains of *Klebs. oxytoca*, which is indole positive, may be misidentified as *Esch. coli*. Like other *Klebsiella*, it is naturally resistant to ampicillin.

3. Non-lactose-fermenting coliforms isolated from faeces

Tests are needed to decide as quickly as possible whether non-lactose fermenters isolated from faeces are *Salmonella* or *Shigella*. Table 5.6 lists the results of overnight screening tests which indicate the need for agglutination tests. It is uneconomical to do routine serological tests without a biochemical screen and may mislead because there is considerable overlap of antigens between different species of coliforms.

A MacConkey agar, or CLED culture for purity and an agar slope to provide growth for serological tests, will be needed in addition to the screening test media.

All strains resembling *Salmonella* or *Shigella* must be identified serologically and by further biochemical tests (API 20E) to confirm without doubt a clinical diagnosis of infection or to recognize a carrier. A positive screen and slide agglutination test (see below) is sufficient evidence for a preliminary report. The presence of a particular species of *Salmonella* or

Shigella does not preclude other species of these pathogens because mixed infections in enteritis caused by food poisoning are not uncommon.

Salmonella

Salmonellae are widespread pathogens of vertebrates, including man. They are usually isolated from faeces, urine or blood but they may be found in other sites, such as pus from osteitis, or from a chronically discharging wound in a salmonella carrier. *Salm. typhi* attacks only man. Biochemically *Salm. typhi* resembles *Shigella* in producing no gas from sugar fermentation but conforms to the majority of its genus in other respects. It is the most pathogenic of all coliforms; infection can be caused by small numbers of bacilli, and laboratory infection has often been recorded although not widely publicized. Great care must be taken when handling it in serological tests.

Arizona, which cause enteritis, mainly in animals, are now classified as a subspecies of *Salmonella* and will be recognized by API 20E.

Serological identification of *Salmonella*

All isolates giving expected reactions of this genus (see Table 5.6) should be tested without waiting for the result of further biochemical tests. Both speed and economy are served by doing slide agglutinations in the appropriate order, using polyvalent sera and those specific for O and H antigens.

Table 5.6   Biochemical screen for non-lactose-fermenting coliforms

	Glucose*	Sucrose*	Indole	H$_2$S*	Urease[†]	Oxidase
Salmonella	A(G)	(AG)	–	+	–	–
Shigella[‡]	A	–	V	–	–	–
Escherichia	A(G)	(AG)	+	–	–	–
Edwardsiella	AG	–	+	+	–	–
Citrobacter	AG	(AG)	V	V	V	–
Hafnia alvei	AG	–	–	–	–	–
Serratia	A(G)	A(G)	–	–	–	–
Morganella	AG	–	+	–	+	–
Proteus	AG	(AG)	V	+	+	–
Providencia	A(G)	(AG)	+	–	V	–
Pseudomonas	A	–	–	–	–	+
Chromobacterium	(A)	–	–	–	–	+
Acinetobacter	(A)	(A)	–	–	(+)	–
Alkaligenes	–	–	–	–	–	(+)
Yersinia enterocolitica[‡]	A	A	V	–	+	–

A = acid; G = gas; V = reaction variable; () = some strains negative.
*Kligler's medium (page 317).
†Christensen's medium (page 318).
‡See text.

Procedure
The strain is tested by slide agglutination with the polyvalent O serum which reacts with strains in groups A to G, provided agglutination is not blocked by Vi antigen, which can be checked by testing all negative strains against *Salm. typhi* Vi serum. The Vi antigen is possessed by various Enterobacteriaceae; a positive result in the absence of other diagnostic criteria is therefore of little significance. Strains which prove negative to both polyvalent O and Vi serum are unlikely to be members of the salmonella group.

Method
Emulsify a small amount of growth from the agar slope in a large loopful of saline on a clean glass slide without spreading the drop. The emulsion must be absolutely smooth and of medium opacity. Add one small loopful of specific serum and mix without spreading. Positive agglutination should be visible to the naked eye by the time the fluids are well mixed; late results are disregarded. Discard the slide immediately into disinfectant. Slide agglutination is potentially dangerous   because when carelessly handled the emulsion of living organisms will contaminate the bench. Therefore place the slide on a large black tile, which can be disinfected afterwards, and lift the loop from the emulsion edgeways to avoid an aerosol due to release of surface tension when it leaves the drop.

In practice, strains are tested against several specific sera for slide agglutination, some of which prove negative and so there is no need for an additional saline control of the suspension. Such a control must, however, be included when all tests prove positive. A small additional loopful of saline is added instead of serum.

Positive results with the polyvalent O serum indicates a *Salmonella* and the next step is to test with sera prepared against O antigens of the individual salmonella groups. In Britain the most useful sera are those reacting with factors 4 and 5, group B; with 6 and 7, group C; with 8, group C_2; with 9, group D; and with 3, 10, 15 and 19, group E.

When biochemical reactions are typical of *Salm. typhi* the polyvalent sera are omitted and the strain is tested directly against *Salm. typhi* O serum, factor 9, and salmonella H specific serum which reacts with flagella antigen d. It must be remembered that a non-motile Vi strain may react with neither of these, but such strains are rare.

When positive results are obtained with any isolate, test it next against polyvalent H (non-specific) and H (specific and non-specific) sera. When a good result is obtained with the latter serum and a feeble or negative one with the non-specific serum, the organism is in the specific phase and will react with the appropriate H specific serum. Turn to the Kauffmann–White table of salmonella antigens and test it again with H specific serum of the organisms in the appropriate group.

Example: the following results might be obtained by slide-agglutinating a strain isolated from faeces.

Polyvalent *Salmonella* species O	+	Polyvalent H (specific and	
Group B factor 4	+	non-specific)	+
Group C factor 7	–	Polyvalent H non-specific	–
Group C$_2$ factor 8	–	*Salm. paratyphi B* H antigen b	–
Group D factor 9	–	*Salm. typhimurium* H antigen i	+

The tests first made against O sera have placed the organism in group B. The polyvalent H serum reactions show that it is in the specific phase; therefore it must be tested with H sera prepared for the specific antigens in group B, the commonest in Britain being *Salm. paratyphi* B and *Salm. typhimurium*. It is a waste of time and serum to test it in the first place with sera prepared for H antigens not found in members of this group.

Diagnostic sera sometimes give a positive slide test with rough non-virulent variants and with other coliforms which are not stable in suspension; moreover, this instability may not be demonstrable in a saline suspension on the slide. When this occurs with the polyvalent O serum, a false positive preliminary report may be sent.

False positive slide agglutination

Slide agglutinations will not always be satisfactory for final identification unless all non-specific antibody has been absorbed from the sera to prevent false reactions. Tube agglutinations should be set up with each serum which gives a positive slide test. If the strain is agglutinated by the specific serum diluted to the titre marked on the bottle, and the saline control of the suspension is satisfactory, identification has been made. When, in the example given, only the polyvalent sera agglutinate the bacillus to titre, it is probably a member of one of the rarer groups with an antigen in common with those of group B.

Tube agglutination tests
Apparatus required
Standardized killed bacterial suspension.
Specific antisera (obtainable from Wellcome Diagnostics).
50 dropper pipettes.
Dreyer's agglutination tubes, or round-bottomed 1 × 7.5 cm tubes.
Water bath controlled at 50°C.

Suspensions
Living suspensions give good reactions in agglutination tests but they are dangerous to handle. There is no rapid way of killing a suspension which leaves it agglutinable by both H and O sera. It is therefore customary to make two killed suspensions, one for H and one for O agglutination tests.

For H agglutination add a few drops of formalin to an over-night broth culture of the organism. Adjust the suspension to the required density about 250 × 10^6 per ml, with saline.

For O agglutination wash the growth off the agar slope with 1 ml saline and transfer the fluid to a clean tube or screw-capped bottle. Heat in a boiling water bath for 5–10 minutes, than add sufficient saline to make a standard suspension as above.*

Method

Set up five agglutination tubes for each serum to be tested. Make twofold serum dilutions 1:10 to 1:160 (10 drops serum dilution plus 10 drops bacterial suspension is sufficient volume for the test). After adding the suspension the final serum dilutions will be 1:20 to 1:320, a range which will include the titre of the diagnostic serum. One control tube, containing saline without serum, is required for each suspension to check autoagglutinability of the bacilli.

Incubate in a 50°C water bath. (Convection currents will mix serum dilution and suspension in narrow Dreyer's tubes if three-quarters of the tube contents are immersed.) Read after 4 hours. When the results are negative, stand the tubes on the bench overnight and read next morning.

H agglutinations can be read after 2 hours in the water bath but it is worthwhile to reincubate for the full time if the 2-hour reading is negative. It is important to read agglutination tests in a viewing box in a bright light with a dark background. Under these conditions standard agglutination is seen by the naked eye as clumping of the bacilli, which fall to the bottom of the tube, with clearing of the supernatant fluid. Traces of agglutination and very fine complete O agglutination may be seen only with the aid of a hand lens. The test is a quantitative one and a false negative result may be seen unless the suspension is of standard opacity and the dilutions are made carefully with pipettes of comparable size held vertically while dropping.

The titre of the serum is marked on the bottle; it is normally at least 250. In most cases freshly isolated strains react well and all serum dilution tubes will show standard agglutination. When the titre is less than 160 the result is unsatisfactory. (See page 117.)

Difficulties encountered in the identification of salmonellae
Positive O and negative H agglutination in a non-motile culture
Procedure

Inoculate from a young peptone water culture a semisolid (about 0.5%) nutrient agar plate near the periphery and incubate. Flagellated bacteria will spread across it and subcultures made from the spreading edge will be motile. It may be necessary to repeat the subcultures several times before a satisfactory result is obtained. Alternatively, a Craigie's tube (see below) without antiserum can be employed.

Culture in the non-specific phase

This shown by positive agglutination with the polyvalent H non-specific serum and a negative or feeble result with H specific serum. It is then necessary to set up a Craigie's tube.

---

*Compare with McFarlane's opacity tube No. 1 (Obtainable from Difco). The opacity is such that print is just readable through the suspension.

Procedure
Pour some sloppy (0.5–1%) nutrient agar into a sterile 15 × 2.5 cm tube. Before it sets, mix with it three or four drops of H non-specific serum and place in the middle a piece of sterile glass tube protruding above the level of the medium. When the agar has set, seed the culture into the middle of the glass tube and incubate. As the majority of bacteria in the culture are in the non-specific phase they will be agglutinated by serum, but those in the specific phase will be unaffected and will multiply and find their way to the surface of the agar outside the central tube. Subcultures made from this surface will give positive results with specific sera. It may be necessary to repeat the Craigie tube culture several times before the non-specific culture will give rise to bacilli in the specific phase.

Positive slide agglutination with more than one group serum.
There are antigens common to several groups; for example, factor 12 is common to groups A, B and D, therefore a strain of *Salm. typhimurium* possessing this antigen may give positive slide agglutination with three group sera. The results of the tube agglutination tests will indicate to which group the organism belongs since only an organism possessing a large proportion of the factor specific to the group is likely to be agglutinated to titre. Sometimes, however, positive results are obtained with O sera from groups with no diagnostic common antigen. In this case the reaction may be due to a common antigen not recorded in the Kauffmann–White scheme or to a non-specific antigen reacting with non-specific antibody originally present in one of the sera (as a result of naturally occurring coliform infection in the rabbit from which the serum was taken). Tube agglutination almost always shows a low titre with such reactions but occasionally high titres are encountered. It is therefore very important to perform tube tests to check all positive slide tests and not to be satisfied unless both H and O sera react to titre with the unknown strain. Other enterobacteria giving positive non-specific reactions can easily be mistaken for members of the salmonella group.

Tube agglutination negative or positive in low titre only
Procedure
Retest from a fresh agar slope subculture, using a carefully standardized suspension.

If the repeated tube agglutination tests are still unsatisfactory the organism is most unlikely to be a member of the group but it cannot be excluded on this limited serological evidence alone. Much more detailed examination, using sera not available in hospital laboratories, is necessary to exclude rare *Salmonella*. A preliminary report may be sent that a bacillus, probably not a *Salmonella*, is under investigation. In addition to the routine tests, it is worthwhile to inoculate equally two peptone water tubes, incubate one and leave the other in the dark on the bench. If growth at room temperature (as judged by opacity) is heavier, the strain is not a *Salmonella*. A room temperature agar slope culture will sometimes reveal pigment formation when the incubated cultures remain unpigmented, which again excludes a *Salmonella*.

Tube agglutination satisfactory with O but not with H sera when the culture is motile and in the specific phase
The strain is probably one of the rare members of the group and is sent to a reference laboratory for further tests.

Biochemical tests positive, slide agglutination tests negative
Freshly isolated strains of *Salm. typhi* often have Vi antigens which may mask the O agglutination. Occasional strains therefore which give the biochemical reactions of *Salm. typhi*, are non-motile and are not agglutinated by specific O and H sera, are tested by slide agglutination with Vi serum. Vi antigen is not specific and its presence cannot be taken as evidence that a coliform bacillus is *Salm. typhi* unless biochemical tests are typical. Confirmation of identification by a reference laboratory will then be required.

Atypical strains of *Citrobacter freundi* may masquerade as *Salmonella*. These were previously called Ballerup–Bethesda. They will be recognized by API 20E tests.

Shigella

Shigellae are human and primate enteric pathogens, but are harmless to other vertebrates. They are almost always isolated from faeces but, like faecal commensals, can contaminate wounds or other sites in a carrier. They are rarely isolated from urine and, unlike *Salmonella* do not cause urinary or generalized invasive infection. When the screening tests (see Table 5.6) are positive for *Shigella*, serological tests should be made forthwith. *Sh. sonnei* is a late lactose fermenter but will appear non-lactose fermenting after overnight incubation. However, if there is delay in examining the cultures it must be borne in mind that this species may appear as a lactose-fermenting coliform and colonies from desoxycholate citrate, or other selective primary medium, must be screened.

Plesiomonas shigelloides is antigenically similar to *Sh. sonnei* but is of doubtful pathogenicity (see page 73). It will be recognized by API 20E.

Procedure
Test the growth on the agar slope culture for slide agglutination with shigella antisera. The minimal sera required for routine use are polyvalent flexner (composite specific and group), polyvalent boyd, *Sh. sonnei, Sh. dysenteriae* type II (*schmitzi*) and *Sh. dysenteriae* type I (*shigae*); *Sh. newcastle* is agglutinated by the polyvalent flexner serum. *Sh. alkalescens* and *Sh. dispar* are of very doubtful pathogenicity and are now excluded from this group.

When slide agglutination is strongly positive with one of the appropriate antisera, send a preliminary report and check the result with a tube agglutination test as described for *Salmonella*. The suspension is made by scraping growth from the agar slope into saline, adjusting the opacity to about 250×10^6 organisms per ml* and adding a drop of formalin. When the strain is agglutinated to titre the final report can be sent. When slide agglutination is feeble or negative the strain is probably not a dysentery bacillus. Results of the API 20E tests will enable *Shigella* to be excluded.

Esch. coli is closely related to *Shigella* and atypical non-lactose-fermenting, non-gas-producing strains may cause confusion. These are the formerly classified Alkalescens Dispar group and will be recognized by API 20E.

Difficulties encountered in the identification of shigellae
1. Positive slide agglutination but low titre agglutination in the tube test (1:80 or less.)
Subculture to broth and incubate overnight. Then heat in a boiling water bath for 30 minutes; adjust the opacity of the suspension as before and retest.

2. Biochemical tests persistently positive in the absence of agglutination
Procedure
Seed the peptone water culture on blood agar and MacConkey agar to test for purity. One or both of these plates will probably reveal a contaminant. Even when none appears, pick a single well isolated colony from the blood agar plate and repeat the biochemical tests. A contaminant may fail to survive competition with a coliform bacillus and die, having caused confusion by fermenting some of the sugars during its short lifetime.

Repeat the Gram-stain from growth on the blood agar plate. Members of the *Bacillus* genus, the aerobic spore bearers, can be mistaken for dysentery bacilli if they lose the power of retaining Gram's stain. They can usually be excluded from the dysentery group by their motility or spore formation, but a poorly staining, non-motile, non-sporing strain may cause confusion. API kits cannot be expected to perform satisfactorily when inoculated with a contaminated culture or an inappropriate species.

Edwardsiella tarda is an occasional cause of febrile diarrhoea (Okubadejo and Alausa, 1968). Its colonies are smaller than most coliforms and it is normally sensitive to penicillin.

The remaining species in Table 5.6, with the exception of *Yer. entero-colitica*, (page 128), can be disregarded when isolated from faeces.

4. Non-lactose fermenting coliforms isolated from specimens normally sterile

Escherichia and *Citrobacter* have been mentioned under 'Lactose fermenters'. The non-lactose-fermenting variants have no special significance when isolated from non-faecal specimens.

Hafnia alvei may contaminate wounds or pressure sores but it is believed to be harmless to man.

*See footnote, page 116.

Serratia marcescens is notorious for its red pigment, but strains isolated from infected patients are likely to be non-pigmented. Infection is rare except in hospital patients who may suffer from urinary, respiratory, meningeal or septicaemic infection. Endotoxic shock and endocarditis have been reported (Wilson *et al.*, 1983). Antibiotic-resistant *Serratia* may become endemic in hospitals (Wilfert *et al.*, 1970). *Serratia liquefaciens* (previously *Enterobacter liquefaciens*) is less often isolated. Unlike most other coliforms, *Serratia* are resistant to polymyxins.

Proteus

This genus is now confined to two species, *Prot. mirabilis* and *Prot. vulgaris*. They are found frequently in human and animal faeces. *Prot. vulgaris* is more likely to produce β-lactamase than *Prot. mirabilis* and therefore tends to be more antibiotic resistant. All *Proteus* species are resistant to polymyxins. They make isolation of other bacteria in mixed cultures very difficult because swarming from only one *Proteus* colony can cover the whole plate culture, leaving no visible edge, and its presence may be hard to recognize. It is one reason why MacConkey agar, which inhibits swarming, is a useful primary medium.

Inhibition of swarming
Numerous methods have been described. They depend either on drying the surface of the medium or on inhibition of motility by chemical agents; neither is entirely satisfactory. In practice, success is often achieved by judging, from the Gram-stained smear of the specimen and of the pool of primary growth, which fastidious bacteria are likely to be present and using media containing antibiotic which will inhibit *Proteus* without affecting the fastidious pathogen. (The same problem is encountered with swarming clostridia.) One of the advantages of primary antimicrobial susceptibility tests by the disk method is that a few colonies of an important pathogen may be rescued from a zone cleared by a drug to which it is resistant. *Proteus* is normally sensitive to nalidixic acid and sometimes to aminoglycosides. CLED medium for the isolation of urinary pathogens (page 38) prevents swarming and is less inhibitory than MacConkey agar.

Typing
Swarming can be used to recognize identical strains of *Proteus* by the Dienes phenomenon. Strains isolated from a suspected episode of hospital infection are spot inoculated round the edge of a culture plate with one strain in the centre; seven strains per plate is appropriate. Identical strains will show no line of demarcation at the edge of the swarming area (Skirrow, 1969). Serological, bacteriocine and phage typing can also be employed to characterize strains.

Morganella

Morganella morgani (*Proteus morgani*) is non-swarming and antigenically distinct from *Proteus* which it resembles in some of its biochemical reactions, notably urease production and phenylalanine deamination. It is also related to *Providencia*. It does not normally cause severe infection and is usually isolated from urine or from wounds contaminated with faecal organisms. It is resistant to β-lactam antibiotics and polymyxins.

Providencia

This genus resembles *Proteus* in deaminating phenylalanine and in resistance to polymyxins but *Providencia* species are indole positive and do not always produce urease. They produce little gas in sugar fermentation and do not normally swarm. There are three species: *Prov. rettgeri* (previously *Prot. rettgeri*), *Prov. alcalifasciens* and *Prov. stuarti*. They are not antigenically homogeneous, but can be phage typed or bacteriocine typed to distinguish between members of the same species in epidemics. Strains highly resistant to antimicrobials cause hospital infection; isolation from urine or wounds of patients outside hospital is rare.

Pseudomonas

The bacilli are sometimes slightly curved, and cultures, except *Ps. maltophilia*, are oxidase positive and attack sugars oxidatively, unlike Enterobacteriaceae. They are widespread in nature and capable of growth on very simple media. Many strains will grow in dilute antiseptic solutions. Cetrimide agar (page 315) is used to select *Pseudomonas* in epidemiological investigations.

Two species cause specific diseases in animals and sometimes in man. *Ps. pseudomallei* causes glanders in horses and *Ps. mallei* is the cause of melioidosis in various animals in tropical regions and sometimes serious infection in human contacts. They can be identified by biochemical reactions, API 20NE (non-enteric), and by the Strauss reaction in guineapigs (see Stokes and Ridgway, 1980).

Ps. aeruginosa is common in human and animal faeces but seldom causes infection in healthy people. In hospitals, however, its natural resistance to many antimicrobials and its ability to grow in solutions used for treatment make it difficult to control. Its sensitivity to polymyxin does not impede its spread because this toxic antibiotic is seldom used. Hospital infection of urine, wounds and eyes occurs; also generalized infection including septicaemia, meningitis and osteomyelitis. Isolation from the external auditory meatus and from sputum, especially in patients with tracheostomy, is common, but may signify contamination rather than infection. Typical strains produce green pigment (pyocyanin) but this is not always seen. Other species, *Ps. cepacia* and *Ps. maltophilia*, are occasional causes of hospital infection. Precise identification is important for the control of epidemics; API 20NE is the first step after screening.

Typing, employing serological, bacteriocine and phage typing methods, is undertaken in reference laboratories.

Other non-fermenting Gram-negative bacilli

These are widespread in nature and are often isolated as contaminants from human specimens; they can be identified by API 20NE. *Chromobacterium violaceum* occasionally causes severe septicaemia with internal abscesses (Groves *et al.*, 1969). *Acinetobacter* species are short, stout and non-motile. They are sometimes coccoid and may be mistaken for *Neisseria* but are oxidase negative. They have been isolated from human pus, blood and cerebrospinal fluid but are of doubtful pathogenicity.

Alkaligenes species are also probably harmless. They may resemble *Bord. bronchiseptica* but are urease negative and do not agglutinate mammalian erythrocytes.

Flavobacterium species are found in soil and food. *Flavo. meningosepticum* is a rare cause of meningitis in hospitalized patients, usually neonates.

Antibiotic sensitivity patterns

Coliform bacteria have proved to be capable of developing antibiotic resistance most efficiently. They can do this in a variety of ways but that which has caused most widespread resistance is their ability to transfer resistance to several antibiotics simultaneously by sexual conjugation when genetic material is passed from a donor resistant strain carrying an R (resistance) factor to a sensitive recipient strain and to a proportion of their progeny. This probably happens rarely *in vivo* but the consequences are dramatic since the resistant cells are able to withstand treatment by any of several antibiotics and are at an immediate advantage leading to the replacement of sensitive strains by them in the hospital environment. Fortunately, when antibiotics are withdrawn the advantage is removed and within weeks or months the R factor tends to be lost and strains revert to sensitivity. Identification markers such as lactose fermentation and indole production are also transferred in this way but in this case no biological advantage is gained and these strains remain rare. Difference in genus is no bar to transfer of R factors; for example, *Salmonella* can receive resistance from *Escherichia*.

Of the genera categorized as 'coliform', *Escherichia, Salmonella* and *Shigella* are by nature the most sensitive, being susceptible to all the antibiotics normally used against Gram-negative bacteria. In hospital patients susceptibility is more likely than resistance to indicate identity, except for polymixin (mentioned under individual genera above), which is rarely used in therapy and to which resistance is not easily acquired. A lactose-fermenting coliform from urine which is susceptible to ampicillin is much more likely to be *Esch. coli* than *Klebsiella, Enterobacter* or *Citrobacter*, and it may be reasonable to confirm identity by lack of growth on

Simmons' citrate agar (Cowan and Steel, 1974) without the expense of API tests.

Parvobacteria

This name is given to six genera of small non-sporing, mainly non-motile, Gram-negative aerobic bacilli, which grow comparatively poorly on blood agar and poorly or not at all on MacConkey's bile salt agar. Only one species, *Y. enterocolitica*, is capable of growth outside the human or animal body (except in culture).

The term 'parvobacteria' (signifying their small microscopic and colonial appearance) is convenient, because they resembles each other on first isolation, as the coliforms do. Table 5.7 lists the genera included and their important characteristics. They may be isolated from blood, cerebrospinal fluid, serous fluids and infected discharges. Differentiation from coliforms is usually clear but occasionally small colony variants of coliform bacilli are encountered, which at first sight may be mistaken for parvobacteria. Their true nature is revealed by their ability to form gas in sugar fermentation, and on repeated subculture they yield a few large typical colonies on MacConkey agar.

Table 5.7 Parvobacteria

Genus	Haem*	Motility	AnO$_2$ growth[†]	MacConkey agar[‡]	Acid in carbo-hydrates	Oxidase	Catalase
Haemophilis	(+)	−	+	−	+	(+)	(+)
Bordetella	−	(+)	−	(+)	−		(+)
Brucella	−	−	−	[+]	−	−	+
Pasteurella	−	−	+	−	+	+	+
Yersinia	−	(+)	+	+	+	−	+ +
Francisella	Grows on Dorset's egg medium (see text)						

() = variable; [] = after long incubation.
*Haemolysis of horse blood agar.
†Strict anaerobic.
‡See *Note* on page 88.

Most parvobacteria are fastidious and daily subculture on highly nutrient blood agar, or on the medium of first isolation, is needed to ensure survival during investigation. Exceptions are *Bord. bronchiseptica*, *Pasteurella* and *Yersinia*. API tests (page 111) can be used in the identification of these less fastidious species. Parvobacteria grow poorly anaerobically; some are strict aerobes. The addition of 5–10% CO$_2$ enhances growth and may be essential for primary isolation (see below).

Haemophilus

All species are fastidious. They can be differentiated by their need for growth factors which, unlike most other bacteria, they are unable to

Table 5.8 *Haemophilus*

Species	Requires			Pathogenicity	
	X	V	CO_2	Acute pyogenic	Other
H. influenzae	+	+	−	+	+
H. aegyptius	+	+	−	+	
H. parainfluenzae	−	+	− +	−	+
H. ducreyi	+	−	− +	−	+
H. aphrophilus	− +	− +	+	−	+

synthesize. X factor is needed for iron metabolism and is derived from haemoglobin. V factor is a co-hydrogenase present in tissue.

Haemophilus, seen in Gram-stained smears of specimens, are small coccobacilli which stain poorly. Dilute carbol fuchsin will stain them better than other red dyes. In culture, pleomorphism is common, with long, serpent and large coccoid forms. The addition of 5–10% CO_2 enhances growth and is essential for the primary isolation of some strains (Table 5.8).

Encapsulated *H. influenzae* Pittman type b causes acute, sporadic meningitis and epiglottitis, mainly in children. The type b antigen can be detected in body fluids of infected patients (see page 35). Non-capsulated strains are frequently found in exacerbations of chronic bronchitis and bronchiectasis and in otitis media and nasal sinusitis. As they are normal inhabitants of the upper respiratory tract, it may not be easy to assess their pathogenic role, especially in patients treated with penicillin which will eliminate *Str. pneumoniae* but not *Haemophilus*.

H. parainfluenzae is commonly isolated from sputum and throat swabs and is a rare cause of sore throat. Haemolytic strains may be mistaken, at first sight, for streptococci. This is also the most likely species to be found in pus outside the respiratory system.

Haemophilus has been studied extensively and can be divided into a variety of subspecies. In clinical microbiology this serves no useful purpose because it throws no light on the potential pathogenicity of non-capsulated strains. Differentiation into *H. influenzae* and *H. parainfluenzae* as judged by the need for growth factors is sufficient identification. Haemolysis tends to be unstable and does not signify pathogenicity.

The need for X and V growth factors can be demonstrated by a satellitism test. Blood agar* and nutrient agar plates are inoculated with the test organism in parallel streaks about 1 cm apart. A spot of a staphylococcus culture is then seeded between the streaks. (The standard *Staphylococcus* employed as control for antibiotic sensitivity tests is suitable.) The plates are incubated overnight. On blood agar there is plenty of X factor. When the strain needs V factor the bacteria near the staphylococcus will be favourably placed; they will therefore form larger

---

*Routine defibrinated horse blood agar (page 311) is so highly nutritive for haemophilus that satellitism may not be seen. Oxalated horse blood agar is more suitable for this test. Strains needing traces only of X factor may grow on some kinds of nutrient agar.

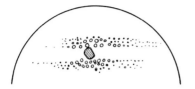

Fig. 5.3   Satellitism test.

colonies than those at the periphery (see Fig. 5.3).

In plain nutrient agar there is no haemin, therefore strains needing X factor will not grow on it; those needing V but not X will again show large satellite colonies round the staphylococcal growth (Fig. 5.3). In mixed cultures satellitism may be seen on the original blood agar culture. When the colonial and microscopic appearance of the satellite is typical there may be no need to test it further; it can be labelled an haemophilus. The advantage of this satelletism method is that a suitable staphylococcus is a reliable producer of V factor, which is highly labile, and no positive control is required.

An alternative method is to place commercially prepared paper disks, impregnated with X or V factor, on a nutrient agar plate inoculated with the test strain. X factor is stable but a control *Haemophilus* requiring V factor must be tested to ensure the potency of the V factor disk. V factor diffuses much more easily than X factor. If disks are placed too close together, the V factor may diffuse beyond the X factor disk, leading to satelletism apparently due to X rather than V factor.

Blood agar contains small amounts of V factor, enough for the isolation of *H. influenzae* in pure culture. If the medium is unusually rich in it, or if the strain needs comparatively little, the satellitism test may fail. Need for the growth factor is then tested by inoculating four peptone water tubes, one containing V factor, one with X factor, one with both and one with neither. The tubes are inoculated from growth on blood agar, care being taken not to scrape up any of the medium. They are incubated overnight. (For preparation of the growth factors, see Stokes & Ridgway 1980.) As the opacity after overnight culture is not always easily seen, a control set of uninoculated tubes is incubated for comparison. This also checks the sterility of the added growth factors.

H. aegyptius, the Koch–Weeks bacillus, causes epidemic conjunctivitis, rare in Britain. *H. aphrophilus*, an inhabitant of the mouth, is a rare cause of subacute endocarditis.

H. ducreyi causes genital soft sore. Some strains grow on horse blood agar, but scrapings from the floor of an ulcer should be seeded on freshly prepared 3 per cent nutrient agar containing 20–30 per cent defibrinated fresh rabbit blood (in addition to the routine cultures) when a laboratory diagnosis is attempted. For media for primary isolation, see Hannah and Greenwood (1982). The bacilli may be pleomorphic, showing bipolar staining or chain formation.

Table 5.9 *Bordetella*

	Primary growth on nutrient agar	Motility	Pathogenicity to man
Bord. pertussis	–	–	+ +
Bord. parapertussis	+	–	+
Bord. bronchiseptica	+	+	?

Bordetella

The three species are isolated from the respiratory tract of man and animals. They are all obligatory parasites and pathogenic (Table 5.9).

Bord. pertussis causes whooping cough and *Bord. parapertussis* caused mild whooping cough in some countries (not Britain). *Bord. bronchiseptica* is primarily an animal respiratory pathogen but is occasionally isolated from man. On primary culture (see page 61) *Bord. pertussis* resembles *H. influenzae* but, on further incubation, colonies increase in size and develop the typical pearly appearance. It is not dependent on X or V factors but it needs a highly nutrient medium without peptone for primary isolation (see page 313). On Bordet–Gengou or charcoal agar the colonies are 0.5–1 mm in diameter after 4 days' incubation. Identification is by agglutination with specific antiserum. Specific antigens are unusually labile; they can be altered by culture on different media. Therefore a negative agglutination test is not significant unless the strain used in preparation of the specific antiserum was cultured on medium similar in composition to that on which the strain to be tested was grown (Lacey, 1960).

Difficulty may be encountered with autoagglutinable strains. On subculture such strains may become smooth, or it may be possible to suspend the organism in saline, allow agglutinated particles to settle and then to obtain a satisfactory tube agglutination test (see page 115) with the smooth supernatant.

Brucella

All species are intracellular parasites of man and animals. Properties of the three human pathogens, which cause undulant fever, are listed in

Table 5.10 *Brucella*

	Animal host	Need for 5–10% CO_2	Growth in the presence of standard dyes		
			Thionin	Basic fuchsin	Pyronin
Br. melitensis	Goats and sheep (mainly)	–	+	+	–
Br. abortus	Cattle	+ +	--	+	+
Br. suis	Swine	–	+	–	–

Table 5.10. In Britain *Br. abortus* is much the commonest cause of undulant fever. The organism can be isolated from the blood of patients during one of the bouts of pyrexia. On first isolation, growth in an atmosphere containing 5–10% CO_2 is essential. Identification of the organism as a member of the genus is easily made by lack of sugar fermentation, inability to grow under strict anaerobic conditions and agglutination with specific antisera. Differentiation into the different species, however, is not a simple matter because antigenically they are very similar.

In addition, tests for H_2S production and agglutination with absorbed sera are of value. It is possible to divide these species into a number of biotypes, which aids epidemiological studies (Wilson *et al.*, 1983). Treatment of the patient is the same for all brucella infections, so identification of the species is not a matter of urgency.

Brucella may be isolated from contaminated material by culture on blood or liver agar plates screened with penicillin, or a guinea-pig may be inoculated intramuscularly with the test material; after 6 weeks, autopsy will reveal signs of infection and the organism can be recovered in pure culture from the spleen. The guinea-pig serum will usually show brucella agglutinins from the second week after inoculation.

Pasteurella

These are parasites of man and of animals. The only medically important species is *Past. multocida* (*septica*), which inhabits the respiratory tract of domestic and other animals; infection can often be traced to contact with them.

Colonies on blood agar resemble *Neisseria* and may be mistaken for them when bipolar staining is marked. It is commonly isolated from bite wounds and sometimes from sputum, where it probably plays no part in infection. In addition to properties listed in Table 5.7, it is indole positive and produces acid but no gas from sucrose. When in doubt, identity can be confirmed by using API 20NE for non-enteric Gram-negative bacilli.

Yersinia

The three species of this genus are parasites of man and of animals and cause characteristic diseases. They are identified by biochemical, serological and bacteriophage reactions. *Y. pestis* and *Y. pseudotuberculosis*, originally classified as *Pasteurella*, resemble each other biochemically and serologically. The antigenic structure of *Yersinia* is complex, they cross-react not only with each other but also with members of other genera (see below).

Y. pestis causes bubonic plague and may be imported to Britain from endemic areas in India or China. The pneumonic form is unlikely to be encountered, but *Y. pestis* may be isolated from pus from enlarged lymph glands (bubo). Identification is best carried out at a reference laboratory.

Y. pseudotuberculosis is well known as a guinea-pig pathogen giving rise to autopsy findings resembling those which result from infection of

Myco. tuberculosis, as its name implies. Natural infection of these and other rodents, kept as pets, may lead to accidental ingestion and human abdominal lymphadenitis. The bacillus can be cultivated from the cut surface of glands removed at operation, the patient having been suspected of acute appendicitis. The glands are reddish in colour, swollen and soft, and can be recognized by the surgeon as likely to be infected with *Yersinia*. Cultures overnight on blood agar yield a few non-haemolytic colonies 0.5-1 mm in diameter. API 20E biochemical tests for enteric bacteria include *Yersinia* and identification can be confirmed by agglutination with specific antisera. There are several types, but almost all human infections are due to type 1. The patient's serum may also agglutinate a known suspension. Some types of *Y. pseudotuberculosis* have antigens in common with *Salmonella* of groups B and D.

Y. enterocolitica, also a parasite, can live in the environment, especially in water. At 22°C it is motile, but not when incubated at 37°C; it grows better at the lower temperature. It will grow slowly at 4°C and this property can be used to select it from contaminated material. It causes enteritis, mesenteric lymphadenitis, septicaemia and secondary immuno-logical reactions (e.g. arthritis). In patients with iron overload, virulence is enhanced and severe generalized infection is seen (Chiu *et al.*, 1986). Biochemically it can be identified by API 20E. It is antigenically distinct from the other two species and some strains cross-react with *Brucella*. Isolation is most likely from faeces. It produces acid from sucrose (with small smounts of gas when incubated at 22°C) and will be recognized as a non-lactose fermenter in screening tests for coliforms (see Table 5.6). It is unlike pathogenic coliforms, as it is a coccobacillus and prefers low-temperature growth. Its presence does not necessarily imply infection.

Francisella

F. tularensis causes tularaemia in jack rabbits and ground squirrels, and occasionally in man. It should be considered as a possible cause of fever in a patient newly arrived from an endemic area. It is related to *Y. pestis* and *Brucella* but sufficiently unlike these to be classified as a separate genus. It was first isolated on Dorset's egg medium, but prefers a coagulated egg yolk medium. In specimens it is a very small, encapsulated Gram-negative bacillus, but in culture it is extremely pleomorphic. It is very liable to cause laboratory infection, and identification should be undertaken in a reference laboratory.

Campylobacter and Vibrio

Campylobacter

The medically important species of this large genus have only been studied widely since selective methods for their isolation (page 73) became available (Skirrow, 1977). They are vibrio-like, curved, highly motile, Gram-negative bacilli, microaerophilic and thermophilic (42°C). They are

Table 5.11   *Campylobacter* pathogenic to man

Species	Resistance to nalidixic acid	Hippurate hydrolysis	Urease production
Camp. jejuni	(−)	+	−
Camp. coli	−	−	−
Camp. laridis	+	−	−
Camp. pylori	+	−	+

(−) = usually negative.

fastidious and do not attack carbohydrates. They are a common cause of acute enteritis and occasionally invade the blood stream. Unlike other enteric pathogens, they are sensitive to erythromycin.

Two species, *C. jejuni* and *C. coli*, are commonly associated with human enteritis (Table 5.11). A third species, *C. laridis*, is occasionally found. Recently *C. pylori* was discovered in Australia to be associated with acute gastritis, and possibly with peptic ulceration (Marshall and Warren, 1984). It resembles *Campylobacter* more than any other genus; it is highly sensitive to erythromycin and other antimicrobials but is not yet firmly classified (Goodwin *et al.*, 1986).

When isolated from individual patients with enteritis, typical microscopic and colonial appearances on the selective medium and inability to grow in air at 37°C are sufficient identification for *Campylobacter*. Further investigation throws no light on pathogenicity, prognosis or treatment. Full identification and typing of epidemic strains is essential, however, if sources of infection are to be discovered. Biotyping, serological and bacteriophage methods have all been described (Bolton *et al.*, 1984).

Vibrio

These are Gram-negative, often curved, motile organisms found in fresh and salt water. Epidemics are caused when species infective to man pollute drinking water or food. Control is achieved by public health methods to prevent this.

In Britain, selective media are employed for their isolation from faeces of patients with enteritis newly arrived from endemic areas (page 74). Typical colonies can be identified using API 20E (page 111) and by agglutination with specific antisera. *Vibrio cholerae*, either classic or El Tor, or *Vibrio parahaemolyticus*, which lives in salt water and may contaminate sea food are the most likely isolates. Since they are rarely encountered, confirmation of identification by a reference laboratory is desirable.

Spore-bearing bacilli

The spore bearers are divided into two genera: *Bacillus*, which is aerobic, and *Clostridium*, which is anaerobic. They are found in air, water, soil, house dust, faeces and wounds. The anaerobes are more important in medicine and will be considered first.

Clostridia

The degree of anaerobiosis necessary for growth varies with different species. Some, such as *Cl. tetani*, are very strict anaerobes; others, such as *Cl. perfringens (welchi)*, are capable of growth in the presence of small amounts of oxygen. All the medically important species except *Cl. perfringens* are highly motile and tend to swarm on blood agar. (For prevention of swarming, see page 120.) They are usually found in mixed infection, either in pus from deep and lacerated wounds or from the uterus. Many discharges infected with anaerobes have a foul odour. The odour is caused by the breakdown of dead tissue by comparatively harmless proteolytic species. The four most dangerous species, *Cl. perfringes, Cl. novyi (oedematiens)*, *Cl. septicum* and *Cl. tetani*, produce no foul smell and may be found in odourless discharges.

Pathogenicity depends on the production of very powerful toxins. If conditions are not suitable for the production of these toxins, clostridia are harmless. Potentially pathogenic species may be isolated from surface wounds of patients without toxic symptoms.

Spore formation aids isolation because other bacteria can be killed by heat, leaving the spore bearers viable. Moreover, since all spores are not equally heat sensitive, it is sometimes possible to separate one spore bearer from another less resistant by suitably heating either liquid cultures or the original material. When the presence of clostridia is suspected either from the appearance of the stained film or from the nature of the lesion, the routine method is amplified. The original material is seeded on a neomycin blood agar and also onto Nagler's medium (see below). When all cultures and smears have been made, the remainder of the material is heated in a tube in a boiling waterbath and cultured on blood agar (in air and anaerobically) and into cooked meat broth after 5, 10 and 20 minutes' heating.

Cl. perfringens rarely spores and is more likely to be recovered from the original anaerobic plate culture or from the cooked meat broth. It can be identified after overnight incubation by the Nagler reaction. The original material, or a suspected colony, is seeded on egg yolk medium (page 318). When *Cl. perfringens* grows on it the α-toxin, which is lecithinase, diffuses into the medium and changes the fat in the egg yolk, forming a cloudy halo round each colony. This reaction can be specifically inhibited by antitoxin.

Method (after Hayward, 1941)
Dry an egg yolk medium plate for the Nagler reaction in the incubator for an hour and spread about five drops of antitoxin* over one half of its surface. Seed the material for culture so that the pool of inoculum covers

*Polyvalent therapeutic antitoxin can be used, provided there is not too much preservative in it.

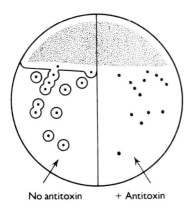

No antitoxin   + Antitoxin

Fig. 5.4   Nagler reaction.

part of both areas and spread it out on both halves of the plate; then incubate it anaerobically overnight (Fig. 5.4).

If toxin-producing *Cl. perfringens* is present, colonies about 1–2 mm in diameter of Gram-positive non-sporing bacilli will be found on both halves of the plate. Those on the untreated half will be surrounded by cloudy haloes due to the presence of α-toxin. No haloes will be seen on the antitoxin-treated half because the toxin is neutralized. Provided there are no spores and the organism is an anaerobe, the reaction is specific and the presence of *Cl. perfringens* can be reported without further tests. *Cl. bifermentans* gives a positive reaction but can be recognized by its spores. Some aerobic bacilli show cloudy zones and closely resemble *Cl. perfringens* when grown anaerobically on blood agar. When growth of the organism is profuse on the original anaerobic plate culture, it can be assumed to be an anaerobe if no similar bacilli are found on the aerobic culture. When growth is scanty, lack of it on the aerobic culture may be due to sampling error and it is then necessary to subculture to prove that the organism is incapable of aerobic growth, before a final report can be sent.

All these clostridia produce toxins which are lethal to mice and guinea-pigs. With the exception of *Cl. perfringens*, which is identified by the Nagler reaction, they are finally identified and proved virulent by inoculating two animals with cooked meat broth cultures, one being protected with specific antitoxin (see Stokes and Ridgway, 1980).

Enterotoxic *Cl. perfringens*

Food poisoning is caused when meat contaminated with *Cl. perfringens* spores is cooked insufficiently to kill the spores and is then allowed to stand at room temperature for some hours. The spores germinate to form a 'cook-meat culture' which, when eaten, causes abdominal cramps and diarrhoea (Hobbs *et al.*, 1953). The strains are poorly haemolytic on horse blood agar, but are Nagler positive. (For investigation and epidemiology, see page 291.)

Table 5.12   Clostridia which are known human pathogens

	Spores	Lactose	Glucose	Sucrose	Maltose	Pathogenicity
Cl. perfringens (welchi)	OS	AG	AG	AG	AG	Gas gangrene (food poisoning)
Cl. novyi (oedematiens)	OS	–	AG	–	AG	Gas gangrene
Cl. septicum	OS	AG	AG	–	AG	
Cl. histolyticum	OS	–	(A)	–	(A)	
Cl. tetani	RT	–	–	–	–	Tetanus
Cl. botulinum	OS	(AG)	AG	–	AG	Food poisoning
Cl. difficile	OS	–	AG	–	–	See text

OS = oval subterminal; RT = round terminal; A = acid; G = gas.

Cl. botulinum is a rare cause of toxigenic food poisoning in adults (see page 69). It has now been implicated as a cause of serious generalized infection of infants when it colonizes the gut and produces toxin *in vivo*; the mode of infection is obscure (Turner *et al.*, 1978). This infective form of botulism is rare in adults (Chia *et al.*, 1986).

Fermentation reactions of clostridia (Table 5.12), are tested in peptone water sugars, either incubated anaerobically or each one containing a sterile iron bar or nails which are nearly as long as the column of fluid. They will reduce Eh sufficiently for the most strict anearobes. Clostridia often metabolize indicator, so fresh sterile indicator must be added to each tube before reading. Equivocal results are common, and prolonged incubation or repeated tests may be required. For the use of gas-liquid chromatography in identification, see page 269.

Cl. difficile: This strictly anaerobic, toxigenic, Gram-positive bacillus can be isolated from the faeces of about 40 per cent of normal infants and occasionally from normal adults; numbers too small for isolation may often be present (Larson *et al.*, 1978). Colonies on primary culture plates give yellow-green fluorescence when examined under a Wood's ultraviolet lamp. One of its end products of metabolism is isocaproic acid.

The toxin is neutralized by *Cl. sordelli* antitoxin as well as by its homologous antitoxin. Its presence in culture or in faecal specimens may be established by cytotoxicity tests in tissue culture or by counter-current immunoelectrophoresis (Welch *et al.*, 1980). The toxin is associated with necrotizing enterocolitis and with antibiotic-associated diarrhoea. *Cl. difficile* certainly plays a role in these conditions, but the mode of pathogenicity and its epidemic potential in hospital patients are at present unclear. Identification of the toxin is more important than that of the bacterial species. Non-toxigenic *Cl. difficile* are harmless. Typing methods for epidemiological studies have been reported (Tabaqchali *et al.*, 1984).

Antibiotic sensitivity patterns

Pathogenic clostridia are at present sensitive to penicillin and other β-lactam antimicrobials. Although they are normally sensitive to macrolides, lincomycin and tetracyclines, acquired resistance to these drugs is increasing. Like all anaerobes, they are sensitive to metronidazole and resistant to aminoglycosides. They are sensitive to vancomycin, which is given orally in the treatment of necrotizing enterocolitis.

Bacillus

Members of this genus are often encountered in wounds, particularly after road accidents, in discharges from chronic ulcers and from other sites likely to be contaminated with soil and dust. They also occur as air-borne contaminants on solid media. Microscopicaly they are large, usually square-ended, Gram-positive bacilli, sometimes showing spores. Only one species, *B. anthracis*, is an habitual human pathogen; the others are usually considered to be harmless to man. They should not, however, be lightly dismissed on this account as they have been known to cause human infection. Easily tested points of difference between *B. anthracis* and other members of the group are as follows. *B. anthracis* is non-motile, capsulated, grows in long chains, forms no turbidity in broth, forms inverted fir tree growth in gelatin, with slow liquefaction, and is pathogenic to laboratory animals. Animal inoculation should only be performed by designated reference laboratories, because of the risk of disseminating spores. Other spore-bearing aerobes may show one or two but not the majority of these characteristics. Occasionally they lose their ability to retain Gram's stain and may be mistaken for coliforms. They form acid but no gas in a variety of sugar media and all the common species are indole negative. Although *B. cereus* is no more infective than other species it is a cause of food poisoning. An enterotoxin is produced when it is allowed to grow in cooked rice which, having been exposed to air, is kept warm, sometimes for many hours to serve to customers in restaurants (Mortimer and McCann, 1974).

Non-sporing anaerobic bacilli

These, mainly Gram-negative, bacilli include numerous species which are commensals in the colon, mouth and vagina of man and animals. For the most part they live in symbiosis with their host but sometimes invade tissue, especially abnormal tissue, and cause abscesses and septicaemia. Their infectivity may be enhanced by synergism with other microbes (Mackowiak, 1978).

Bacteroides

This genus contains many species and is the most numerous of the intestinal flora. *Bact. fragilis* is the most likely pathogen. Although it is isolated from abdominal abscesses and wounds much more frequently than any other species, it comprises only about 10 per cent of commensal strains (Duerdin, 1980). It is also isolated from abscesses in other sites, including lung and brain. Pathogenicity is related to the possession of polysaccharide capsules seen in freshly isolated strains (Kasper, 1976). When seen in smears of pus, *Bact. fragilis* is a small Gram-negative bacillus often seen in large numbers and usually accompanied by other organisms, especially anaerobic cocci. The capsules are not usually visible but may be seen in an indian ink preparation of a freshly isolated culture. (For colonial appearance, see page 87.) It can be identified by biochemical and serological tests, but in an individual patient this often serves no practical purpose. Proof is needed that it is, indeed, an anaerobe. It can then be labelled *Bacteroides* species. If capsules are seen, this is sufficient indentification of *Bact. fragilis*. For further identification tests, see Duerdin *et al.* (1980).

Among the other species, *Bact. melaninogenicus* is easily recognized by its action on blood, which colours its colonies black. It is most often isolated in mixed culture from abscesses in the mouth or genital tract. *Bact. ureolyticus (corrodens),* also found in oral abscesses, is recognizable by its ability to corrode the surface of agar media. It is a strict anaerobe.

Antibiotic sensitivity patterns

Like other anaerobes, *Bact. fragilis* is sensitive to metronidazole and resistant to aminoglycosides. It produces β-lactamase which neutralizes a large variety of β-lactam antibiotics. Its susceptibility to other antimicrobials is variable; it acquires plasmid-mediated resistance. Gram-negative anaerobic bacilli, unlike most aerobic Gram-negative bacilli, are resistant to nalidixic acid.

Fusobacterium and *Leptotrichia*

Fusobacterium differs from *Bacteroides* in being spindle shaped and naturally sensitive to penicillin. Their ecology is similar.

Fus. necrophorum is the most likely pathogen. It is usually filamentous and pleomorphic, but may resemble *Bacteroides*. Pathogenicity is caused by exotoxins. It is a slow-growing strict anaerobe and is often highly susceptible to exposure to oxygen; many strains are haemolytic. It is indole and H_2S positive, catalase negative and produces DNAase; *n*-butyric and propionic acids are major metabolic products. It is much less commonly isolated than *Bact. fragilis*. It causes calf diphtheria and occasionally necrobacillosis in man which begins with sore throat; septicaemia with lung abscess follows (Moore-Gillon *et al.*, 1984). *Fus. necrophorum* is sensitive to penicillin, metronidazole and most other antibiotics, but resistant to aminoglycosides. Necrobacillosis is potentially lethal; diagnosis and treatment are urgent.

L. buccalis is synonymous with Vincent's fusiform bacillus. It is the only species of *Leptotrichia*. Isolation is seldom attempted. For diagnosis of Vincent's angina, see page 54.

Anaerobic, non-sporing Gram-positive, or Gram-indeterminate bacilli may also be encountered. They belong to the *Corynebacterium* and *Lactobacillus* genera. They are seldom human pathogens.

Listeria and *Erysipelothrix*

These are Gram-positive non-sporing aerobic bacilli. They can exist in a rough or smooth form and resemble each other colonially and morphologically. When seen in smears of specimens they may be mistaken for diphtheroids. They are widespread in nature and well established animal pathogens. When inoculated into rabbits they cause mononucleosis; they are penicillin sensitive. Differentiation can be achieved by the following tests. *List. monocytogenes* is β-haemolytic on blood agar, grows at 4°C, hydrolyses aesculin, is catalase positive and is motile. It is also resistant to aminoglycosides. *Ery. rhusiopathiae* is α-haemolytic and negative in the other tests. Although *Listeria* cross-reacts in serological tests with other microbes, it is antigenically distinct from *Erysipelothrix*. *Listeria* is more important medically and will be considered first.

List. monocytogenes can spread directly from farm animals to man, but epidemics are more likely to be caused by contaminated food – e.g. milk (Fleming *et al.*, 1985) or coleslaw (Schlech *et al.*, 1983). The organism survives for long periods and is one of the few pathogens which can mutiply at 4°C. Contamination of chickens bought for consumption in the home is common (Hurley, 1983). Infection in adults resembles a mild flu-like illness or may be symptomless. It is followed by carriage in faeces and sometimes in the vagina. In adults it also causes meningitis which, because it results in a monocytic cell reaction, may be mistaken for tuberculous meningitis. It is essential to make the correct diagnosis because *List. monocytogenes* is penicillin sensitive and recovery is likely if treatment is prompt. Infection during pregnancy may result in uterine sepsis and fetal death. The infant may be infected either *in utero* or postnatally and is likely to suffer meningitis, with or without septicaemia. *List. monocytogenes* is considered to be the second most important cause of neonatal meningitis (Bortolussi, 1984).

It would be valuable to have a specific antigen–antibody test for serological diagnosis in suspected infection in pregnant women, but this is not yet available. Serological and phage-typing techniques have been employed in epidemiology.

Ery. rhusiopathiae causes erysipeloid in man. It can be recovered from tissue, or tissue fluid, taken from the edge of the lesion (see page 83). When the conditon is suspected the material is seeded into 0.2 per cent glucose broth in addition to the routine media. Septicaemia is common in animals and is rarely encountered in man. Agglutination tests are of value in diagnosis.

Legionella

These are highly fastidious, small, Gram-negative bacilli unrelated to any other genus. *L. pneumophila* was the first species to be discovered, in the USA in 1976. There are at least six species and they differ from each other sufficiently for it to be suggested that there should be a family

Legionellaceae comprising three genera, *Legionella*, *Tatlockia* and *Fluori-bacter* (Garrity *et al.*, 1980).

The species which are associated with respiratory disease in man are *L. pneumophila*, *L. dumoffi* and *L. micdadei*. *L. pneumophila* is oxidase and catalase positive, urea negative, produces brown pigment on suitable media, hydrolyses hippurate and liquefies gelatin. There are at least six serotypes, distinguishable by direct immunofluorescence staining. Other species may or may not produce oxidase, do not hydrolyse hippurate and are serologicallly distinct. Culture of specimens in hospital laboratories is not often successful, the diagnosis of legionella pneumonia being achieved by other means (page 260). Therefore identification is best undertaken in a reference laboratory.

Antibiotic sensitivity

All species, except *L. micdadei*, form β-lactamase. *In vitro* they are susceptible to erythromycin, rifampicin, chloramphenicol and cefoxitin, and to some aminoglycosides. They are resistant to polymyxins, vancomycin and clindamycin, which can be employed in selective media. *Legionella* species multiply intracellularly and are likely to survive therapy by antimicrobials which fail to penetrate cells.

Antibiotic-screened medium is essential when attempts are made to isolate *Legionella* from the environment. Their growth in water is related to the presence in it of amoebae. Unlike many highly fastidious bacteria, they survive well outside the body.

Miscellaneous

Eikenella

Eikenella corrodens is a small, slender, slow-growing Gram-negative aerobic bacillus forming a matt colony about 0.5 mm diameter which 'corrodes' the surface of blood agar. It is found fairly frequently in mixed culture and sometimes in pure culture in patients who have received antimicrobial treatment. Its colonial and microscopic appearances are typical and, as its pathogenicity is doubtful, no more detailed identification is usually required. However, it could be mistaken for *Haemophilus aphrophilus*, a rare cause of bacterial endocarditis, or *Bacteroides corrodens*, a strict anaerobe.

Gardnerella

G. vaginalis is a small non-motile, non-capsulated, fastidious, Gram-variable bacillus. It is seen in very large numbers adherent to squamous epithelial (clue) cells in smears of high vaginal swabs in leucorrhoea and cervicitis. It has finally been given a genus of its own because it is insufficiently close to *Haemophilus*, *Corynebacterium* or *Lactobacillus* with which it has previously been classified. The precise role of *G. vaginalis* in bacterial vaginosis is unclear. Various groups of anaerobes are also implicated, but their role, too, is uncertain. The diagnosis of bacterial vaginosis is essentially clinical. Three out of the following four criteria are accepted as a basis for diagnosis: vaginal pH >4.5, thin vaginal discharge, clue cells (see below) and a fishy amine odour (detected by the addition of 10% potassium hydroxide to the secretion on a glass slide). *G. vaginalis* can be isolated from vaginal secretions in the absence of symptoms, hence a routine search for this organism is not helpful. When alerted by the presence of clue cells or numerous bacilli resembling *Gardnerella* in the original smear, the organism can be identified by spreading the specimen heavily on human blood agar screened with nalidixic acid and polymyxin B (page 312). *G. vaginalis* will be seen after 48 hours' incubation in air plus 5–10% CO_2 as small grey colonies with diffuse β-haemolysis. The organism is resistant to sulphonamide but sensitive to metronidazole. It is further identified by the hippurate hydrolysis test.

Hippurate hydrolysis test
Method
Emulsify a large loopful of pure culture in 0.4 ml distilled water in a small capped test tube.

Add 0.2 ml ninhydrin solution and leave at room temperature (22–25°C) for 2 hours. (Ninhydrin solution is poisonous.)

The development of a purple-red colour indicates the presence of glycine produced by hippurate hydrolysis, i.e. a positive test. A positive control organism must be used for comparison.

Lactobacilli

These organisms live in the intestinal canal and vagina, and appear to be harmless. Most of them prefer a medium more acid than that used in diagnostic work, so they are seldom isolated. Döderlein's bacillus is a member of this group. It is often seen in cervical and vaginal smears as a large Gram-positive bacillus, and it may appear on blood agar cultures as minute non-haemolytic colonies. Other varieties of lactobacilli are found in cervical and wound swabs; they are non-motile, Gram-positive bacilli with straight parallel sides which tend to form chains. They are catalase negative, and some species are strict anaerobes.

Mycoplasma

These differ from bacteria in having no rigid cell wall, and from viruses in being able to grow in cell-free medium. They resemble the L-forms of bacteria. They have been known to cause fatal pleuropneumonia in cattle for many years. There are various species, markedly host specific.

Mycoplasma pneumoniae, the cause of primary atypical pneumonia, is very difficult to isolate; culture as a method of routine diagnosis is not practicable. A sample of blood must therefore be taken early in the infection if a reliable serological diagnosis is to be made without undue delay (see Chapter 10). In man the genital species *Mycopl. hominis* is most easily grown. It can be isolated on defibrinated horse blood agar provided the sample is not allowed to dry (transport medium preserves it well). The medium must be fresh and remain moist, and be incubated from 2 to 5 days. Growth is equivalent in moist air plus CO_2 and anaerobically but the minute non-haemolytic colonies are often more easily seen on the anaerobic culture because moisture is more easily preserved. It can be isolated from blood in puerperal infection and from pus in pelvic sepsis. It is an occasional cause of urinary infection where it appears in significant numbers associated with pus cells, like other urinary pathogens. Small numbers can be isolated from the urethra and genital tract of healthy people. It has occasionally been isolated from more distant sites – e.g. pleural fluid (Stokes, 1955).

Because of its lack of cell wall, microscopic examination by scraping colonies off the medium with a loop reveals nothing recognizable; a different technique is required.

Method
Sterilize a glass coverslip by flaming. When cool, place it on the surface of the medium over the colonies to be examined and press down gently. Then lift it with forceps (flamed and cooled), taking great care not to slide it on the surface of the medium. The colonies will adhere to it, leaving minute pits in the agar. Lightly flame the coverslip to fix the preparation. For ease of handling, lay the coverslip, colonies uppermost, on a glass slide and seal the edges with molten paraffin wax; it can then be stained. The colonies are Gram-negative sponge-like structures with minute bacilliform and coccoid bodies at the periphery. Normal bacterial colonies consist entirely of bacilli or cocci, but L-forms may resemble mycoplasma.

Mycoplasma hominis is resistant to penicillin and erythromycin; it also withstands thallous acetate (1.25 mg/100 ml), which can be used in selective media. It is sensitive to lincomycin, tetracycline, chloramphenicol and aminoglycosides. Typical morphology and stability on inhibitor-free medium (L-forms tend to revert to their normal appearance) are sufficient for a preliminary report. Species identification, when required, is best carried out in a reference laboratory.

Ureaplasma urealyticum (T-mycoplasma) probably causes a proportion of cases of non-chlamydial non-gonoccal urethritis, but it can also be isolated from the normal genital tract of sexually active persons. Colonies are too small to see with a hand lens and produce no opacity in liquid medium, their growth is recognized by a change in pH shown by indicator incorporated in the culture medium (Taylor Robinson *et al.*, 1969). Until there is firm evidence of their importance in medicine there is no need to attempt culture in diagnostic laboratories.

M. genitalium, which resembles *M. pneumoniae*, may also cause urethritis and pelvic inflammatory disease (Tulley *et al.*, 1981; Møller *et al.*, 1984).

Streptobacillus (Actinobacillus) moniliformis

This organism is a branching, Gram-variable, non-motile, non-acid-fast, pleomorphic bacillus. It lives in the upper respiratory tract of rats and can be isolated from the blood in one type of rat-bite fever (the other type is caused by *Spirillum minus*) and from the blood of patients suffering from Haverhill fever (Shanson *et al.*, 1983). In liquid culture it shows long branching filaments, some of which break up to form bacilli or cocci in chains which stain irregularly, Gram-positive and Gram-negative forms appearing in the same field. Most strains grow with difficulty on blood agar but when subcultured from the original blood broth will appear after 3–4 days' incubation as minute translucent colonies. Growth on solid medium is usually found to consist of comparatively short and almost diphtheroid forms. Sometimes large rounded bodies are found, and the bacilli may show central or terminal swellings. It is recognized by its extreme pleomorphism and slow growth. It is most difficult to maintain in culture.

Spirochaetes

Spirochaetes are widespread in nature; they resemble bacteria but are motile without possessing flagella. There are three genera important in medicine: *Treponema* which are anaerobes, *Borrelia* which are microaerophilic and *Leptospira* which grow in air.

Treponema cause world-wide chronic disease in man. *Tr. pallidum* causes syphilis, *Tr. pertenue* yaws and *Tr. carateum* pinta. These species are so closely related that they are indistinguishable apart from their pathogenic effect. Virulent strains cannot be cultivated but they may be seen in specimens from lesions, where they can be identified by specific immunofluorescence. Cell debris can closely resemble spirochaetes under dark-ground or phase-contrast microscopy. The inexperienced are unwise to make a preliminary report of their presence on this evidence alone.

Tr. vincenti can be cultivated with difficulty, but for the diagnosis of Vincent's angina see page 54.

Borrelia species resemble bacteria; they are Gram-negative and microaerophilic. Unlike spirochaetes, their antigens can change during infection and isolation is therefore important in diagnosis. *Borr. recurrentis* causes European relapsing fever. It may be seen in blood from acutely ill, febrile patients, preferably in its motile state by phase-contrast or dark-ground illumination, but also in blood films and can be isolated using special media (Kelly, 1971). It survives in clotted blood for some days.

Tick-borne erythema chronicum migrans (ECM) is caused by *Borr. burgdorferi*. The infection may progress to cause neurological symptoms or myocarditis. Generalized infection is described as Lyme disease (Kahan *et al.*, 1983). Serological tests can be employed in diagnosis.

Leptospira are carried by animals and infect man by direct contact or by water polluted with animal urine. The spirochaete enters through skin lesions which may be inconspicuous, or via intact mucous membranes.

They have close-set primary coils not disturbed by their flexible movement. They are aerobic and can be grown in Fletcher's medium containing rabbit serum (page 318). Although leptospirosis is more often diagnosed serologically, when a patient is seen early in infection and has not received treatment, blood culture is the most rapid method of diagnosis. Blood, and, after a few days, urine, may be highly infective. There are unlikely to be sufficient spirochaetes in specimens to be able to see them, but they can be recognized in cultures viewed by dark-ground or phase-contrast microscopy. They are actively motile and are often hooked at the ends or make buttonhole loops.

Two species are recognized, *L. interrogans*, which includes the parasites and potential pathogens and *L. biflexa* which is saprophytic. *L. interrogans* has a number of serotypes, two of which are likely to be encountered in Britain. Type *icterohaemorrhagiae* carried by rats causes Weil's disease (infective jaundice) but less than half of those infected are jaundiced; it is the most dangerous. Type *canicola* carried by dogs is usually a milder infection but may cause meningitis. Leptospira give rise to a polymorphonuclear cell reaction.

Spirillum minus is not a true spirochaete; it has rigid spirals but also flagellae. It is a natural parasite of rats and causes rat-bite fever in man. (See also *Streptobacillus moniliforms*, page 139.) For further information, see Wilson *et al.* (1983).

Chlamydia, Coxiella and Rickettsia

These small Gram-negative, intracellular bacilli cannot be grown in artificial media. Tissue culture is undertaken in reference laboratories and is outside the scope of this book.

Antibody tests for *Chlamydia*, using patient's serum, are generally unreliable (see page 259) but it is possible to confirm a clinical diagnosis by specific identification in cell-containing discharges, using polyclonal and monoclonal antibody tests which recognize chlamydial antigen (see page 270). *Chlam. trachomatis* is the most common cause of non-gonococcal urethritis. It is a major cause of pelvic sepsis in women and causes ophthalmia neotatorum and paratrachoma as well as classic hyperendemic trachoma.

Chlam. psittaci is primarily a bird pathogen but causes severe respiratory disease in man when it enters the lung by inhalation. Diagnosis is by serological tests (page 254). Some strains may be primary human pathogens (Grayston *et al.*, 1986).

Rickettsia and *Coxiella* are maintained in arthropods and animals, and infect man by contact with them. *Cox. burneti* causes Q fever and is also found in culture-negative endocarditis. Diagnosis is serological. There may be no history of contact with animals.

Rickettsia species cause fevers of varying severity, given different names in different parts of the world. Epidemic typhus is now rare. There is an antigenic cross-reaction with *Proteus*, made use of in the Weil–Felix agglutination test, which employs *Proteus* suspensions, for preliminary diagnosis. Final identification is made in reference laboratories because of the scarcity of specific antigen. For further information and differentiation between these three genera, see Wilson *et al.* (1983).

References

Anaerobic Laboratory Manual, 4th edn (1977) Ed. by L.V. Holdeman, E.P. Cato and W.E. Moore. Virginia Polytechnic Insitute, Backsburg, VA

Baird-Parker, A.C. (1974) In: *Bergey's Manual of Determinative Bacteriology* 8th edn, P. 478. Ed. by R.E. Buchanan and N.E. Gibbons. Williams and Wilkins, Baltimore

Bayston, R. and Higgins, J. (1986) *Journal of Clinical Pathology* **39**, 654

Bickham, S. and Jones, W. (1972) *American Journal of Clinical Pathology* **57**, 244

Birch, B.R., Keaney, M.G.L. and Ganguli, L.A. (1984) *Journal of Clinical Pathology* **37**. 1289

Blair, E.B., Emerson, J.S. and Tull, A.H. (1967) *American Journal of Clinical Pathology* **47**, 30

Bolton, F.J., Holt, A.V. and Hutchinson, D.N. (1984) *Journal of Clinical Pathology* **37**, 677

Bortolussi, R. (1984) *Clinical and Investigative Medicine* **7**, 213

Castle, D., Kessock-Philip, S. and Easmon, C.S.F. (1982) *Journal of Clinical Pathology* **35**, 719

Chia, J.K., Clark, J.B., Ryan, C.A. and Pollack, M. (1986) *New England Journal of Medicine* **315**, 239

Chiu, H.Y., Flynn, D.M., Hoffbrand, A.V. and Politis, D. (1986) *British Medical Journal* **292**, 97

Clinicopathological Conference (1966) *British Medical Journal* **i**, 93

Cowan, S.T. and Steel, K.J. (1974) *Identification of Medical Bacteria*. Cambridge University Press, Cambridge

Duerdin, B.I. (1980) *Journal of Hygiene Cambridge* **84**, 301

Duerdin, B.I., Collee, J.C., Brown, R., Deacon, A.G. and Holbrook, W.P. (1980) *Journal of Medical Microbiology* **13**, 231

Elek, S. (1949) *Journal of Clinical Pathology* **2**, 250

Fleming, D.W., Cochi, S.L. and MacDonald, K. (1985) *New England Journal of Medicine* **312**, 404

Garrity, G.M., Brown, A. and Vickers, R.M (1980) *International Journal of Systematic Bacteriology* **30**, 609

Goodwin, C.S., Armstrong, J.A. and Marshall, B.J. (1986) *Journal of Clinical Pathology* **39**, 353

Grayston, J.T. Kuo.C. Wang, S. and Altman, J. (1986) *New England Journal of Medicine* **315**, 161

Groves, M.G., Strauss, J.M., Abbas, J. and Davis, C.E. (1969) *Journal of Infections Disease* **120**, 605

Hale, J.H. (1951) *British Journal of Experimental Pathology* **32**, 307

Hannah, P. and Greenwood, J.R. (1982) *Journal of Clinical Microbiology* **16**, 861

Hayward, N.J. (1941) *British Medical Journal* **i**, 811.

Hobbs, B.C., Smith, M.E., Oakley, C.L., Warrack, G.H. and Cruickshank, J.C. (1953) *Journal of Hygiene Cambridge* **51**, 75

Holmes, B. and Dawson, C.A. (1985) *Journal of Clinical Pathology* **38**, 937

Holmes, B., Willcox, W.R., Lapage, S.P. and Malnick, H. (1977) *Journal of Clinical Pathology* **30**, 381

Hurley, R. (1983) *Clinics in Obstetrics and Gynaecology* **10**, 75

Johnson, W.D. and Kaye, D. (1970) *Annals of the NY Academy of Sciences* **174**, 568

Kahan, A., Dougados, M., Vannier, A. and Amor, B. (1983) *Lancet* ii, 174

Kasper, D.L. (1976) *Journal of Infectious Diseases* **134**, 59

Kelly, R.T. (1971) *Science* **173**, 443

Lacey, B.W. (1960) *Journal of Hygiene Cambridge* **58**, 57

Larson, H.E., Price, A.B., Honour, P. and Borellio, S.P. (1978) *Lancet* i, 1063

Leading Article (1977) Lancet ii 803

Leading Article (1985) *Lancet* ii, 1403

Leinonen, M., Luotonen, J., Herva, E., Valkonen, K. and Makela, P.H. (1981) *Journal of Infectious Diseases* **144**, 570

Mackowiak, P.A. (1978) *New England Journal of Medicine* **298**, 83

McLeod, D.T., Ahmad, F., Capewell, S., Croughan, M.J., Calder, M.A. and Seaton, A. (1986) *British Medical Journal* **292**, 1103

Marshall, B.J. and Warren, J.R. (1984) *Lancet* i, 1311

Maxted, W.R.(1948) Lancet ii 255

Møller, B.R., Taylor-Robinson, D. and Furr, P.M. (1984) *Lancet* i, 1102

Moore-Gillon, J., Tak, H.L., Eykyn, S.J. and Phillips, I. (1984) *British Medical Journal 288*, 1526

Mortimer, P.R. and McCann, G. (1974) *Lancet* i 1043

Okubadejo, O.A. and Alausa, K.O. (1968) *British Medical Journal* iii, 357

Parker, M.T. and Ball, L.C. (1976) *Journal of Medical Microbiology* **9**, 275

Petts, D.B. (1984) J. *Clinical Microbiology* **19**, 432

Public Health Laboratory Service Monograph No. 5 (1974) *Laboratory Methods* HM Stationery Office, London

Report of Research Committee of the British Thoracic Society and PHLS (1987) Quarterly Journal of Medicine New Series 62 No. 239 p 195

Report of Study Group (1977) *British Medical Journal* i, 131

Rowe, B., Taylor, J. and Bettelheim, K.A. (1970) *Lancet* i, 1

Shanson, D.C., Gazzard, B.G., Midgley, J. and Dixey, J. (1983) *Lancet* ii, 92

Schlech, W.F., Larigue, P.M. and Bortolussi, R.A. (1983) *New England Journal of Medicine* **308**, 203

Skirrow, M.B. (1969) *Journal of Medical Microbiology* **2**, 471

Skirrow, M.B. (1977) *British Medical Journal* ii, 9

Stokes, E.J. (1955) *Lancet* i, 276

Stokes, E.J. and Ridgway, G.L. (1980) *Clinical Bacteriology*, 5th edn. Edward Arnold, London

Tabaqchali, S., Holland, D., O'Farrell, S. and Silman, R. (1984) Lancet i, 935

Taylor, J. and Charter, R.E. (1952) *Journal of Pathology and Bacteriology* **6**, 729

Taylor Robinson, D., Addey, J.P. and Goodwin, C.S. (1969) *Nature* **222**, 274

Thomas, C.G.A. and Hare, R. (1954) *Journal of Clinical Pathology* **7**, 300

Tulley, J.G., Taylor-Robinson, D., Cole, R.M. and Rose, D.L. (1981) *Lancet* i, 1288

Turner, H.D., Brett, M.D., Gilbert, R.J., Ghosh, A.C. and Lieberschertz, H.J. (1978) *Lancet* i, 1277

Welch, D.F., Menge, S.K. and Matsen, J.M. (1980) *Journal of Clinical Microbiology* **11**, 470

Wellstood, S. (1982) *Journal of Clinical Microbiology* **15**, 226

Wilfert, J.N., Barrett, F.F., Ewing, W.H., Finland, M. and Kass, E.H. (1970) *Applied Microbiology* **19**, 345

Williams, R.E.O., Rippon, J.E. and Dowsett, L.M. (1953) *Lancet* i, 510

Wilson, G.S., Miles, A.A. and Parker, M.T. (Eds.) (1983) *Topley and Wilson's Principles of Bacteriology Virology and Immunity*, 7th edn, vol. 2. Edward Arnold, London

6

Investigation of Chronic Infections

Laboratory diagnosis of chronic infection cannot often be achieved by the methods so far described. Onset is often insidious and the patient is seldom investigated early in the infection. Granuloma, rather than purulent lesions, develop which are usually deep-seated and suitable specimens may be difficult or impossible to obtain. Moreover, stimulation of specific antibody is poor and attempts to detect antigens in specimens are often unhelpful because they may be absent or non-specific. Furthermore, the true nature of a chronic lesion is often masked by the presence of secondary invaders which are more easily cultivated and may, indeed, contribute to symptoms. When they are eliminated by treatment, improvement, but no cure, ensues.

Chronic infection may be caused by one of a variety of organisms. The investigation of fungal and protozoal diseases, which are often chronic, need special techniques which are described in Chapters 7 and 8. *Treponema pallidum* cannot be cultivated and the serological diagnosis of syphilis is dealt with in Chaper 10. The remaining important causes of granulomatous lesions are the mycobacteria and actinomyces. Of these, mycobacteria, especially *M. tuberculosis*, are much the most important, and investigation of tuberculosis will be described first.

Tuberculosis

Prevention of laboratory infection

Although antimicrobial treatment and control by public health measures have reduced dramatically the number of tuberculous patients needing investigation, this has not much affected the risk of infection to hospital staff (of all grades) who come in contact with them or handle their specimens before diagnosis and treatment. The following rules for handling all sputa and other specimens likely to be tuberculous are followed:

1. The laboratory worker must be tuberculin-positive.

2. All specimens and cultures must be handled in a safety cabinet (Collins *et al.*, 1974).

3. Specimens must be shaken without wetting the caps of bottles – e.g. on a vortex or other mechanical mixer.

4. A tube or bottle to be centrifuged must first be wrapped in a selfseal plastic bag to contain spilt material if the tube should break; a sealed bucket must be used.

5. Acid-fast bacilli are resistant to disinfectants; therefore glassware must be heat treated. Boiling for 5 minutes is effective but autoclaving may be convenient. Pipettes must be discarded with their tips under fluid (hypochlorite cleaning fluid 2,000 ppm chlorine) to prevent an aerosol when the teat is removed. Disposable pipettes and loops are preferred.

6. The cabinet must contain a discard jar for pipettes and a burner. Other equipment should be kept outside until required.

7. A separate room should be provided for work on tuberculous material.

8. Autopsy on patients with known active tuberculosis should not be undertaken. Staff working in the autopsy room must be tuberculin positive.

Three types of investigation are employed to aid diagnosis: microscopic examination, culture and a skin test for hypersensitivity to tuberculin. Methods of selective culture and biochemical identification tests have improved greatly. Animal inoculation is costly, hazardous and relatively inefficient; it is therefore obsolete for the routine diagnosis of tuberculosis and for the identification of *M. tuberculosis* in medical laboratories (Yates *et al.*, 1978).

Microscopic examination

This is a test to aid *clinical* diagnosis; the microbiologist does not assume that the bacilli he sees are *Myco. tuberculosis* (see Chapter 1). *Laboratory* diagnosis can be made only by culture, and takes several weeks. Because of this delay, microscopy plays an unusually important part. The value of a positive finding depends on the probability that there are no acid-fast bacilli, other than tubercle bacilli, in the specimen; this varies with different types of specimen. The chance of finding harmless acid-fast bacilli in sputum is slight and microscopy is therefore of great value; gastric juice, urine and faeces fairly often contain them and a diagnosis made on the strength of positive microscopy alone is therefore not satisfactory and needs confirmation by further tests. A source of error which must be avoided is contamination of solutions or glassware, either with saprophytic acid-fast bacilli, which are sometimes found in dust and tap water, or with the dead bodies of tubercle bacilli from previous positive specimens and cultures. Acid-fast bacilli, unlike most other bacteria, retain their structure and staining properties after death. They may adhere to glass, survive the cleaning process and be washed off into subsequent specimens. The following rules are adopted to avoid the grave risk of false positive reports from this cause.

1. As far as possible, all specimens are sent in disposable cartons.
2. New glass slides are used for smears.
3. Stains are made up in distilled water and dropped from bottles onto the slides or a mechanical device is used, and properly maintained, to

avoid the risk of transfer of bacilli between slides.

4. Blotting paper is cut in small squares and each piece is discarded after the whole of its surface has been used.

5. Centrifuge tubes, test tubes and bottles used for tuberculous material are immersed in 50% nitric acid* for 2 hours after sterilization and ordinary cleaning. They are then washed free of acid, dried, sterilized and marked to be used for TB only.

6. Marked bottles and caps are used to hold media for the culture of tubercle bacilli. They are kept entirely separate, and should be of a different shape, from those in which specimens are collected.

Methods

There are two methods in general use at the present time: the classic Ziehl–Neelsen method followed by examination under ordinary illumination, and the fluorescence method in which the bacilli are stained with a dye which fluoresces in shortwave light. The principle of both methods is to demonstrate the unique power of acid-fast bacilli to retain strong stains after decolorization with acid and alcohol. In laboratories where ten or more examinations are made daily the fluorescence method is to be preferred. The staining process is quicker and simpler than Ziehl–Neelsen's method, the bacilli appear bigger and the whole area of the smear can be scanned in less than 5 minutes with the 16mm objective once experience has been gained. The method lends itself to mechanization because no heating is required. A good optical system well maintained and a dark room (or part of a room) for examination of the slides is, however, essential; without this the classic Ziehl–Neelsen method is preferred. The requirements for fluorescence microscopy of acid-fast bacilli and for immunofluorescence (see Chapter 10) are different. The same microscope and light source can be employed, but because the reliability of these methods depends on optimum optical conditions a separate microscope is, in practice, essential for each. Constant changing of the system when only one microscope is available is impracticable. In searching for acid-fast bacilli a wide field is essential in order to cover a large area quickly under low magnification, and therefore a bright field condenser must be employed.

Ziehl–Neelsen stain

1. Flood the slide with strong carbol fuchsin and heat gently till steam rises. Add more stain when necessary and keep steaming fron 5–10 minutes but do not allow it to boil.

2. Wash in tap water (from a freely flowing tap which is in frequent use).

3. Decolorize alternately with 25% sulphuric acid and 95% alcohol until no more colour comes away.

4. Wash in tap water.

5. Counter stain with Loeffler's methylene blue for 3 minutes.

*The acid lasts indefinitely, more is added to replace gradual loss.

Fluorescence microscopy for acid-fast bacilli

Materials:

Microscope with lamp built into the stand.
Iodine-quartz tungsten bulb (Tomlinson, 1967) 100 watt.
Aplanat condenser (preferably oiled).
5 mm thick, blue PY filter to cut out all but shortwave light.
Yellow filter in eyepiece.
Eyepiece, either $\times 8$ or $\times 10$.
Par-focal objectives 16 mm and 4 mm.

Auramine–phenol stain for fluorescence method

1. Flood the slide with auramine phenol for 4 minutes.
2. Wash well in tap water.
3. Flood with acid–alcohol–decolorizer for 4 minutes.
4. Wash.
5. Counter-stain with potassium permanganate for 30 seconds.

Films of sputum, or other material, made on glass slides are stained with auramine phenol, a yellow dye which fluoresces in shortwave light. Acid-fast bacilli retain the dye after decolorization with acid-alcohol. The advantage of fluorescence is that the stained bacilli appear larger and are more easily seen, particularly in specimens such as pus, urine deposits and cerebrospinal fluid deposits where background fluorescence is slight. In sputum, examination by this method has been shown to yield a higher proportion of positives than by conventional methods (Wilson, 1952). Using the 16 mm objective acid-fast bacilli appear as bright points of light which, when examined with 4 mm objective, are seen to be typically shaped bacilli. Confidence can be gained initially by marking the position on the slide and re-examining after overstaining with the conventional Ziehl–Neelsen method. The only disadvantage is that a positive smear must be examined with each batch of slides to ensure that the microscope is set up correctly. An unstained positive slide should be included so that both the stain and optics are checked. Negative results should not be reported without a satisfactory control.

Originally a mercury vapour lamp was thought to be essential for optimal fluorescence but an iodine-quartz tungsten lamp* has been found to be equally good for most purposes, cheaper and easier to use. It also has a longer life and does not give off so much heat; when turned on it is instantly ready for use.

The positive slide is first examined. A grease pencil mark is made on its upper surface to encircle the area of the stained smear. A drop of oil is placed on the condenser and the slide is lowered into position so that there is an oil seal between slide and condenser. The low power objective is then focused until the grease pencil mark can be seen. The field inside it is then

*100 W, Atlas A1/215.

examined for acid-fast bacilli. The unknown specimens are then focused in the same way and examined by scanning the field in strips until the whole area within the grease pencil mark has been viewed or until acid-fast bacilli have been seen. When experience has been gained, most fluorescent debris seen in sputum can be recognized as such under the low power so that time is not wasted by continually taking a closer look with a high power lens. An oil immersion objective is not required.

Concentration of specimens
Concentration for microscopy only
Liquid, non-purulent specimens are centrifuged at 3000 r.p.m. for 30 minutes. The deposit is examined as concentrated as possible because acid-fast bacilli are likely to be few (see also under individual specimens).

Sputum, thick pus and gastric juice: add 2 parts of 4% sodium hydroxide to 1 part of the specimen. Incubate for 1 hour or more, until fluid. Centrifuge.

Faeces: saprophytic acid-fast bacilli are common in faeces and virulent bacilli are very scanty in tuberculosis. The examination of faecal specimens for *M. tuberculosis* is therefore considered to be a waste of time and materials (Grange, 1983a).

Concentration for culture and microscopy
None of the many concentration methods is ideal because all the chemicals employed to kill contaminating organisms also damage living tubercle bacilli to some extent. Strong chemicals such as sodium hydroxide and sulphuric acid kill contaminants in a short time but the tubercle bacilli will also suffer unless exposure to them is accurately timed. Sputum is particularly difficult to treat because time must be allowed for liquefaction and for the chemical to penetrate to all the contaminating organisms. As the consistency of specimens is extremely variable, no rule can be made for the time each is to be treated. It is a matter of judgement, and the tendency is to overtreat the specimen so that contaminated cultures are avoided. In routine work careful timing is very difficult to achieve, and a slow acting substance not too lethal to tubercle bacilli is preferred for sputum, gastric juice and large samples of pus. Treatment of different types of specimens is considered in detail later.

Culture

A laboratory diagnosis, independent of clinical findings, cannot be made until *M. tuberculosis* has been cultured. A negative culture is of more value than negative microscopy alone because, as in other infections, cultures are frequently positive when no organisms can be found in the stained film.

Culture of uncontaminated material presents no difficulty. Contaminated specimens such as sputum, laryngeal swabs, gastric juice, pooled specimens of urine and pus from secondarily infected wounds are treated to kill the non-acid-fast bacilli and to concentrate the specimen before culture. Slightly contaminated specimens can be cultured successfully on selective medium (Mitchison *et al.*, 1973) (see page 315). Löwenstein–Jensen (L–J) medium is employed for the human type of *M. tuberculosis* but Stonebrink's pyruvate egg medium is reqired for bovine strains, which are inhibited by glycerol, and will support the growth of human strains which fail to grow on L–J medium (Stonebrink, 1958). Hughes (1966) found that cultures of sputum from 5 of 99 tuberculous patients yielded growth only on pyruvate egg and confirmed that when, for economy, only one medium can be used this is the medium of choice.

Specimens needing treatment to get rid of contaminating organisms and others such as cerebrospinal fluid which the microbiologist has reason to think might be accidentally contaminated should be cultured on selective medium. Non-purulent fluids which are unlikely to be contaminated should, in addition, be cultured in Kirschner's liquid medium, which can also be introduced into the original container to allow any bacilli remaining there to grow when the bottle is incubated. Tubercle bacilli tend to adhere to each other in clumps in specimens, which makes sampling error great and reduces the chance of success when few bacilli are present. Moreover, an egg will occasionally contain bacterial inhibitors, and media must therefore be prepared from large batches of eggs and well homogenized to dilute any inhibitor which may be present.

The media are seeded heavily and the caps are screwed on tightly to prevent evaporation; moist medium is essential for the growth of tubercle bacilli. The cultures are inspected weekly and those sterile after 8 weeks' incubation are discarded unless acid-fast bacilli have been seen in the original smear, in which case they are incubated for a further month. Occasionally growth appears very late, particularly from specimens from treated patients. Growth of human strains on egg media can be expected within 2–3 weeks but may be delayed for much longer, even from material not exposed to chemotherapy. Negative 3-month cultures indicate either that the bacilli seen are dead, which is likely in a treated patient, or that they are opportunist mycobacteria incapable of growth at 35–37°C. Cultures should therefore be transferred to a 30°C incubator for a further 3 months with weekly inspection. Equipment contaminated with dead but visible bacilli (see page 144), inferior culture media or too rigorous preculture treatment are likely causes of failure to isolate when acid-fast bacilli have been seen.

Procedure for different types of specimens
Sputum
Examine each specimen for acid-fast bacilli before treatment. When they are seen in one sample, culture this sample; do not risk dilution with further samples which may be negative. Deposits from up to three samples with negative microscopy can be pooled for culture. The concentrated pool should then be examined for acid-fast bacilli.

Method
Add an equal volume of 10% crystalline sodium triphosphate solution to

sputum in its container. Shake on a vortex mixer and incubate overnight (18 hours). Measure 2 ml of the now liquefied sputum into a centrifuge bottle or tube, preferably disposable, containing 20 ml acidified sterile distilled water (35 ml of 1 M HCI in 1 litre distilled water). Mix again on the vortex mixer, then place the bottle or tube in a self-seal plastic bag and centrifuge at 3000 r.p.m. for 20 minutes. Decant the supernatant and, using a pipette, distribute the deposit over the surface of one pyruvate egg and one L–J slope. Incubate in the sloped position for the first week. When three samples are to be pooled, mix the deposits from each of the three bottles in one of them before inoculating the medium and prepare a slide of the material for microscopic examination.

Cerebrospinal and non-purulent serous fluids
Break up any clot by shaking with sterile glass beads. Pleural fluid can be prevented from clotting by adding 2 drops of 20% sodium citrate per 10 ml fluid (Grange, 1983b). Centrifuge at 3000 r.p.m. for 30 minutes; retain the original bottle. Remove the supernatant fluid with a sterile pipette. Make two smears, one as concentrated as possible, for examination for acid-fast bacilli and another for Gram-stain.

When no bacteria are seen in the Gram-stained smear and there are few or no polymorphonuclear cells, it can be assumed that other bacteria are absent. Culture the remains of the deposit without treatment on the following media: L–J, selective Middlebrook's medium, pyruvate egg, Kirschner's liquid medium. Add Kirschner's medium, using sterile precautions, to the specimen bottle and incubate to culture any acid-fast bacilli clinging to the glass.

When bacteria are seen in the Gram-stained smear it is not often necessary to culture for tubercle bacilli, but when this is required add 1 drop of 5% sulphuric acid to the deposit, hold for 20 minutes at room temperature and inoculate media as above using a pipette and sterile precautions. Finally, wash out the centrifuge tube with Kirschner's medium to collect any remaining bacilli.

Purulent serous fluids and pus
Gram-stain and culture overnight for other microbes, refrigerating the specimen meanwhile; examine a smear for acid-fast bacilli.

When the Gram-stained smear and culture show no contaminants, inoculate the refrigerated sample directly to the media described above for non-purulent fluids. When bacteria are seen, the overnight cultures yield growth and culture for mycobacteria is still required, add an equal volume of 5% sulphuric acid to not more than 2 ml pus in a centrifuge tube. When a swab only is provided submerge it in 2 ml of the acid, rubbing as much of the specimen as possible off the swab against the side of the centrifuge tube. Mix on a vortex mixer and stand at room temperature for 20–40 minutes depending on the degree of contamination. Add 16 ml sterile distilled water, squeeze as much liquid as possible out of the swab against the side of the tube before removing it and centrifuge at 3000 r.p.m. for 20 minutes. Remove the supernatant fluid and culture the deposit on the media recommended above but omit Kirschner's medium because the risk of contamination of a liquid culture is great.

Swabs from chronic ulcers

A swab received from a chronic ulcer should be examined for acid-fast bacilli in addition to the Gram-stained smear. The presence of acid-fast bacilli, or the absence of any other likely pathogen, indicates the need for low temperature culture after suitable treatment to get rid of contaminants. Cultures should be made on L–J and pyruvate egg media and incubated at 30°C. If no low temperature incubator is available, cultures can be left in the dark at room temperature. *M. marinum* and *M. ulcerans* will grow at the lower temperature but poorly, if at all, at 37°C (see page 153).

Acid-fast bacilli may be from BCG vaccination. The strain is an attenuated bovine *M. tuberculosis*: it has recognizable properties and can be identified by the experienced.

Urine

1. *Early-morning specimen.* Three consecutive early-morning specimens are collected in wide-mouthed screw-capped jars which have either been specially treated and marked for this purpose (page 145) or are disposable. Each is delivered to the laboratory on the day of collection. (When delay is unavoidable, they are refrigerated.) Mix well and centrifuge 20–30 ml at 3000 r.p.m. for 30 minutes; discard the supernatant fluid. Make two smears from the deposit – one for methylene blue stain (in order to see contaminants) and the other, a concentrated smear, for auramine or Ziehl–Neelsen stain. Examine the methylene blue-stained smear. Add to the deposit 2 ml of 5% sulphuric acid and hold at room temperature for 10, 20, 30 or 40 minutes according to the number of bacteria seen in the methylene blue-stained smear. Add 16 ml sterile distilled water, mix and then centrifuge for 30 minutes. Distribute the deposit between a pyruvate egg slope, an L–J slope and a selective medium slope.

2. *Ureteric catheter specimens*: treat as recommended for cerebrospinal fluid.

Tissue

Grind in a Griffith's tube (see Fig. 3.2, page 43), using sterile sand when necessary, or process in a stomacher. Then treat the emulsion as described for pus.

Gastric juice

The examination is made when patients cough but can produce no sputum; the small quantity coughed up is involuntarily swallowed and can be recovered from the stomach. The resting gastric juice is sucked out through a stomach tube early in the morning. If little fluid is available the stomach may be washed out with a small amount of water or sodium bicarbonate solution. On reaching the laboratory the gastric juice is treated as sputum. All specimens are cultured because of the unreliability of diagnosis by microscopy alone. When delay in examination is unavoidable, the specimen is refrigerated because tubercle bacilli do not survive well in the presence of active enzymes.

Laryngeal swabs
These are taken as an alternative to the examination of gastric juice from patients who cough but can produce no sputum. It is particularly useful method for outpatients. Swabs are prepared on strong wire applicators as in Fig. 6.1 and moistened in sterile water just before use.

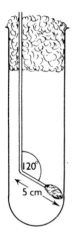

Fig. 6.1   Laryngeal swab.

Method
Wrap a strip of lint round the patient's protruded tongue, hold it gently and ask him to breathe through his mouth. Pass the tip of the swab through the mouth and over the back of the tongue, until the long straight part of the applicator lies along its surface. The sampling end should now be in the larynx and the patient will cough. It is best to take two swabs on each occasion because the material for culture is very scanty. The specimen is treated immediately by the method described for pus swabs, omitting the Gram-stain and blood agar cultures. Microscopy for acid-fast bacilli is also omitted because all the material on the swab is needed for culture.

Note. The sampler must protect his face with a transparent visor because he is in the direct line of fire of the patient's cough. One can be cheaply made by clipping washed, old x-ray film to a head band; after sampling, the film is discarded and replaced with a fresh piece.

Examination of cultures
The human type of tubercle bacillus grows on egg medium as pale

cream-coloured, rough, crumb-like colonies which are difficult to emulsify. Bovine strains grow slowly and often appear on pyruvate egg medium only; their growth is usually smoother and more confluent. Slopes should always be examined with a hand lens to avoid missing growth which is sometimes difficult to see through the bottle glass. *M. tuberculosis* (human type) grows on L–J medium between the temperatures of 30 and 39°C aerobically after 2–8 weeks incubation. Strains appearing after 4 weeks are often from treated patients. It is a non-chromogen, produces niacin and catalase (except isoniazide-resistant strains, which are catalase negative). For further tests of identification, see Yates *et al.,* (1978).

It is important to check that colonies of acid-fast bacilli are not saprophytes. The saprophytic bacilli grow rapidly, usually within a few days; they are often pigmented and they are capable of growth at room temperature and on plain nutrient agar. The growth is therefore sub-cultured to another egg medium slope and left in the dark at room temperature and also to a nutrient agar slope which is incubated. When these cultures are sterile after a week's incubation and the microscopic morphology is typical of *M. tuberculosis* a preliminary report may be sent. Identification of all strains first isolated from a previously undiagnosed patient should be confirmed, preferably in a reference laboratory. Antimicrobial sensitivity tests may be required, although doubt has been thrown on the value of routine testing (Grosset, 1978). Sensitivity testing techniques need careful monitoring and should be undertaken only by those experienced in them. Cultures must not leave the laboratory until growth is present on two slopes, one to remain in case the one sent is lost.

Pathogenic mycobacteria other than *M. tuberculosis*

Acid-fast bacilli are sometimes isolated from the sputum of patients who are not clinically suffering from tuberculosis or who have very mild symptoms. Although some species of tuberculoid mycobacteria, notably *M. avium (intracellulare)*, can cause chronic and even fatal infection, these are rare and patient-to-patient spread is extremely unlikely. They seldom, if ever, infect previously healthy people. (The incidence is increasing because of the greater number of people suffering from immunosuppression.) They are often resistant to antituberculous drugs, and identification is essential to prevent those without symptoms being submitted to the rigours and cost of antituberculous treatment. The help of a reference laboratory is essential because hospital laboratories cannot gain experience of these uncommon infections and special facilities for incubation at various temperatures are needed. Two species are occasionally found in sputum and two from chronic ulcerating lesions.

M. avium subspecies *intracellulare* is the most important in medicine. This species is primarily pathogenic to birds and has a wide range of growth temperature, from 25 to 43°C. Only *M. avium* itself grows well at

43° (Grange, 1983c). The colonies tend to be smooth and the bacilli shorter than *M. tuberculosis*.

M. kansasi, also isolated from sputum, causes mild symptoms or none. It usually grows within 2 weeks, the bacilli are longer than *M. tuberculosis* and may be barred. It is usually photochromogenic (pigmented when exposed to light). It can be isolated from water (McSwiggan and Collins, 1974).

M. ulcerans was discovered in Australia. It causes an important disease in Africa, buruli ulcer. It grows very slowly at between 31 and 34°C. It is isolated from skin granuloma in hot damp climates. Buruli ulcer causes serious deformity unless prevented by excision.

M. marinum (balnei) lives in swimming baths and aquaria. It enters the skin through minor abrasions and causes swimming-pool granuloma, which tends to heal spontaneously; it resembles *M. kansasi* culturally. For identification, see Grange and McIntyre (1979).

Tuberculin test

Numerous methods for testing hypersensitivity to tuberculin have been described. The graded intradermal (Mantoux) test is reliable and has been used extensively in epidemiological surveys in many countries. Two antigens are available. *Old tuberculin (OT)* is derived from glycerol broth cultures as described by Koch. *Purified protein derivative (PPD)*, also derived from liquid cultures, gives fewer side effects when a high concentration (1 : 100) is tested. The antigen in these preparations is partly denatured by the heating needed in preparation. Endotuberculins, prepared from disrupted living bacilli and sterilized by filtration, have been used (Stanford *et al.*, 1975). Burulin, prepared from *M. ulcerans* in this manner is highly specific.

The value of the test depends on the antibody status of the population tested. In Europe, where tuberculosis is regularly diagnosed and BCG vaccination is practised, and in Asia and Africa, where tuberculosis is rife, the test is not helpful in adults, a high proportion of whom will be positive without active disease. In the USA, where infection is rare and BCG is not normally given, a positive result at any age is significant.

Method

Adults are injected intradermally in the forearm with 0.1 ml of 1 : 10 000 dilution which raises a bleb about 1 cm in diameter; no control is necessary. The result is read between 48 and 72 hours and is positive if there is a patch of *oedema* at the site of inoculation at least 5 mm in diameter; erythema alone is of no significance. Reactions occurring on the first day which fade rapidly are non-specific. When the result is negative the test is repeated in the other forearm using the 1 : 1000 dilution. Alternatively, a multiple puncture test can be performed (see below).

Patients with erythema nodosum, who are likely to be highly sensitive, are tested initially with weaker dilutions, one in a hundred thousand or even one in a million. The consequences of giving too large a dose to a hypersensitive patient are serious and include necrosis of the skin at the site of inoculation, general symptoms with fever and sometimes increased size of the tuberculous lesion.

It is very difficult to remove traces of tuberculin from glass syringes. If a syringe which has previously held a strong dilution is used for injecting a weak dilution, an unpleasantly strong reaction may follow in a very sensitive patient. Disposable syringes and needles are ideal for hyper-sensitivity tests.

Interpretation

A positive result indicates that the tissues have been invaded by the tubercle bacillus some time previously and is useful in the diagnosis of tuberculosis in children under 5 years, who are normally negative unless they have received BCG. It gives no indication of the activity, size or site of the lesion.

A negative result almost excludes tuberculosis of more than 2 months' duration at any age, unless the patient has received steroids. Patients with acute fresh lesions and those with longer standing but rapidly progressive disease may fail to react, but a negative multiple puncture tuberculin test in patients with active chronic tuberculosis is extremely rare.

The multiple puncture test (Heaf and Rusby, 1959) is ideal for screening large numbers of patients attending weekly clinics who are expected to be tuberculin negative or are newly converted after BCG vaccination. One drop of a special preparation of PPD is spread on the forearm and injected into the skin by releasing a 6-bladed 'gun' over the area. The method is painless and the result can be read any time between the third and the seventh day. The 'gun' is sterilized between patients by flaming. The blades can be set in either of two positions so that they are effective in adults and can be made to penetrate less deeply for children. In highly sensitive patients an unpleasantly severe reaction results and the site of inoculation may be visible as six small red papules for months or even years. Therefore when a positive result is likely, in adults from endemic areas or in suspected infection, the graded Mantoux test is preferred. Those failing to react to the 1 : 10 000 intradermal dose can safely be retested by the multiple puncture technique.

A low grade positive tuberculin test can result from infection by other mycobacteria. When this is suspected it may be possible to obtain antigen prepared from strains of tuberculoid bacilli known to invade human tissue. A more pronounced reaction can be expected with the homologous antigen than with PPD in any patient who is chronically infected.

Leprosy

Mycobacterium leprae can be seen in scrapings of the nasal mucosa in the lepromatous form of the disease and in sputum when the lungs are affected. They are acid-fast bacilli which can be stained by the Ziehl–Neelsen or by the fluorescence method as described for tubercle bacilli. They are less strongly acid-fast than *M. tuberculosis* and must not be overdecolorized. In nasal scrapings the bacilli are very numerous and mostly intracellular, the cells appearing stuffed with them. Diagnosis by skin biopsy is also successful and is carried out when nasal scrapings are negative. They are differentiated from *M. tuberculosis* by their inability to grow on egg medium or to infect guinea-pigs.

Tests for reagin in the diagnosis of syphilis are often positive in leprosy, particularly in the nodular type of the disease.

Actinomycosis and nocardiosis

Actinomycosis is a rare chronic granulomatous disease caused by Gram-positive branching bacilli with a tendency to form fungus-like colonies in tissue. These organisms have been separated into two genera: *Actinomyces* species which are obligatory parasites, and *Nocardia*, which enter the tissues accidentally from the environment and cause disease, mainly in those malnourished or immunosuppressed. Despite their morphological resemblance to fungi, their chemical composition and their sensitivity to antibacterial but not to antifungal drugs place them with the bacteria.

Actinomyces

The cause of typical human actinomycosis is *Actinomyces israeli*. It is an obligate human parasite and has been isolated from the mouth of patients not suffering from the disease, so its presence in a culture is not proof of actinomycosis in the patient. It is associated with salivary calculi and is probably the most common cause of their formation. The factors which determine the onset of the disease in a previously healthy human carrier are unknown. When the organism multiplies in tissues they respond by forming a granuloma which enlarges, penetrates the surrounding tissues, whatever their nature, and finally reaches the surface, where it appears as a hard mass with discharging sinuses. The usual sites of infection are the jaw, the caecum or the lungs. Spread by the blood stream is rare but actinomycotic cerebral abscess has been recorded as a complication of the pulmonary form of the disease.

The discharge is seldom profuse and in order to obtain a good sample the whole of the inner dressing is sent to the laboratory in a sterile screw-capped bottle. A swab taken from the sinuses is usually rich in contaminating organisms and poor in material from the deep part of the granuloma which is most likely to yield a positive culture.

Macroscopic and microscopic examination

Using sterile forceps and scissors, remove the part of the innermost layer of the dressing which is most heavily contaminated with pus and place it in a 30 ml screw-capped bottle containing 5–10 ml peptone water. (Saline may interfere with the viability of delicate microbes.) Shake well and examine the fluid for actinomycotic granules. They are colonies of *Actinomyces israeli* which have developed in the tissues. They are about 0.2–1 mm in diameter, yellowish and oily in appearance. Remove one with a Pasteur pipette and squash it between two glass slides; separate the slides and Gram-stain. Fresh granules are soft and easily emulsified but old ones may be calcified. If no soft granules can be found, it is necessary to treat calcified ones with dilute hydrochloric acid before staining. The organism is seen as a tangled mass of Gram-positive branching mycelium with Gram-negative clubs at the periphery; the appearance is typical and diagnostic of actinomycosis.

Culture

Material from old lesions may be sterile or yield only contaminants, but there is usually no difficulty in recovering the organism from young active lesions. When soft fresh granules are found, they are washed three times in saline to remove contaminating organisms and are then cultured on two blood agar plates, incubated in air plus 5–10% CO_2 and anaerobically plus about 10% CO_2. When no granules are found the fluid is cenrifuged and the deposit is cultured in the same manner. *Actinomyces israeli* is incapable of growth in air, which distinguishes it from the many harmless aerobic species which sometimes contaminate wounds. Growth is usually visible on the anaerobic culture after 3 days' incubation as 0.5–1 mm yellowish crumb-like colonies which sometimes tend to adhere to the medium and may not be very easily emulsified. Gram-stained films from cultures reveal a very different appearance from the colonies found in tissues. The organism is mainly bacilliform and resembles diphtheroids, for which it may easily be mistaken. The arrangement, however, is a little different because many bacilli lie in V or Y forms and careful search usually reveals a few filaments showing false and occasionally true branching; it is non-acid-fast.

A. eriksoni is a rare cause of pulmonary actinomycosis. It does not form granules in tissue, but in other respects resembles *A. israeli* (Georg *et al.*, 1965).

A. israeli is sensitive to penicillin but treatment is not always successful. Penetration to the organism in granulomatous lesions is difficult and surgery combined with prolonged penicillin treatment is often necessary. Other organisms may also play a part. *Actinobacillus actinomycetem-comitans,* a Gram-negative, penicillin-resistant bacillus is regularly present. Tetracycline is active against both and may succeed. Rifampicin in pulmonary actinomycosis is reported to have a rapid effect (King and White, 1981).

Actinobacillus actinomycetemcomitans is a pathogen in its own right; it lives in the mouth and is occasionally isolated from the blood in subacute endocarditis. It grows as well aerobically as anaerobically, and resembles *Haemophilus aphrophilus* (King and Tatum, 1962).

Nocardia

Members of this genus resemble *Actinomyces* but are aerobes. They cause granulomatous infections of animals and man but are not obligatory parasites. They are normally sensitive to sulphonamides but resistant to penicillin and many other antimicrobials (Curry, 1980).

N. asteroides causes a tuberculosis-like pulmonary infection, sometimes activated by steroid therapy and immunosuppression. The organism is weakly acid-fast; it is unlikely to withstand decolorization employed for tubercle bacilli. The Gram-stain shows typical filamentous, Gram-positive, branching bacilli. For culture, contaminants can often be eliminated by incubation at 40–50°C (Curry, 1980). Laboratory diagnosis is important because antituberculosis treatment is inappropriate. *N. asteroides* is also an animal pathogen, causing farcy in cattle and sometimes granuloma of the udder. The organism has been found in milk (Grange, 1983a).

Madura disease is a chronic granulomatous infection, usually of the foot (in labourers who wear no shoes) in hot countries. Actinomycetes or fungi (page 163) may be identified from the lesions. In India *N. madurae* is the main cause. In South America the disease, which is clinically similar, is caused by *N. brasiliensis*. For further information on *Nocardia*, see Mishra *et al.*, (1980). Other species of *Actinomyces* and *Nocardia* occasionally infect man and many are animal pathogens (Wilson *et al.*, 1983).

References

Collins, C.H., Hartley, E.G. and Pilsworth, R. (1974). *The Prevention of Laboratory Acquired Infection.* Stationery Office, Public Health Laboratory Service Monograph, No. 6. HM London

Curry, W.A. (1980) *Archives of Internal Medicine* **140**, 818

Georg, L.K., Robertstad, G.W., Buckman, S.A. and Hicklin, M.D. (1965) *Journal of Infectious Diseases* **115**, 88

Grange, J.M. (1983 a–c) In: *Topley and Wilson's Principles of Bacteriology, Virology and Immunity*, 7th edn. Ed. by G.S. Wilson, A.A. Miles and M.T. Parker. Edward Arnold, London. a and b: vol. 3, p. 43; c: vol. 2, p. 82

Grange, J.M. and McIntyre, G. (1979) *Journal of Applied Bacteriology* **47**, 285

Grosset, J. (1978) *Bulletin Union Internationale contre la Tuberculose* **53**, 200

Heaf, F. and Lloyd Rusby, N. (1959). *Recent Advances in Respiratory Tuberculosis*, p. 62. Churchill, London

Hughes, M.H. (1966) *Journal of Clinical Pathology* **19**, 73

King, E.O. and Tatum, H.W. (1962) *Journal of Infectious Diseases 111*, 85

King, J.W. and White, M.C. (1981) *Archives of Internal Medicine 141*, 1234

McSwiggan, D.A. and Collins, C.H. (1974) *Tubercle* **55**, 291

Mishra, S.K., Gordon, R.E. and Barrett, D.A. (1980) *Journal of Clinical Microbiology* **11**, 728

Mitchison, D.A., Allen, B.W. and Lambert, R.A. (1973) *Journal of Clinical Pathology* **26**, 250

Stanford, J.L., Rook, G.A.W., Convit, J., Godal, T. *et al.*, (1975) *Journal of Experimental Pathology* **56**, 579

Stonebrink, B. (1958) *Acta Tuberculosea Scandinavica* **35**, 67

Tomlinson, A.H. (1967) *Immunology* **13**, 323

Wilson, M.M. (1952) *American Review of Tuberculosis* **65**, 709

Wilson, G.S., Miles, A.A. and Parker, M.T. (Eds.) (1983) In: *Topley and Wilson's Principles of Bacteriology, Virology and Immunity,* 7th edn, Vol. 2, pp.14 *et seq.* Edward Arnold, London

Yates, M.D., Collins, C.H. and Grange, J.M. (1978) *Tubercle* **59**, 143

7

Fungal Infections

R.J. Hay

Introduction

Mycology is becoming increasingly important in diagnostic microbiology laboratories because modern therapy has increased the risk of fungal disease. Fungi, with few exceptions, are less efficient at initiating infection than are bacteria or viruses, and in temperate climates the only common fungal diseases in previously healthy people are the superficial mycoses, especially ringworm, and vaginal or oral thrush. In mixed infections the bacteria will be easily recognized in the laboratory but the fungal pathogens may be overlooked until elimination of the bacteria fails to effect a cure. The true state of affairs may be suspected if hyphae or yeasts are seen in the Gram-stained smear. Correct laboratory diagnosis is needed to ensure optimum treatment.

Opportunist infections by microbes resistant to antimicrobials are frequent in hospital patients; among these fungi are common. They have the advantage of being naturally resistant to most antibacterial drugs, and their relative lack of ability to evade natural defences ceases to be a disadvantage when patients at risk have debilitating disease or immunosuppressive treatment. Infection caused by fungal commensals may start superficially, rapidly become systemic and, unless promptly treated, overwhelm patients and cause their death. The symptoms usually resemble those of other generalized infections and laboratory diagnosis is essential.

Fungi cause a number of diseases with distinctive clinical features, some

Table 7.1 Fungal Infections

Superficial mycoses	Dermatophytosis Superficial candidosis Pityriasis versicolor Onychomycosis	
Subcutaneous mycoses	Mycetoma Chromomycosis Sporotrichosis	
Systemic mycoses	*Pathogens:*	histoplasmosis, coccidioidomycosis, paracoccidioidomycosis, blastomycosis
	Opportunists:	aspergillosis, systemic candidosis, mucormycosis, cryptococcosis

of which closely mimic other conditions such as tuberculosis. Table 7.1 lists the fungal infections of man. The superficial mycoses are relatively common and have a worldwide distribution. By contrast, the subcutaneous infections such as mycetoma and chromomycosis are rare and largely confined to the tropics and subtropics. Systemic mycoses include respiratory infections, such as histoplasmosis, which affect individuals without underlying disease and have a limited geographic distribution.

Diagnostic methods

The principal methods of laboratory diagnosis in mycology are direct microscopy, culture, serology and histopathology; except in allergic diseases such as allergic bronchopulmonary aspergillosis, skin tests have little diagnostic value.

Direct microscopy

This technique can be applied to scrapings of skin, nail clippings, sputum or fluid samples. As most fungi are relatively large (over 2 μm in diameter), staining is not always necessary. Material is softened in 10% aqueous potassium hyroxide and examined using a light microscope with the condenser racked down. A mixture of Parker blue-black ink and 30% potassium hydroxide (1:1) may be useful to demonstrate *Malassezia furfur* in pityriasis versicolor as well as some nail pathogens. Both take up the stain immediately. Fungi are usually Gram-positive but they often appear indistinct with a Gram-stain. The periodic acid–Schiff (PAS) stain is preferable. Heat-fixed smears are covered with 0.5% periodic acid solution for 5 minutes, rinsed in distilled water and then placed in Coleman's Feulgen reagent for 15–20 minutes. The pink colour appears after washing in running tap water for 10 minutes.

Culture

Most fungi grow well at 25–28°C. The medium most suitable for isolation is Sabouraud's dextrose agar (SDA) (1% mycological peptone, 4% dextrose and 1.5% agar) containing chloramphenicol (0.005%) or penicillin (20 mg/l)/streptomycin (40 mg/l). But many pathogenic fungi, including *Candida albicans*, will grow on blood agar. For skin surface samples the addition of 0.05% cycloheximide (Actidione) will suppress the growth of saprophytic fungi. It will also inhibit some pathogenic yeasts and is particularly useful for the isolation of dermatophytes. For special purposes, such as the identification of dimorphic fungi, enriched media such as brain–heart infusion agar may be necessary.

On primary isolation, many fungi grow slowly and, although in some cases it is possible to identify organisms within 48 hours, in many infections cultures have to kept for up to 4 weeks. A higher temperature (37°C) is used for some special tests and a few organisms such as *Trichophyton verrucosum*, the cause of cattle ringworm, show a preference for this temperature.

The identification of fungi is based on their colonial morphology, pigmentation and microscopic appearances. It is useful to tease out a fragment of the culture on a glass slide in a drop of lactophenol cotton blue using two mounted needles. Fungi can usually be classified into one of two morphological forms. The yeasts produce smooth colonies and are unicellular organisms which reproduce by budding. Mould fungi tend to form large, often downy, colonies and the organisms form chains of joined cells – hyphae. Some fungi are dimorphic; i.e. they exist in either phase under different conditions. In human infection the yeast-like phase is found in specimens, and identification can be achieved only by examining mould-like colonies in culture and producing conversion to the yeast phase *in vitro* by culture on enriched media. Fungal recognition is not easy and it is advisable in many cases to refer to a laboratory manual (Clayton and Midgley, 1985; Koneman and Roberts, 1985).

Serology

Serodiagnosis is useful in systemic fungal infections and has both diagnostic and prognostic value. Most commercially produced systems detect antibody and can be difficult to interpret in opportunistic infections. For cryptococcosis an antigen-detection system is used. Generally, serodiagnostic tests are best referred to specialized laboratories.

Superficial mycoses

Although the superficial mycoses usually have characteristic clinical appearances, in most cases the diagnosis can be confirmed by direct microscopy or culture of swabs or skin scrapings. Skin scrapings are best taken with a solid (banana) scalpel which is not as sharp as a knife with disposable blades. If scrapings have to be sent by post, they should be folded in paper or card; thick black paper is ideal. With infected nails, it is useful to sample both the nail plate and the subungual debris.

Dermatophytes (ringworm fungi, tinea)

The dermatophyte fungi are moulds which infect the keratinized layer of skin, the stratum corneum, hair and nails. Dermatophytosis is relatively common and includes diseases such as athlete's foot (tinea pedis) and scalp ringworm (tinea capitis). Some dermatophytes are transmitted from man to man (anthropophilic) whilst others are transferred from animals to man (zoophilic). As the latter are usually primary host specific, their recognition is important because this identifies the likely source.

This is particularly important in children with scalp ringworm (tinea capitis) where small epidemics may follow infection with dermatophytes such as *Trichophyton violaceum* which can be transmitted from child to child.

Epidemics in childhood caused by *Microsporon audovini* are no longer seen.

Taking of specimens

Scrapings should be taken if possible from the active margin of lesions. If small vesicles or blisters are present the roof is a useful source of material. In the scalp, infected hairs are usually broken and, in some cases, fluoresce green under a filtered ultraviolet (Wood's) light. The latter is useful for screening patients and for selecting hairs for culture.

Direct microscopy

Dermatophyte hyphae are usually clearly visible and pass right across epithelial cell borders. This distinguishes them from many artefacts such as 'mosaic fungus' which can be seen to follow the edge of cells. Scalp hairs should be carefully examined to see where the organisms form chains of specialized spores – arthrospores. Ectothrix fungi form arthrospores on the outside of the hair shaft whereas endothrix organisms form them within the hair itself. This may give a preliminary identification of the source of the organism.

Culture

Dermatophytes grow well, but slowly, if implanted into Sabouraud's dextrose agar (SDA) incubated at 25–28°C. They are usually identifiable in 10–14 days. The pattern of the formation of specialized spores, microconidia and macroconidia, is important in recognition as well as colonial morphology and pigmentation. For full identification, reference to a specialized handbook is usually necessary (e.g. Rebell and Taplin, 1970). The principle characteristics of the most common dermatophytes are shown in Table 7.2

In some cases it is necessary to grow organisms on special media or use nutritional tests for identification (Philpot, 1977). For instance, *Microsporum canis* forms macroconidia best on sterile boiled rice grains. As it is not always possible to distinguish the various sporing cultures, a further technique is often used – the slide culture.

Slide cultures

A 1-cm SDA block is cut from a sterile plate and transferred to a sterile microscope slide resting on a bent glass rod in a Petri dish. Small fragments of the test colony are inoculated using a mounted needle into the four sides of the block, which is then covered with a coverslip sterilized by briefly flaming in a Bunsen. A few drops of water are added to the dish which is then covered and incubated at 25–28°C. After 7–14 days the agar block is discarded and the coverslip is placed in lactophenol blue on a fresh glass slide. Likewise a drop of stain is placed on the used glass slide which is covered with a fresh coverslip. The mycelium which adheres to either glass surface usually shows the characteristic microscopic morphological appearances, which may be lost if needle mounts are used.

Table 7.2 Characteristics of common dermatophytes

	Source	Hair invasion	Wood's light	Cultural features	Spores
Trichophyton rubrum	Man	very rare	NA	White fluffy, red to yellow pigment on undersurface	Few long macroconidia; microconidia ±
T. mentagrophytes	Animal	Rare, ectothrix	Neg.	White fluffy to white with powdery centre	Many microconidia
T. interdigitale	Man			Reverse may be brown	Some long macroconidia
T. verrucosum	Cattle	Ectothrix	Neg.	Slow growth – white granular	Chlamydospores
T. violaceum	Man	Endothrix	Neg.	Violet to purple, smooth	
Microsporum canis	Cats, dogs	Ectothrix	Pos.	White – but yellow pigment in most isolates	Thick-walled pointed macroconidia
Epidermophyton floccosum	Man	very rare	NA	White to buff or buff/yellow pigment	Club-shaped macroconidia

NA = not applicable.

Pityriasis versicolor

Pityriasis versicolor is a common skin disease caused by the lipophilic yeast *Malassezia furfur*. Affected areas are covered with hypo-or hyper-pigmented scaly patches. The organisms form into clusters containing round or ovoid yeasts and short fat hyphae. These can be demonstrated in skin scrapings although it is often helpful to use the Parker stain (page 159). Culture is difficult and unnecessary.

Onychomycosis

Nail infections may be caused by fungi other than dermatophytes such as *Aspergillus* species, *Hendersonula toruloidea* or *Scopulariopsis brevi-caulis*. When culturing nails it is advisable to use two plates of SDA – one containing cycloheximide, the other without – as cycloheximide inhibits many of these organisms.

Because these fungi are often environmental contaminants, it is usually necessary to obtain positive cultures on several different occasions before their presence can be regarded as significant.

Subcutaneous mycoses

Subcutaneous mycoses are rare and are largely confined to the tropics or subtropics. They include mycetoma, chromomycosis and sporotrichosis. Mycetoma (Madura foot) is caused either by species of actinomycetes or by fungi, many of which are pigmented. Perhaps the most important aspect of the laboratory recognition is the correct collection of samples. The organisms form into aggregates or grains within sinuses which discharge onto the skin surface. Grains can often be found by opening a sinus which is 'pointing' (pustular) with a sterile needle and the organisms are expelled with the pus and serous material. Grains are small particles up to 1 mm in diameter which may be white, black/brown or red. They should be washed in sterile saline before plating onto SDA.

The direct microscopy of mycetoma grains is useful. If they are gently crushed in 20% potassium hydroxide the filaments composing the grains can be distinguised. If they are greater than 2μm in diameter they are likely to be fungi. For practical purposes, actinomycete filaments in such preparations are not distinguishable under the $\times 40$ objective.

Systemic mycoses

The opportunistic mycoses include diseases such as systemic candidosis, aspergillosis and cryptococcosis. The interpretation of laboratory tests may be difficult, particularly where the organisms are normal commensals (e.g. *Candida albicans*). By contrast the systemic infections caused by pathogens such as *Histoplasma capsulatum* or *Coccidioides immitis* are more amenable to laboratory investigation.

Candidosis

Fungi of the genus *Candida* cause a variety of superficial as well as systemic infections. *Candida albicans*, the most common cause of the disease, is a normal commensal of the mouth, gastrointestinal tract and vagina. The superficial diseases include oral and vaginal candidosis (thrush), paronychia and some forms of intertrigo. Systemic infections vary in clinical presentation according to the site of infection and condition of the patient. For instance, they may be restricted to a single site such as urine or peritoneum (after secondary infection of peritoneal dialysis fluid) or be more widely disseminated through all body organs in a neutropenic patient. Specific forms of systemic candida infection may also occur following heart valve surgery (endocarditis) or prolonged intravenous catheterization in non-immunosuppressed patients. The usual pathogen is *Candida albicans*. However, *C. tropicalis* (in neutropenics), *C. parapsilosis* (in endocarditis) and other species may be found. *Torulopsis glabrata*, a related organism, may also cause septicaemia.

Direct microscopy

This is generally useful in superficial mycoses; yeasts, pseudohyphae and hyphae can be distinguished. Although invasion by candida is normally associated with hyphal formation, this may be absent, particularly if only a small amount of material is available for examination. Conversely, hyphal formation may occur *in vitro*, particularly if a specimen such as a sputum sample takes 6–12 hours in transit between patient and laboratory. Hence the presence or absence of hyphal formation may be an unreliable indicator of invasion if taken in isolation.

Cultural identification

Candida albicans grows readily on many media, including SDA and blood agar. Its growth may be suppressed by the presence of certain Gram-negative bacteria such as *Pseudomonas* species. In systemic infections, blood cultures are often negative. Whilst attempts have been made to improve the yield with a variety of techniques from arterial sampling to use of hypertonic media, the eventual isolation rate is seldom significantly raised. The failure probably reflects the comparative infrequency of candidaemia during the course of a systemic infection. The most useful approach is to use two consecutive blood culture samples 12–24 hours apart. Vented bottles containing biphasic media (e.g. SDA plus SD broth) are helpful.

The simplest identification method is the germ tube test (Mackenzie, 1962). Very small quantities of a colony are inoculated into 0.2 ml of mammalian serum (horse, human) in small plastic tubes. These are incubated for 3 hours at 37°C. At this stage a small loopful of serum is examined microscopicaly for the presence of small germ tubes originating from yeast cells. This phenomenon is seen with *C. albicans*, although some other species such as *C. tropicalis* may form germ tubes if the serum is left for 6 hours or longer.

Table 7.3 Assimilation reactions of yeasts

	Glucose	Maltose	Sucrose	Lactose	Cellibiose	Galactose
Candida albicans	+	+	+	+	+	+
C. tropicalis	+	+	+	−	+	+
C. pseudotropicalis	+	−	+	+	+	+
C. parapsilosis *	+	+	+	−	−	+
C. guilliermondii†	+	+	+	−	+	+
C. krusei	+	−	−	−	−	−
Torulopsis glabrata	+	−	−	−	−	+
Cryptococcus neoformans‡	+	+	+	−	±	+

*Does not form germ tubes.
†Assimilates ramnose.
‡Produces urease.

This test is sufficient for identification. However, in systemic infections it may be necessary to carry the process further if a non-*albicans* species of *Candida* is suspected. Sugar assimilation or fermentation tests using media containing 2–3 per cent sugar can be employed. For most practical purposes a commercial system (e.g. API Laboratory Products Ltd) is the most convenient (for technique, see manufacturer's enclosure). The assimilation patterns of common isolates are shown in Table 7.3. Finally, morphological identification is best carried out on cornmeal agar. A heavy inoculum of yeast is streaked across a plate containing the medium and a coverslip is placed over one end. The area is examined under low power after 24–48 hours' incubation at 25–28°C and small rounded chlamydospores are seen at the tips of hyphal branches. Chlamydospores seldom form at 37°C.

Serodiagnosis

The serological recognition of candida infections is potentially useful in systemic infections. However, the interpretation of results is difficult because exposure to the organism is widespread and hence most individuals have antibodies. Serological tests are most helpful in endocarditis or postsurgical infections when sequential samples can be analysed. Details of antigen preparation and serological methods are available in monographs such as that of Mackenzie *et al.* (1980).

An alternative is the detection of circulating candia antigen. Whilst most tests ranging from enzyme-linked immunosorbent assay (ELISA) to gas-liquid chromatography (GLC) are still research procedures, there is at least one commercial kit (from Immutech Ltd) based on the agglutination of antibody-coated latex particles.

Aspergillosis

Aspergillus species cause a variety of infections from pulmonary disease to otitis externa. Usually *Aspergillus fumigatus* is the cause but in infections of pulmonary cavities (aspergilloma) other species may be found. The

Table 7.4   Results of laboratory tests in different forms of aspergillosis

	Direct microscopy	Culture	Serology	Skin test
Allergic bronchopulmonary aspergillosis	±	+	Mod. +	+ +
Aspergilloma	±	+	Strong +	–
Invasive aspergillosis	+	+	Weak + or –	–

laboratory recognition of aspergillus infections relies on direct micros-copy, repeated isolation of the organisms and serology.

Identification of aspergilli

Most *Aspergillus* species grow rapidly on SDA and produce a downy mycelium with characteristic pigmentation and morphology. The iden-tification of the organism depends on the colonial morphology and pigmentation and production of conidial heads (Raper and Fennel, 1965). The most common organism, *A. fumigatus*, produces rapid cottony growth with grey-green pigmentation. Conidia (spores) are produced on a columnar-shaped spore head and are usually less than 4 μm long.

Serology can be accomplished using a commercial test system (e.g. Mercia Diagnostics Ltd) or with antigens used as for candidosis (see above).

The relative usefulness of different laboratory tests in forms of aspergi-llosis is shown in Table 7.4.

Cryptococcosis

Cryptococcus neoformans is an encapsulated yeast which invades via the respiratory route and causes disseminated disease, including meningitis. Cryptococcosis is seen particularly in patients with diseases associated with T-lymphocyte abnormalities such as lymphoma, AIDS, sarcoidosis, systemic lupus erythematosus and in patients on corticosteroids. The organism is associated in nature with pigeon droppings but is not a human commensal. Isolation of *C. neoformans* from clinical material should be regarded as significant. One of the most useful tests is the use of India ink to visualize the capsule of organisms in cerebrospinal fluid, and is recom-mended because the organisms are the same size as lymphocytes.

India ink preparation

A drop of material such as cerebrospinal fluid is mixed with an equal volume of India ink on a glass slide, covered with a coverslip and examined. The cell outline of *C. neoformans* can be seen but there is a clear halo of varying width around this where the capsule has repelled the opaque medium. Some macrophages can produce a similar phenomenon, so the slide should be carefully scanned for budding yeasts. Alternatively, nigrosin can be used as the stain.

Other diagnostic procedures

C. neoformans grows best at 30–31°C and may appear slowly on primary isolation. Colonies on SDA are white to yellow and may appear mucoid. India-ink-stained smears from the colony will show the capsule. *C. neoformans* produces urease and this forms the basis of a simple test. The yeast is grown on glucose peptone agar containing 10% by volume of a 20% aqueous solution of urea and phenol red indicator. The latter changes colour as the organism splits urea. Sugar assimilation can also be used for identification using the API system (see p. 164 and Table 7.3).

A slide agglutination test for the presence of capsular antigen in CSF or serum employing antibody-coated latex particles (from Immutech Ltd) is useful (Prevost and Newell, 1978). However, false positive and false negative reactions are seen and, unless tests are being performed regularly, it is best to send material to a reference centre.

Mucormycosis (systemic zygomycosis)

Systemic infections with zygomycete fungi can occur in neutropenic or severely ill diabetic patients. The infections are often characterized by tissue infarction. The fungi are readily isolated on SDA and produce characteristic round spore-bearing structures, sporangia. The colonies are rapidly growing and fill a plate with cottony mycelium covered by brown or dark dots – the sporangia. Fungi of the genera *Rhizopus, Absidia* and *Rhizomucor* are usually implicated.

Other systemic mycoses

Systemic infections caused by other pathogens such as *Histoplasma* or *Coccidioides* are normally confined to defined endemic areas unless they are imported in a patient who has visited such an area. Because they are infections of the respiratory route in healthy people, cultures are particularly hazardous to handle in the laboratory. If these organisms are suspected, isolation should be carried out using tubes not plates, and all manipulations should be performed in a safety cabinet.

Histoplasmosis

Histoplasma capsulatum is a respiratory pathogen which causes pulmonary or disseminated infection in endemic areas of the Americas, Africa and the Far East. The organism can be isolated from soil, particularly in the presence of bird or bat droppings. Most individuals inhaling the organism develop no signs of infection but can be shown to be sensitized by skin testing with histoplasmin. More rarely, acute or chronic pulmonary or more widely disseminated infections result. Generalized infection can be fatal.

H. capsulatum is a small dimorphic yeast 2–3 μm in diameter. It is difficult to recognize in clinical material with potassium hydroxide treatment. However, use of Giemsa stain may highlight organisms in host macrophages. The organism can be isolated from sputum or, in generalized infections, bone marrow. It grows on SDA or blood agar. Primary growth is slow and may take up to 6 weeks at 25–28°C. As stated previously the cultures should be handled in a safety cabinet. The isolates produce tuberculate (spiny) round macroconidia but, as these are also seen in some non-pathogenic fungi, it is necessary to convert the mycelial form into yeast phase. This can be done by inoculating brain–heart infusion agar and incubating slopes at 37°C. Phase transformation occurs over a 2-week period. Alternatively, suspect cultures can be inoculated intraperitoneally into mice which are then sacrificed 4–6 weeks later.

Serological tests (complement fixation, immunodiffusion) can be carried out in reference centres.

Coccidioidomycosis

Coccidioimycosis is respiratory infection which occurs in arid regions of the southern USA, Central and South America. It is caused by the organism *Coccidioides immitis*. Occasionally it is isolated from travellers who have visited an endemic area. As with histoplasmosis, exposure results in asymptomatic sensitization in most individuals but, rarely, disease may be caused. Primary symptomatic infections are associated with flu-like symptoms and, on occasions, erythema nodosum or erythema multiforme. Chronic cavitating pulmonary disease or infection disseminated to meninges, skin, bones or joints may occur.

C. immitis produces a characteristic *in vivo* phase, the spherule which is a large circular structure up to 100 μm in diameter filled with endospores. These can be seen in smears of pus or sputum treated with potassium hydroxide as well as in histological material. Cultures should be handled with extreme caution in a safety cabinet because the growth is a nondescript fluffy white to yellow mould producing large numbers of arthrospores. Tubes should be used in preference to plates. Identification of *C. immitis* is best accomplished by a reference centre, and tubes should be sealed, packed in screw-capped metal tubes within adequately sealed wood or cardboard containers. The suspected diagnosis should be carefully recorded on the information for the receiving laboratory.

Serological tests (complement fixation, immunodiffusion) can be carried out in reference centres, and are useful diagnostically and prognostically.

References

Clayton, Y.M. and Midgley, G. (1985) *Medical Mycology*, Gower Medical Publishing, London

Koneman, E.W. and Roberts, G.D. (1985) *Practical Laboratory Mycology*. Williams and Williams, Baltimore

Mackenzie, D.W.R. (1962) *Journal of Clinical Pathology* **15**, 563

Mackenzie, D.W.R., Philpot, C.M. and Proctor, A.G.J. (1980) *Basic serodiagnostic methods for diseases caused by fungi and actinomycetes*. PHLS Monograph series, 12. HM Stationery Office, London

Philpot, C.M. (1977) *Sabouraudia* **15**, 141

Prevost, E. and Newell, R. (1978) *Journal of Clinical Microbiology* **8**, 529

Raper, K.B. and Fennel, D.J. (1965) *The Genus* Aspergillus. Williams and Williams, Baltimore

Rebell, G. and Taplin, D. (1970) *The Dermatophytes: their recognition and identification*. University of Miami Press, Coral Gables, Florida

8

Diagnostic Parasitology

A.H. Moody

The increasing ease and speed of travel between countries of the temperate, tropical and subtropical zones in recent years has brought the possibility of encountering medically important parasitic infections into most district hospitals. *Giardia lamblia* is increasingly recognized as a cause of enteritis in Britain (Jephcott *et al.* (1986)). In addition, opportunistic infection by protozoa of immunodeficient patients means that diagnostic parasitology is no longer the preserve of the reference laboratory only, but an important function of hospital microbiology laboratories.

Although medical parasitology is essentially a subspecialty within microbiology, it utilizes many procedures and techniques which are commonly employed in other pathology disciplines and these are described, when appropriate, for specific parasitic diagnosis.

The parasitology laboratory

Special equipment needs within a microbiology department (see also Chapter 2) include:

Electric mixer
Coplin jars, to hold stains
Eyepiece micrometer and calibration slide
Microscope with high quality substage condenser
Brass wire sieve 100 mm diameter, 425 μm mesh (4 inch 40 mesh Endecotts Ltd, see Appendix). A nylon mesh coffee strainer can be used.

The laboratory should be well ventilated and preferably extracted to the outside of the building to prevent build-up of fumes from the use of ether and formalin solutions. Naked Bunsen burners should not be used in the vicinity. Access to a class 1 protective cabinet should be available.

Microscopic measurement

Micrometer measurement of protozoan cysts and helminth ova is an essential diagnostic criterion for parasitology.

Calibration of an eyepiece micrometer is accomplished using a pre-calibrated slide which has a length of 1 mm divided into one hundred divisions etched on it. Each slide division is equal to 10 μm and, by comparing the eyepiece micrometer to the slide markings, the number of eyepiece divisions equivalent to a specific number of slide divisions can be determined. From this can be calculated the micrometer value of each eyepiece division.

Example:

Slide micrometer = 1 mm = 100 divisions of 10 μm each
Using $\times$ 10
objective   10 eyepiece divisions = 10 slide divisions
     1 eyepiece division = 10 μm
Using $\times$ 40
objective   40 eyepiece divisions = 10 slide divisions
     1 eyepiece division = 2.5 μm

Examination for intestinal parasites

Collection and preservation of faecal samples

A wide-mouthed screw-capped jar is needed to collect 50–100 g samples. Helminth ova may continue to develop at room temperature but both ova and protozoan cysts can be satisfactorily recovered up to 24 hours after voiding. Beyond this time, and for postal specimens, several grams of faeces are emulsified in preservative. Either 10% formalin or polyvinyl alcohol (PVA) solution is suitable because they do not interfere with staining and concentration techniques. Unformed or liquid faeces or those containing blood and mucus may also contain viable trophozoites which will die within 1 hour of passage, in the cold, and be unrecognizable. Fresh mucosal scrapes from the rectum also need urgent attention. They must be collected on the premises and be delivered within 15 minutes to the laboratory. Trophozoites can be preserved by fixation in faecal smears.

The distribution of ova and cysts in a single motion is uneven. Random sampling of single specimens will retrieve less than 50 per cent of potential parasites in light infections. Increasing the sampling to three on consecutive days will increase the recovery potential by 75–100 per cent. As many as six samples may be necessary for some protozoal infections such as giardiasis. Selective sampling of unformed faeces, those containing blood, mucus and any segments or adult worm is helpful.

Preservation methods

1. *Formed faeces*: Emulsify 1 part faeces in 3 parts preservative.
2. *Unformed faeces* (or those with blood and mucus): fix faecal smears, while still moist, in Schaudinn's fluid for 30 minutes.
3. *Fresh mucosal scrapes*: Process as for unformed faeces.

Table 8.1 lists the trophozoite stages of parasites and their diagnostic stages of development commonly encountered in faeces.

Table 8.1   Diagnostic stages of parasites commonly encountered in faeces*

Helminths

Adult worms	Segments (proglottids)	Rhabditiform larvae
Ascaris lumbricoides *Enterobius vermicularis*	*Taenia saginata* *Taenia solium* *(Diphyllobothrium latum)* *Inermicapsifer* spp. *(Dipylidium)*	*Strongyloides* spp. (Hookworm)

Ova

Nematodes	Trematodes	Cestodes
Ascaris lumbricoides Hookworms *Trichuris trichiura*	*Schistosoma mansoni* *Fasciola hepatica* *(Clonorchis sinensis)*	*Taenia* spp. *Hymenolepis nana* *Hymenolepis diminuta*

See also Fig. 8.2.
It is not uncommon to see objects that can be confused with helminths in faeces; e.g.
1. Hairs – larvae have defined internal structure (mouth, oesophagus, gut)
2. Seeds/Pollens – ova are symmetrical, with regular size and shell, and they may be embryonated.

Protozoa

	Amoeba	Flagellates	Ciliates
Trophozoites	*Entamoeba histolytica* (haematophagus) *Entamoeba coli*	*Giardia lamblia* *Chilomastix mesnili* *Trichomonas hominis* *(Enteromonas hominis)*	*Balantidium coli*
Cysts	*Entamoeba histolytica* *Entamoeba coli* *Entamoeba hartmanni* *Iodamoeba bütschlii* *Endolimax nana*	*Giardia lamblia* *Chilomastix mesnili*	*Balantidium coli*
Oocysts	*Isospora belli* *Cryptosporidium*		

See also Fig. 8.1a–h.
Confusion in diagnosis usually relates to the failure to measure sizes of cysts accurately and to note internal contents (see Table 8.3.).

*Those given in parentheses are rarely seen in the UK.

Macroscopic and microscopic examination

Normal faecal consistency may vary, according to diet. Most obvious abnormalities are:

1. Pale, frothy, suggestive of excess fat, often seen in giardiasis and tropical sprue.

2. External mucus and blood, seen in amoebic dysentery, bacillary dysentery and inflammatory bowel disease.

3. Unformed or watery faeces containing fresh cellular exudate or erythrocytes. These often contain active protozoan trophozoites (Table 8.2)

Table 8.2 Diagnostic characteristics of trophozoites in faeces

	Size	Motility	Nuclear pattern	Flagella	Other features
Entamoeba histolytica	10–60 μm	Active, directional	As for cyst (Table 8.3)	–	Clear pseudopodia, ingested RBC
Entamoeba hartmanni	5–12 μm	Sluggish	As for cyst (Table 8.3)	–	Blunt pseudopodia, no ingested RBC
Entamoeba coli	20–40 μm	Sluggish, non-directional	As for cyst (Table 8.3)	–	Blunt pseudopodia, small pods, bacteria in endoplasm
Endolimax nana	5–10 μm	Sluggish	–	–	Small blunt pseudopodia
Iodamoeba bütschlii	10–40 μm	Sluggish	–	–	Small blunt pseudopodia
Dientamoeba fragilis (no cyst form)	9–15 μm	Amoeboid, blunt pseudopodia; sluggish	2 nuclei consisting of 3–8 granules only	–	–
Giardia lamblia	9–20 μm	Pear shape, irregular, jerky	2 nuclei	8	Large sucking disc near nuclei
Chilomastix mesnili	6–24 μm	Pear shape, stiff pointed tail, no rotation	–	4	–
Enteromonas hominis	4–10 μm	Oval, jerky rotation	–	1	Flattened side, long posterior flagellum
Retortamonas intestinalis	4–9 μm	Oval, jerky rotation	–	2	Prominent cytostome
Balantidium coli	50–200 μm	Revolving, rapid	–	Ciliated	Many vacuoles; May have RBC ingested, large cytostome
Trichomonas hominis	4–10 μm	Oval, jerky rotation	–	3	Prominent undulating membrane

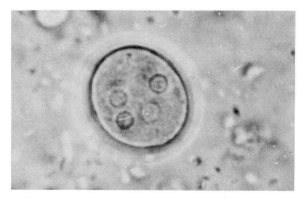

(a1)

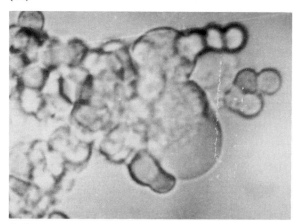

(a2)

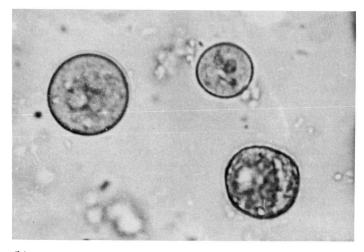

(b)

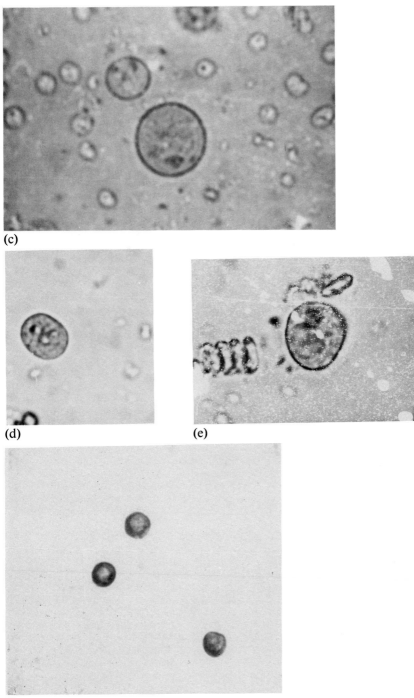

(c)

(d)   (e)

(f)

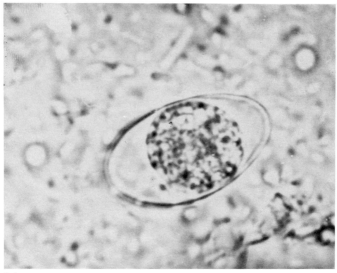

(g)

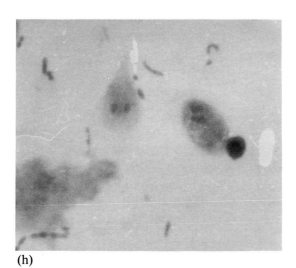

(h)

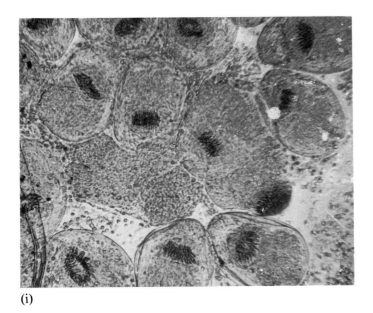

(i)

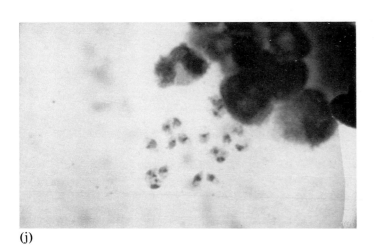

(j)

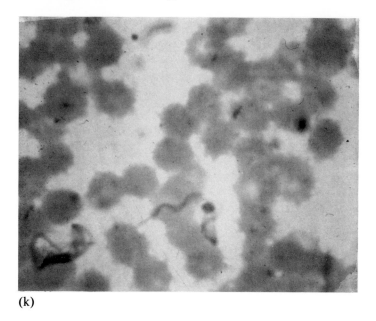

(k)

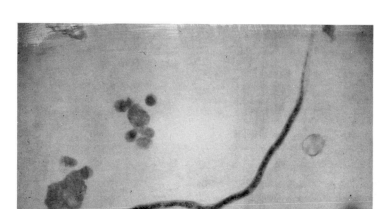

(l)

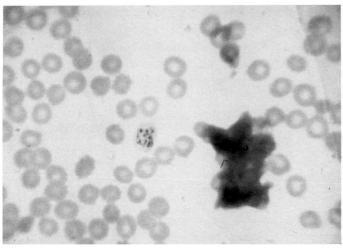

(m)

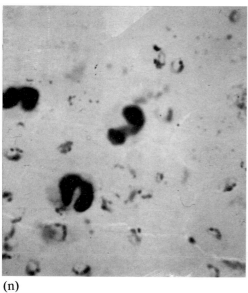

(n)

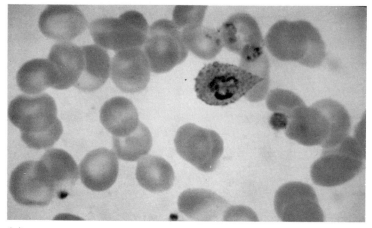

(o)

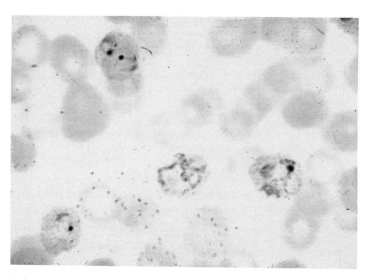

(p)

Fig. 8.1 (a) *Ent. histolytica* – (a1) cyst, (a2) trophozoite; (b) *Ent. coli* – *Ent. histolytica*; (c) *Ent. coli* – *Ent. hartmanni*; (d) *Endolimax nana*; (e) *Iodamoeba butschlii*; (f) oocyst of *Cryptosporidium*; (g) oocyst of *Isospora belli*; (h) *Giardia lamblia* – cyst, trophozoite; (i) protoscolices (hydatid); (j) *Leishmania* amastigotes; (k) trypomastigotes; (l) microfilaria of *Loa loa*; (m) *Pl. falciparum* – preschizont; (n) *Pl. falciparum* trophozoites (thick film); (o) *Pl. ovale* late trophozoite; (p) *Pl. vivax* developing trophozoites.

4. Small 'rice grain' egg sacs of *Inermicapsifer* species may be visible.

All stools showing any of these abnormalities must be examined by direct microscopy after suspension in warm (37°C) saline.

Direct microscopy
Samples for direct microscopy should be not more than 4 hours old (at room temperature) if the characteristic motility of trophozoites is to be seen.

Method
Emulsify 2–3 mg faeces, or selected exudate, in warm (37°C) saline. Using the × 40 objective, scan the suspension for motile trophozoites of ciliates, flagellates or haematophagous amoebae. Note particularly the cellular exudate, which helps to distinguish bacillary and amoebic dysentery from inflammatory bowel disease. Suspensions from amoebic dysentery have fewer pus cells and bacilli than those from bacillary dysentery; macrophages and erythrocytes will also be seen. Samples from inflammatory bowel disease usually contain very large numbers of pus cells and erythrocytes and many mucosal cells; no amoebae and few bacteria are seen. Other observations include fat globules, undigested food and Charcot–Leyden crystals. Ova and cysts may also be seen. Mixed infection is common and *the search must not cease* when one parasitic species is found.

Examine rectal scrapes similarly for the haematophagous trophozoites of *Entamoeba histolytica*. Urgent examination is required, as typical movement is inhibited by drying.

Table 8.2 lists the diagnostic characteristics of trophozoite stages of parasites commonly encountered in faeces.

Concentration techniques for ova and cysts

The Ridley–Allen modified formol–ether concentration method is suitable for detecting the range of ova, cysts and larvae likely to be encountered in a hospital laboratory. The procedure should be carried out in a safety cabinet, preferably with a spark-proof motor for the mixer.

Method

Reagents: 10% v/v formalin in distilled water
              Diethyl ether or ethyl acetate

Suspend approximately 1 g faeces in 10 ml formalin solution in a centrifuge tube. Mix well, using wooden applicators, and pass through a brass wire sieve or a nylon coffee strainer (600 μm pore). Wash the tube. Collect the filtrate into a beaker and transfer to a boiling tube. Add 3 ml ether, or ethyl acetate which is less flammable. Mix well, using an electric mixer, for 15 seconds. Transfer the solution to the original centrifuge tube and centrifuge at 100 **G** (3000 r.p.m.) for 1 minute. Use an applicator to loosen the surface plug of fat and debris, and invert over a discard jar within the cabinet. Use the remaining fluid to resuspend the deposit. Tranfer the deposit to a slide using a glass pipette or by inversion of the tube; open capillary tubes are not recommended. Cover the deposit with a 22 mm² coverslip which provides a suitable depth and distribution of ova, cysts and larvae present when the total area is scanned.

Concentration techniques using flotation methods may prove superior for concentration of specific parasite ova but none gives such adequate overall results.

Staining methods

Staining saline smears of faeces, exudate or deposits can provide useful information for diagnosis or species identification (Tables 8.2 and 8.3).

1. Fix thin saline preparations of faeces while still wet in freshly prepared Schaudinn's fluid. These can be stained by trichrome or iron haematoxylin to demonstrate the chromatin pattern of nuclei in amoebic trophozoites.

2. Allow thin saline preparations of faeces to dry in air. Fix them in methanol for 5 minutes. Stain them (see below) to demonstrate trophozoite stages of flagellates or ciliates, oocysts of cryptosporidia and cellular exudate.

3. Add stains to faecal concentrate suspensions to enhance diagnostic features of cysts (Table 8.3)

Specific staining reactions

1. Eosin 1% in saline at 37°C. This is useful as a negative background for active amoebic trophozoites, shows clear distinction between ecto- and endoplasm.

2. Iodine (equal volumes of Lugol's iodine and 25% acetic acid). When allowed to flow under the coverslip of a concentrated preparation of faeces it provides a graded concentration of dye. It stains glycogen brown and emphasizes nuclear chromatin in amoebic cysts.

3. Burrow's stain (see page 198). When added to faecal concentrations in equal volume it stains chromatoid bodies of *Entamoeba histolytica* cysts deep blue after 24 hours.

4. Modified Field's stain (Field stain A and B from BDH Ltd). Stain methanol-fixed smears by pipetting onto the slide 1 ml of stain B (diluted 1 part to 4 parts distilled water pH 6.8) followed by 1 ml of undiluted stain A. Mix well and leave for 1 minute. Wash with tap water, drain and leave until dry. This is a useful stain for flagellates and amoebic trophozoites.

5. Modified Ziehl-Neelsen stain for coccidia oocysts (*Cryptosporidum* and *Isospora*) species. (Auramine phenol method can be employed, page 146.) Stain methanol-fixed faecal smears with unheated carbol fuchsin for 15 minutes. Decolorize with 1% acid alcohol for 10–15 seconds and counter-stain with 0.4% malachite green.

For more detailed information on staining methods, see Cheesebrough (1981) and Garcia and Ash (1979). Referal to an atlas of human parasito-

Table 8.3 Diagnostic characteristics of cysts in faeces

	Usual size	No. of nuclei	Nuclear chromatin	Glycogen	Chromatoid bodies
Entamoeba histolytica	10–15 μm, round	Mature 4 Immature 1–2	Delicate peripheral chromatin; central karyosome.	Diffuse in young cyst	1–3 bars with blund round ends
Entamoeba hartmanni	6–9.5 μm, round	1–4	As for Ent. histolytica (EH)	As for EH	As for EH
Entamoeba coli	14–30 μm, round	1–8, can be 16	Course peripheral chromatin; large eccentric karyosome	Diffuse in young cyst	Infrequent splintered ends to rods
Endolimax nana	6–8 μm, oval	4	Pinpoint, refractile; no peripheral chromatin	Rarely seen	Small, oval; not diagnostic
Iodamoeba bütschlii	9–14 μm, Irregular	1 (eccentrically placed)	Large eccentric karyosome; no peripheral chromatin	Compact well-defined mass	Not diagnostic
Giardia lamblia	9–14 μm, oval/round	4	Not diagnostic	Refractile axostyle and fibrils	
Chilomastix mesnili	6–10 μm, lemon shape	1	Not diagnostic	Cytostome and fibrils	
Enteromonas hominis	6–8 μm, oval	1–4; staining needed	Not diagnostic		
Isospora belli	40–60 μm, oval, thin wall	Contains 1 or 2 oocysts, each with 4 sporozoites			
Cryptosporidium	4–5 μm, round	Contains 4 sporozoites			
Balantidium coli	50–60 μm, oval/round	1 macro and 1 micro			

logy (e.g. Ash and Orihel, 1984; Yamaguchi, 1981) is recommended; they
will include parasites rarely encountered in Britain.

Cultivation of faeces for parasites

Routine culture of faeces for *Strongyloides* should be made on all
clinically suggestive cases when microscopy is negative.

Charcoal culture method

1. Comminute 10 g faeces in tap water until it forms a thick suspension.
2. Mix in an equal volume of granulated hardwood charcoal.
3. Place a piece of No.1 Whatman filter paper into a Petri dish and
moisten with water.
4. Transfer the faecal/charcoal mixture onto the filter paper and add
water until it glistens. Seal the dish to prevent evaporation.
5. Keep the sealed dish in the dark at room temperature for 5–7 days.
Check daily and replenish with water, if necessary, to keep the culture
moist.
6. After 5 days pipette 2–3 ml water around the filter paper. The transformation of *Strongyloides* and hookworm larvae from rhabditiform to
infective filariform occurs and the larvae will migrate into the water.
Inspect for a further 2 days, using an inversion or dissecting microscope,
for active filariform larvae. If none is seen, formolize the culture and pass
it through a wire sieve. Concentrate the filtrate by the formol–ether
technique and the deposit may reveal scanty larvae.

Amoebae may be cultured using Robinson's medium. This method may
provide a higher yield of amoebae as trophozoites than microscopy alone
(Robinson, 1968).

Jejunal fluid

Sampling of jejunal mucus using the string test (Enterotest capsule,
Hedeco) provides increased sensitivity for the detection of *Giardia* trophozoites and *Strongyloides* larvae (see Fig. 8.2g).

The patient swallows a capsule containing a fine string long enough to
reach the jejunum; the end of it is taped to his face. He lies on his right side
for 4 hours to allow the capsule to reach the jejunum and dissolve. The
string is then removed and sent to the laboratory. On arrival, mucus from
the last 10 cm is squeezed into saline in a centrifuge tube. After centrifugation the deposit is searched for trophozoites of *Giardia lamblia* and
rhabditiform larvae of *Strongyloides* which may not have been seen in the
faecal concentration.

The Crosby capsule provides a small biopsy of jejunal mucosa which
can be dabbed onto a slide. This impression is air dried and fixed with
methanol before staining with modified Field's stain for *Giardia* trophozoites (Fig. 8.1h). Jejunal aspiration may contain ova from parasites in
the bile ducts.

Perianal swabs

Perianal swabs collected early in the morning provide a useful alternative to the National Institutes of Health (NIH) Sellotape method for ova of *Enterobius* (Fig. 8.2e) *Giardia* cysts (Fig. 8.1h) or *Taenia* ova (Fig. 8.2i). The swab is agitated in saline which is centrifuged to concentrate any ova or cysts which may be present.

Examination for invasive parasites

Cerebrospinal fluid (CSF)

Free-living amoebae are recognized as potential agents of severe or fatal disease in man. *Naegleria fowleri*, a free-living amoeba of warm water or thermally polluted areas, may cause fatal primary meningoencephalitis. *Acanthamoeba* species usually cause chronic disease, generally in immunosuppression but can also attack immunocompetent people, causing corneal ulcers or keratitis. Isolation is made on saline or nutrient agar spread with *Esch. coli* and incubated at 37°C.

Purulent CSF may contain *Naegleria* trophozoites in primary amoebic meningoencephalitis.

Tissue

Parasites
Rectal snips

The passage of *Schistosoma* ova through the rectal mucosa makes this a useful examination site for evidence of current or past infection by all species of schistosoma, particularly *S. mansoni* (Fig. 8.2n) and *S. japonicum*. Ova may be seen as complete eggs containing an active miracidium, as shown by flame cell activity. They can also be seen in varying degrees of degeneration or calcification, often surrounded by a granuloma. Four mucosal snips are collected from opposing sites 2 cm into the rectum, using a curettage blade.

Method

Squash the snips between two slides. Examine them under low power magnification, and when ova are seen use higher magnification to confirm flame cell activity.

Cysts

Larval cysts of *Echinococcus granulosus* (hydatid cyst) or *E. multilocularis* are found in various locations, particularly liver, lungs and bony sites. The inner layer of the cyst, being germinally active, produces brood capsules or daughter cysts full of protoscolices. These protoscolices and hooklets can be seen microscopically in material from ruptured or aspirated cysts (Fig. 8.1i). Leakage of cyst fluid gives rise to detectable antibody levels (see page 197).

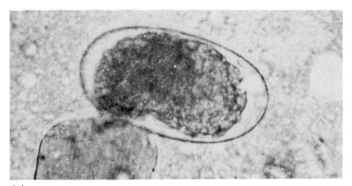

(a)

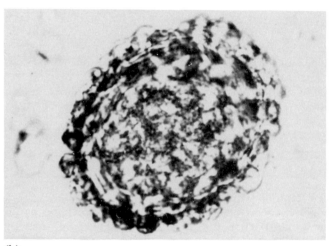

(b)

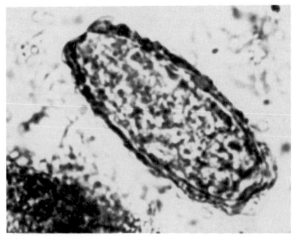

(c)

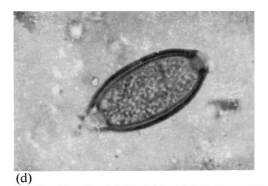

(d)

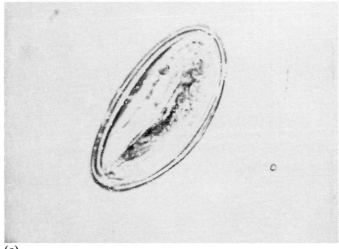

(e)

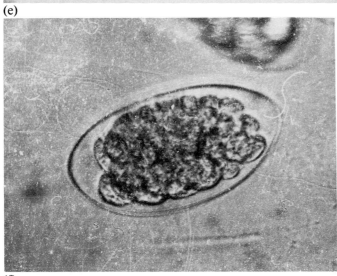

(f)

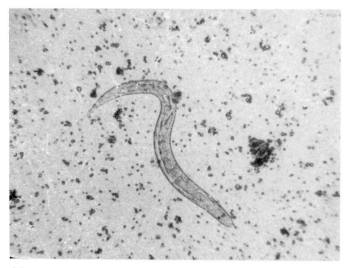

(g)

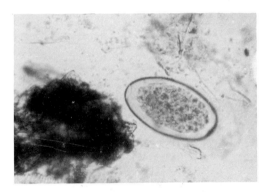

(h)

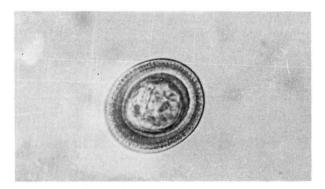

(i)

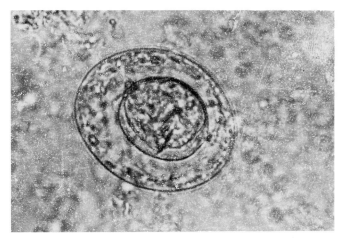

(j)

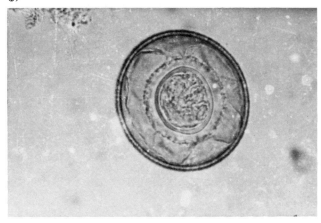

(k)

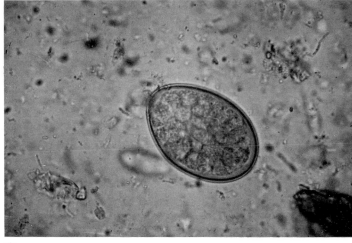

(l)

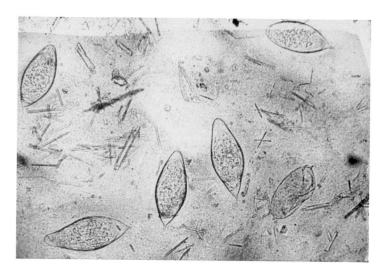

(m)

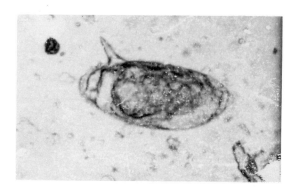

(n)

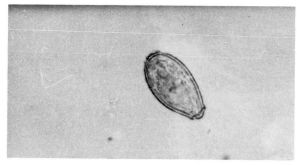

(o)

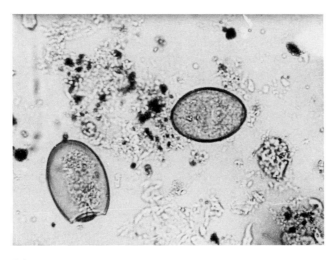

(p)

Fig. 8.2 Helminths: (a) hookworm; (b) fertile *Ascaris lumbricoides*; (c) unfertile *Ascaris*; (d) *Trichuris trichiura*; (e) *Enterobius vermicularis*; (f) *Trichostrongylus*; (g) larva of *Strongyloides* species; (h) *Fasciola hepatica*; (i) *Taenia* species; (j) *Hymenolepis nana*; (k) *Hymenolepis diminuta*; (l) *Diphyllobothrium latum*; (m) *Schistosoma haematobium*; (n) *Schistosoma mansoni*; (o) *Clonorchis sinensis*; (p) *Heterophyes heterophyes*.

Larval cysts of *Taenia solium* cause accidental human infections forming cysticerci in muscle and bone. Diagnosis is serological or histological.

Protozoan cysts in tissue are usually pseudocysts, not having a firm wall. *Toxoplasma gondii* and *Trypanosoma cruzi* both form tissue pseudocysts. These can be diagnosed histologically, but more readily by serology. Free 'zoites' may be seen in pus from brain abscess in disseminated toxoplasmosis of immunocompromised patients.

Sputum

Adult trematode flukes *Paragonimus westermani* growing in pairs in the lung produce rusty haemoptysis. Sputum or faeces may contain ova.

Pneumocystis carinii is an opportunist which causes pneumonia in immunosuppressed patients, including those with AIDS. Impression smears from lung biopsy or bronchial brushings can be stained with Giemsa, or Grocott's modified Gomori silver stain, to reveal collections of up to eight trophozoites in a circular cyst. A monoclonal antibody immunofluorescence test has been developed to detect antigen in bronchoalveolar lavage (Kovacs *et al.*, 1986).

Immunosuppressed patients can develop an overwhelming superinfection of the filariform larvae of *Strongyloides* which appear in large numbers in the sputum. Oocysts of *Cryptosporidium* may also be found.

Urine

Evidence of haematuria, by dipstick, is usual when ova are present. Collect terminal urine samples over 24 hours or take random mid-day samples and centrifuge at low speed (1500–2000 r.p.m.) for 2–3 minutes. Ova of *Schistosoma haematobium* (Fig. 8.2m) may be seen in the deposit. Filter large samples through a 12 μm Nuclepore or Millipore membrane. Examine as described for parasites in faeces. Viability of ova will be shown by activity of the flame cells within the miracidia.

Contaminants may include trophozoites of *Trichomonas vaginalis*, ova of *Enterobius vermicularis* and *Giardia lamblia* cysts.

Chyluria is caused by lymphatic filariasis, particularly by *Wuchereria bancrofti* (W. Pacific) and *Brugia* species. Microfilaria may be found in the urine.

Urogenital specimens

Trophozoites of *Trichomonas vaginalis*, with typical undulating membrane and jerky rotational movement, can be seen from swabs placed in saline or transport medium. Dry smears can be stained after methanol fixation using Giemsa or acridine orange fluorescence.

Blood and tissue

Filariasis

The filarial worms are important causes of disease and morbidity in man. All are arthropod-vector transmitted and the adults are viviparous. The first stage larvae, known as microfilaria, are present in blood or subcutaneous tissue. Differentiation between species of microfilariae is made by comparison of the following features: size, presence or absence of a sheath, nuclear size and extension into tail, location in blood or skin, and periodicity of appearance.

Microfilariae are found in the peripheral blood in *Loa loa* (mid-day periodicity) (Fig. 8.1l), *Wuchereria bancrofti*, *Brugia malayi* (midnight periodicity) and *Mansonella perstans* (non-periodic). Microfilariae of *Onchocerca volvulus*, *Mansonella ozzardi* and *Mansonella streptocerca* are found in skin tissue and are non-periodic. For details of morphological differentiation, see Ash and Orihel (1984) or Yamaguchi (1981).

Because of the periodic nature of microfilariae and the presence of several species in a common area, the standard practice for investigating filarial infections should include staining by several methods, as different species take up stain differently. Microfilariae do not survive well on prepared slides and are best examined locally whenever possible.

Methods
Blood
Collect 10 ml citrated blood between 10:00 and 14:00 hours (day blood) and between 22:00 and 02:00 hours (night blood).

Filter the blood through a 5μm pore Nuclepore polycarbonate

membrane (Sterilin Ltd) holding it in a Swinnex Millipore holder. (The blood is pushed through using a syringe, and blood cells are removed by following with 10 ml saline plus 2 ml air.) Transfer the membrane to a slide, add a drop of saline and cover with a coverslip. Motile microfilariae can then be seen.

When a filter is not available the blood can be lysed by adding 2 ml 1% saponin in saline. After 20 minutes, centrifuge and examine the deposit, which will also contain cell debris.

Skin snips
Collect 1 mg (approximately) skin snips from shoulders, buttocks and calves into saline in a flat-bottom microtitre tray, or directly onto slides for microscopy. Microfilariae will not emerge from the skin immediately and the snips should remain for at least 2 hours at room temperature before viewing.

Stains to show nuclei and sheath

1. Add 1% methylene blue in saline to the wet preparation of the filter.
2. For better differentiation and identification, wash microfilariae from the filter in a small volume of saline. Dry the suspension on a glass slide and fix in methyl alcohol for 5 minutes. Species from the Far East often stain better with Giemsa, but those from Africa usually need heated haematoxylin.

(a) Stain with 4% Giemsa in buffered water, pH 6.8, for 30 minutes. Differentiate in buffered water until nuclei are distinct.

(b) Stain with Delafield haematoxylin at 60°C for 20 minutes. Blue in tap water and differentiate with 0.5% acid alcohol until nuclei are distinct. Sheath and nuclei stain well.

Malaria (Table 8.4; Fig. 8.1m–p)
Diagnosis of malaria is made from peripheral blood, bone marrow aspiration and, occasionally, CSF. At birth, transplacental transfer may occur and parasites may be found in cord blood. Biopsy of various tissues may reveal schizogony stages or deposited haemozoin pigment.

Routinely, thick and thin blood films are prepared from venous or capillary blood. Blood taken at the height of fever will contain the greatest number of parasites. Thick blood films are used for concentration and are prepared by placing 3 or 4 small drops of blood onto the centre of a slide and spreading them evenly over an area of 1 cm². Correct thickness is apparent when bold print is just visible through the smear. This corresponds to 10–15 times concentration.

Staining methods
Thin blood films
Fix in absolute methyl alcohol for 1 minute. Stain with 10% Giemsa (BDH R66) in aqueous phosphate buffer, pH 7.2, for 15 minutes. Malaria chromatin and inclusion dots stain red, cytoplasm blue and pigment yellow/brown (Table 8.4 and Fig. 8.1m–p).

Table 8.4   Differential diagnosis of malaria

	Pl. falciparum	Pl. malariae	Pl. vivax	Pl. ovale
Size of parasitized RBC Variation in shape	Normal None	Small, deeper stained None	Enlarged (reticulocyte) None	Enlarged (reticulocyte) 20% of infected cells may be oval, all show *fimbriation* at periphery of RBC
Inclusions in RBC	Maurer's clefts in developing trophozoite state	Usually not apparent. Fine stippling of RBC may be seen (Ziemann's)	Schüffner dots in all stages. Stippling appears from young trophozoite	James dots. May appear later than *Pl. vivax*
Young trophozoites	Usually fine 'signet ring'. May show cytoplasm and chromatin irregularities	Thick ring, wide chromatin, pigment granules	Ring stage slightly larger than *Pl. falciparum*. Fine stippling. Pigment not obvious	Compact thick ring, no pigment. James dots may not be seen
Developing trophozoites	Cytoplasm vacuolated, chromatin enlarged. Maurer's clefts in RBC	Small cytoplasmic mass with single chromatin and several pigment clumps. May stretch across RBC as 'band' form	Trophozoites show active amoeboid forms, chromatin enlarges, Schüffner dots obvious. Pigment granules may appear	Compact cytoplasm, may show some amoeboid features. Little obvious pigment. James dots present
Pre-schizont	Seen in semi-immune or splenectomized patient and acute clinical. Single large pigment mass, divided chromatin	Small cytoplasmic mass with 2–3 chromatin parts. Pigment in 2–3 clumps	Large condensed cytoplasm, 2 or more chromatin divisions. Schüffner dots. Pigment as 1 or 2 clumps	Compact cytoplasm, divided chromatin, may have few pigment granules but not obvious. James dots
Mature schizont	20–40 merozoites, single pigment mass. Seen in deep capillaries	8–10 merozoites. Regular pattern. Heavy pigment masses	18–24 merozoites with 1 or 2 pigment clumps irregular pattern. Heavy Schüffner stippling	Compact, 8–12 merozoites. Small pigment clumps with irregular pattern. Heavy James stippling
Gametocyte	Seen in *Pl. falciparum* after 10 days. Crescent shape, can 'round up' in EDTA anticoagulant with exflagellation. Pigment and chromatin condensed in ♀, scattered in ♂	Round, occupies $\frac{2}{3}$ of the RBC. Scattered, obvious pigment. Single large chromatin mass	Round, occupies $\frac{2}{3}$ of the RBC. Scattered fine pigment, large chromatin mass	Round, occupies $\frac{1}{2}-\frac{3}{4}$ of the RBC. Scattered pigment, large chromatin mass

See also Fig. 8.1 m–p.

Thick blood films
Stain unfixed dry films by Field's stain A and B solutions (page 198) with a water rinse between the two; a 3-second immersion in each solution is adequate. Erythrocytes will lyse; all diagnostic features of the protozoa are unimpaired.

Plasmodium falciparum is often resistant to chloroquine and other drugs. Protozoal morphology can be affected by non-lethal therapeutic drugs and also by EDTA anticoagulant. The appearance of cytoplasm, chromatin and haemozoin pigment may be altered.

Assessment of the effect of treatment can be made using the parasitaemia evaluation method. Parasites are counted in at least 1000 erythrocytes and expressed as a percentage parasitaemia, which is followed daily until clearance.

Leishmaniasis

Kalar-azar (visceral leishmaniasis) is caused by *L. donovani/infantum*. *L. braziliensis* complex causes mucocutaneous leishmaniasis and the *L. mexicana* and *L. tropica* species cause cutaneous disease.

The amastigote stage seen in man is an intracellular parasite of macrophages in blood and tissue (Fig. 8.1j). The insect and cultivated forms are flagellated promastigote and epimastigote stages. In Giemsa-stained preparations the amastigotes are seen as oval bodies, 2–4 μm, with pale blue cytoplasm, red nucleus and a unique rod-shaped body called the kinetoplast. Diagnosis is made from slit-skin smears or biopsy impressions from cutaneous ulcers. Bone marrow or splenic aspirates and, rarely, liver impressions are examined from patients with visceral leishmaniasis.

Culture is essential for complete diagnosis, and zymodene or DNA probes are used for full identification. Culture media recommended for primary isolation are:

1. Rabbit blood agar slopes with an overlay of distilled water, or 1% glucose saline (sufficient to come halfway up the slope); nutrient diffuses into the fluid to allow growth (NNN medium).

2. Schneider's insect tissue culture medium (Gibco) supplemented with 30% fetal calf serum.

Incubate at 24°C in the dark for 36 hours. Inspect daily for the presence of promastigotes. Continue incubation for at least 10–14 days before reporting a negative result.

Trypanosomiasis

The *Trypanosoma* species pathogenic to man are *T. gambiense* and *T.rhodesiense*, which cause acute and chronic sleeping sickness in Africa, and *T. cruzi*, which causes Chagas' disease in Central and South America. Trypomastigote stages in blood are characterized by their shape, nuclear position, kinetoplast and flagellar appearance. African species are morphologically indistinguishable and have a clear undulating membrane and free flagellum (Fig. 8.1k). *T. cruzi* has no obvious undulating membrane, is curved in a C shape and has a large prominent kinetoplast.

Trypanosoma have a variable surface glycoprotein which they are capable of shedding at frequent intervals, inducing high levels of IgM antibody in blood or CSF. *T. cruzi* does not long remain as a trypomastigote before transforming to an amastigote stage and forming a pseudocyst in tissue, particularly myocardium.

Diagnosis of trypanosomiasis can be made by the examination of:

1. Peripheral blood films processed as described for malaria.
2. Buffy coat preparations where the protozoa may be concentrated.
3. DEA cellulose mini-ion exchange column.
4. Cerebrospinal fluid deposits.
5. Culture in NNN medium (see above, for *Leishmania*).
6. Serum for the presence of circulating antibodies (tests undergoing evaluation).

Toxoplasmosis

Isolation of *Toxoplasma gondii* is not practicable in hospital laboratories, and examination of lymph glands and other tissue is frequently non-specific. Therefore, specific serological tests are needed to confirm histological results. Differentiation between a recently acquired active infection and chronic infection, which is common and unlikely to be related to symptoms, is the problem.

Assay of specific IgM by ELISA using antibody class capture is the method of choice for acute, acquired toxoplasmosis. It is available in reference laboratories, where it has replaced the IgM immunofluorescence antibody test (Hall, 1984). A highly sensitive screening latex test which detects IgG antibody is also available for use in hospital laboratories. (Balfour *et al.*, 1982) (see also page 265).

Serological investigations

Limited availability of antigens makes serological investigation a reference laboratory procedure. For addresses of laboratories undertaking these tests see page 198. All requests should be accompanied by 2 ml serum and an account of the history and physical signs of the patient.

Four types of antibody tests can be employed: immunofluorescence (IFAT), counter-current immunoelectrophoresis (CIEP), cellulose acetate precipitation (CAP) and enzyme-linked immunosorbent assay (ELISA). A brief account of the available tests is given below, listed in alphabetical order.

1a. **Amoebae (Entamoeba histolytica) (IFAT, CIEP, CAP, ELISA).** Antibody is demonstrable in amoebiasis with abscess or amoeboma from about 10 days after infection. Antibody levels return to normal in about 6 months after successful treatment. Intestinal infection may give low or negative values. Serum from cyst passers is usually negative. Some non-amoebic liver diseases can cause false positive results.

CAP antigen is a soluble amoebic extract. The test acts as confirmation for the IFAT. Positive results indicate active infection and the titre rapidly returns to normal after successful treatment.

1b. **Free-living amoebae (IFAT)**. Positive serology to several cross-reacting species (*Naegleria, Acanthamoeba*) is obtained by IFAT.

2. **Cysticerosis (IFAT)**. Cystic larvae in the brain, eye or other tissue give positive results. Adult *Taenia saginata* give negative results.

3. **Fascioliasis (IFAT)**. Antibodies produced are species specific. Cryostat section of *Fasciola hepatica* is the usual source of antigen.

4. **Filariasis (ELISA, IFAT)**. All species of filaria and most infections with migrating *Strongyloides* larvae give rise to a cross-reacting antibody. A single test is therefore sufficient. A specific *Strongyloides* antigen will distinguish antibody caused by this species. Large numbers of microfilariae may absorb antibodies.

5. **Giardiasis (IFAT, ELISA)**. Positive serology reflects the degree of mucosal damage by *Giardia*. Negative serology is often found in mild or asymptomatic cyst passers. Detection of *Giardia* antigen in faeces can be achieved by ELISA (*Green et al.*, 1985).

6. **Hydatid disease (CIEP-specific IgM)**. Positive serology indicates that a cyst has released antigen. The CIEP is a good test for hydatidosis, as there is a highly specific precipitin line which very rarely occurs in other diseases. Serodiagnostic methods are unreliable as tests of cure. Tests, under trial, which are dependent on IgM titres only should be a better guide to disease activity.

7. **Leishmaniasis (ELISA, IFAT)**. Visceral leishmaniasis will produce high titres of antibody in early or high immune cases. Cutaneous forms may give only low or negative values. Some antigens may cross-react with autoimmune antibodies in the IFAT.

8. **Malaria (IFAT)**. For retrospective diagnosis only. There is some specificity between different strains. It is useful for differential diagnosis in tropical splenomegaly syndrome.

9. **Pneumocystis (IFAT)**. In immunodeficient patients, positive values may be seen soon after the onset of infection. A fourfold increase in titre strongly suggests pneumocystis. A negative result does not exclude infection.

10. **Schistosomiasis (ELISA, IFAT)**. Positive values can be expected from 6 weeks after exposure to cercariae. All species cross-react and titres remain high for up to 2 years following treatment.

11. **Strongyloides (filaria ELISA and specific test)**. Only 60–70 per cent react with filaria antigen. A specific *Strongyloides* antigen is more sensitive.

12. **Toxocariasis (ELISA)**. Positive after invasion by visceral larva migrans.

13. **Toxoplasmosis (ELISA, latex screening test)**. See page 265.

14. **Trichiniasis (IFAT)**. Positive from larval invasion. Very specific when *Trichinella spiralis* larvae are used.

Preservative solutions
Formalin: 10% formalin solution v/v is equivalent to 4% formaldehyde solution.

Polyvinylalcohol solution (PVA)
1. Glacial acetic acid   5.0 ml
   Glycerol   1.5 ml
   Schaudinn's solution   93.5 ml
   (2 parts saturated mercuric chloride + 1 part 95% ethyl alcohol)
2. Polyvinylalcohol powder 5.0 g
Heat solution 1 to 75°C before stirring in PVA powder.

Stains
Burrow's stain:
   Thionin   20 mg
   95% ethyl alcohol   3 ml
   Glacial acetic acid   3 ml
   Distilled water   94 ml

Field's stain (modified):
   Field stain A and B (BDH Chemicals Ltd)
Dilute stain B, 1 part to 4 parts distilled water at pH 6.8. Use stain A undiluted.

Addresses of reference laboratories

Department of Parasitology and Amoebiasis Unit
Hospital for Tropical Diseases
4 St Pancras Way
London   NW1 OPE

Department of Parasitology
Liverpool School of Tropical Medicine
Pembroke Place
Liverpool   L3 5QA

Other reference facilities for toxocariasis and toxoplasmosis can be obtained from the handbook of the Public Health Laboratory Service.

References

Ash, L. and Orihel, T.C. (1984) *Atlas of Human Parasitology*, 2nd edn. ASCP Press, Chicago

Balfour, A.H., Fleck, D.G., Hughes, H.P. and Sharp, D. (1982) *Journal of Clinical Pathology* **35**, 228

Cheesebrough, M. (1987) *Medical Laboratory Manual for Tropical Countries*, vol. 1., 2nd edn. Tropical Health Technology, Doddington, Cambs

Garcia, L.S. and Ash, L. (1979) *Diagnostic Parasitology – Clinical Laboratory Manual*, 2nd edn. C.V. Mosby, London

Green, E.L., Miles, M.A. and Warhurst, D.C. (1985) *Lancet* **ii**, 691

Halls, S.M. (1984) *British Medical Journal* **289**, 571

Jephcott, A. E., Begg, N.T. and Baker, I.A. (1986) *Lancet* **i**, 730

Kovacs, J.A., Gill, V., Swan, J.C *et al.* (1986) *Lancet* **ii**, 1

Robinson, G. (1968) *Transactions of the Royal Society of Tropical Medicine and Hygiene* **62**, 285

Yamaguchi, Y. (1981) *A Colour Atlas of Clinical Parasitology*. Wolfe Medical, London

9

Antimicrobial Drugs

The identification of pathogens from clinical material is only part of the task of the clinical microbiologist; the clinician will also require rapid and reliable guidance on antimicrobial chemotherapy. There are a large number of antimicrobial drugs currently available. Garrod *et al.* (1981) state that 'it seems unlikely that any totally new antibiotic remains to be discovered, since those of recent origin have similar properties to others already known'. Whilst it is salutary to reflect on these words, new anti-bacterial agents are continually being marketed, and many others are under development. In our view, the clinical microbiologist must take full responsibility for advising on treatment. He will need to familiarize himself with the effect on bacteria and the advantages and likely toxic effects of the newer agents. The trend in many hospitals is to provide a fixed formulary of drugs regularly stocked by the pharmacy. The clinical microbiologist should therefore be closely involved in the rationalization of the antimicrobial agent stock list. Rational antimicrobial treatment, particularly in hospital, is essential not only for the benefit of individual patients but also to ensure prolonged usefulness of the drugs. The field of antimicrobial chemotherapy is becoming increasingly complex as the nature of diseases caused by micro-organisms changes, especially where modern techniques of therapy result in compromise of the patient's immune system. The principles of antimicrobial chemotherapy are outside the scope of this book and the reader is referred to Kucers and Bennett (1979) and Garrod *et al.* (1981) for further information.

To meet clinical demands, rapid sensitivity tests are essential. However, it must be appreciated that the choice of drug is not solely dependent on the results. When a drug in concentrations higher than is likely to be achieved in body fluids fails in the laboratory to inhibit the growth of a micro-organism, it is unlikely to succeed clinically. The converse is not necessarily true. Many other factors need to be considered; for example, absorption, penetration, *in vivo* inactivation and the role of other bacteria. To these must be added the requirements of route of administration, underlying condition of the patient (e.g. renal or liver failure and immune status) and, on occasion, cost. These factors underline the need for the clinical microbiologist to liaise with his clinical colleagues so that reports related to antimicrobial chemotherapy are relevant to the whole patient, and not simply to the micro-organisms tested (see page 7).

Type of infection
There are three main types of infection that will be encountered.

Acute generalized infection
In general, any drug active against the pathogen in laboratory tests will be effective, provided that adequate doses are given. One exception to this generalization is the typhoid bacillus. This organism is sensitive to various antimicrobial agents in the laboratory (e.g. tetracycline) but clinical response to this and some other agents is unexpectedly poor.

Subacute infections with local lesions
In this situation (e.g. endocarditis) the lesions may be in a part of the body where penetration by antimicrobial agents is difficult to attain. Any drugs proving active against the pathogen in the laboratory will usually provide a short-term improvement in the patient's condition. However, to achieve lasting success, an antimicrobial agent which will penetrate the lesion and *kill* rather than simply inhibit growth of micro-organisms is required. Examples of such agents are the penicillins, particularly benzylpenicillin, and aminoglycosides such as gentamicin. Much has yet to be learned about the penetration of antimicrobial agents in different kinds of septic lesion, but it has been shown that the minimal concentration of penicillin and certain other drugs in tissue fluid from inflammatory lesions is higher than the corresponding blood level.

Chronic deep-seated infections (non-tuberculous)
Treatment with antibiotics alone will not as a rule cure these conditions, even when the microbes causing them are highly sensitive. They are useful in combination with other forms of treatment to prevent generalized spread of infection during surgical procedures, or for inserting into infected cavities after these have been opened and drained. For the latter purpose the pH of the fluid in the cavity is of importance in the choice of drug; for example, the aminoglycosides are relatively inactive in acid solutions and the tetracyclines are unstable in neutral and alkaline solutions.

All infections do not fit neatly into the above categories. Tuberculosis, for example, is usually a chronic deep-seated infection; however, it responds as an acute infection when treated with the correct antimicrobial agents. A parallel with typhoid may be drawn in that drugs such as the tetracyclines, which are active against *Myco. tuberculosis in vitro*, give a poor response clinically.

Site of infection
Meninges
Inflammation of the meninges increases their permeability to antimicrobial agents. Indeed, the appearance of streptomycin in the cerebrospinal fluid (CSF) following intramuscular therapy for miliary tuberculosis may be an early indicator of meningitis. Intrathecal therapy

for meningitis is dangerous and, nowadays, rarely indicated. Frequent lumbar puncture may lead to the introduction of other bacteria (including commensals) which will in themselves cause severe meningitis. Furthermore, the dose of antimicrobial agent needs careful measurement, and mistakes have resulted in severe damage or death from toxicity.

Chloramphenicol, sulphonamides, trimethoprim and modern antituberculous drugs penetrate readily into the subdural space. After the usual oral doses, levels of chloramphenicol in CSF are approximately 50–80 per cent of the blood level, even in the absence of meningeal inflammation. Although penetration by penicillin is relatively poor, in acute meningitis a high dose given frequently by intravenous injection will usually raise the level in the CSF sufficiently to kill the bacteria, thus obviating the need for intrathecal therapy. By testing the fluid against the organism isolated from it in the manner described for serum in endocarditis (see page 232), the adequacy of penetration can be checked. Furthermore, particularly in neonates, it may be necessary to measure drug levels in the CSF (e.g. chloramphenicol) to ensure (1) adequacy of penetration and (2) to avoid toxicity.

Urinary tract
Most antimicrobial agents are concentrated in the urine, sometimes more than a hundredfold. It is often possible, therefore, to treat uncomplicated urinary tract infections successfully when the pathogen is relatively resistant. For example, a low dose – 250 mg – amoxycillin 8-hourly by mouth is sufficient for the treatment of *Esch. coli* cystitis although the minimal inhibitory concentration required for the organism is about 8 mg/1 and much higher doses by injection will be needed for infection at other sites.

In patients with an indwelling catheter the presence of a foreign body (the catheter) in the bladder not only acts as a nidus for infection but also provides a route by which reinfection can readily occur. Many catheter-associated urinary tract infections fail to respond to antimicrobial therapy. Unless there are generalized symptoms, it is better to regard the presence of bacteria as colonization and to withhold treatment. When the catheter is removed and the urine fails to clear, treatment is indicated.

Superficial ulcers and wounds
The local application of antimicrobial agents, in addition to systemic therapy, will sometimes aid the cure of these infections when the organisms are relatively resistant. Such treatment should in general be avoided, and antiseptics or physical methods are to be preferred. The topical application of antimicrobial agents valuable for systemic therapy should particularly be avoided. The patient may become hypersensitive to the drug and will be deprived of its subsequent systemic use. Furthermore, this form of treatment, more than any other, selects bacterial resistance. In wards and departments where gentamicin ointment is often applied, *Staph. aureus* and *Ps. aeruginosa* highly resistant to it can be isolated not only from treated patients but also from their contacts amongst other patients and staff, and from the dust and air. In addition, some of the

strains will also be resistant to the newer aminoglycosides, and it is very difficult to prevent their spread throughout the hospital. Similar remarks apply to the use of topical fucidin for superficial *Staph. aureus* infections in hospital. On the rare occasions when such treatment is justified, the patient should be isolated.

Laboratory control of chemotherapy

The laboratory control of antimicrobial chemotherapy is always desirable and often essential if optimal use is to be made of the numerous agents now available. Purulent specimens from sites normally sterile are tested against appropriate antimicrobial agents on primary culture, a separate sensitivity plate being included (see below and page 213). Primary sensitivity testing of specimens from sites with normal flora are not performed, unless microscopy suggests infection by a single pathogen. Primary sensitivity tests from the throat, faeces or vagina are unlikely to yield useful information, and should be omitted.

A higher degree of therapeutic control may be required in certain infections: for example, bacterial endocarditis. In this condition the clinical microbiologist can provide further important data and should be prepared to respond to the demands which will be made upon him at short notice. In endocarditis, it is usually necessary to find a drug or combination of drugs which will be bactericidal to the infecting agent, not simply inhibitory. Thus, in addition to sensitivity tests, tests of bactericidal activity are required. Tests with the patient's own serum, after treatment has started, against the pathogen isolated, will indicate whether the antimicrobial agents are achieving a sufficient concentration in the serum to give almost complete killing of a moderately heavy inoculum (see page 233). It must be appreciated that the above tests are at best no more than a crude indication of what may be expected to occur *in vivo*. The results need to be interpreted in the light of other known facts, particularly other clinical indicators of the patient's progress. For example, there is little agreement on the timing of serum samples for determination of bactericidal dilution, nor of the result that correlates best (or even at all) with the outcome of therapy. The controversy has recently been reviewed by Weinstein *et al.* (1985) and Mellors *et al.* (1986).

The concentration of a drug in blood and urine after varying doses of different preparations is well known. Provided that there is no evidence of renal failure or impaired absorption, the concentrations in these fluids in an individual can be assumed to follow known pharmacokinetics. Should a pathogen prove to be sensitive *in vitro* to a drug which proves ineffective for treatment, assay of serum or serous fluid may be indicated to determine whether expected levels are in fact attained. Control of dosage is essential when toxic drugs are given to a patient in renal failure. Patients receiving therapy with aminoglycosides or vancomycin should have serum levels determined even when renal function is apparently unimpaired. Both groups of drug may result in ototoxicity, particularly following prolonged therapy, and the aminoglycoides may in addition cause renal damage. Absorption and metabolism of aminoglycosides varies markedly in individuals, and calculation of the dose in mg/kg occasionally leads to underdosing. For estimating potentially toxic levels, the amount of drug in the blood immediately before a dose is due is a more reliable guide than estimation of the peak level. The peak level will vary between individuals and with the route of administration. Useful supplementary evidence can be gained by determining the level of drug in serum 1 hour after intra-venous or intramuscular therapy, particularly with regard to adequacy of dose. However, it must be understood that this convention will not necessarily be a true peak level. Where there is difficulty in controlling drug levels in patients with renal failure, 'peak' and trough levels should be measured to give a more complete picture of drug metabolism.

When treatment is urgent, every effort should be made to obtain spe-cimens for culture before the first dose is given. If this be omitted the chance of making the diagnosis is greatly reduced and the clinician may be left with no alternative but blind antibiotic treatment which is undesirable for both therapeutic and financial reasons.

It is sometimes considered that routine sensitivity tests are unnecessary, as when the pathogen is known the drug of choice is clearly indicated. The number of organisms where this statement is reliable is diminishing. An overnight test may provide evidence of sensitivity before the pathogen has been fully identified. In practice, antimicrobial sensitivity is often a guide to identification. During recent years, *Str. pyogenes, Str. pneumoniae* and *Haemophilus influenzae* resistant to tetracycline have appeared and are no longer uncommon. Penicillin resistance of *Neisseria gonorrhoeae*, and of *H. influenzae* mediated by β-lactamase production, is now well established. Strains of *Str. pneumoniae* showing resistance to penicillin and chloramphenicol have been described. Strains of *Str. pyogenes* resistant to penicillin may yet appear. It is important that sensitivity tests are routinely performed on all pathogens to detect changes in sensitivity to common drugs.

The majority of microbes develop resistance to some drugs very quickly and when they are unable to develop resistance they are replaced by different strains, sometimes of the same species, which are resistant. Resistant organisms can be expected in all the normal bacterial reservoirs of the body within a day or two of the onset of treatment; this change of flora sometimes takes place within a few hours. Staphylococci, coliforms and streptococci, other than *Str. pneumoniae* and *Str. pyogenes*, are frequently resistant to penicillin, tetracycline and other drugs. The fre-quency with which these resistant strains are encountered· is related to the frequency with which the drugs are prescribed in the community sampled.

'Resistance' is not an exact term. Clinically, it implies that a drug used in normal doses cannot be expected to be effective. Resistance thus defined is extremely variable. For example, *Str. faecalis* is 'resistant' to penicillin, requiring a minimal inhibitory concentration (MIC) of 2 mg/1, whereas *Ps. aeruginosa* is 'sensitive' to ticarcillin and requires an MIC of 16 mg/1. Acquired resistance also varies widely. *N. gonorrhoeae*, normally sensitive to 0.06 mg/1 of penicillin, is said to be resistant when the MIC rises to 0.25 mg/1 because a single intramuscular dose used in the treatment of gonorrhoea is no longer effective, although larger and repeated doses often succeed. This kind of resistance is also seen in *Str. pneumoniae*. In contrast, resistance conferred by R factors, especially when caused by the ability to produce enzymes which inactivate antimicrobial agents is of a very much higher order. The MIC often exceeds 128 mg/1, and may be inoculum dependent under laboratory conditions. Tests performed under these circumstances must be interpreted with care. Rapid tests for β-lactamase production are now available and are useful for the early identification of organisms producing the enzyme (e.g. gonococci or *Haemophilus* species. Unless maintained by exposure to one or more of the antimicrobials to which the strain is resistant, transmissible resistance (due to R factors or plasmids) may be lost *in vivo*.

Antibiotic sensitivity tests

Numerous methods are available for testing the sensitivity of bacteria to antimicrobial agents. In the routine diagnostic laboratory there is a need to combine speed with qualitative accuracy. This can be achieved either using impregnated disc diffusion methods or by break-point determination. Disc diffusion methods are most commonly employed. Absorbent discs impregnated with a standardized amount of antimicrobial agent are placed on culture plates preseeded with the organism to be tested. After overnight incubation, the degree of sensitivity is judged from the size of the inhibition zone produced. For break-point determinations, standardized amounts of antimicrobial agent are incorporated into the medium. Organisms are inoculated, and the presence or absence of growth after incubation overnight is related to degree of sensitivity to be expected clinically. This method in theory approaches the ideal for sensitivity testing, but in practice has not yet gained wide acceptance owing to problems with standardization of conditions and concentrations of antimicrobial agent employed. It cannot at this stage be recommended for routine use, but may in the future become the method of choice.

When, to save time, a test is attempted on original material, a separate sensitivity culture is required because of the danger of altering morphology and making identification difficult. A disc diffusion test must be used in this circumstance, owing to the possibility of mixed cultures. Sensitivity tests require special test medium, and discs placed on the diagnostic plates may give misleading results.

Disc diffusion methods

There are a number of ways of performing these tests, three of which have been accepted as sufficiently reliable to give comparable results when performed in different laboratories. They are: the method developed as a result of the International Collaborative Study (ICS) sponsored by WHO, now practised mainly in Sweden (Ericsson and Sherris, 1971); the Kirby–Bauer method adopted officially in the USA (Bauer *et al.*, 1966);

and the comparative method practised in Britain and other countries (Stokes and Waterworth, 1972). The American and Swedish methods depend for interpretation on comparing measured zones with a scale prepared from regression lines relating zone size to minimum inhibitory concentration (MIC). It is therefore mandatory that tests are performed under standard conditions employing a specified medium. Controls are included to check that the medium is working as expected but they are not an essential part of interpretation. In contrast, the comparative method depends on comparison between zones seen with the test organism and those of a known sensitive control cultured in parallel; any sensitivity test medium can be employed.

These three methods have been compared in a single specialist laboratory (Brown and Kothari, 1978a) and in the field (Brown and Kothari, 1978b). None of the methods agreed with an MIC estimation performed in parallel on every occasion and in none of them were zones always reproducible in repeated tests. There were only 7.7 per cent important disagreements between the methods in the field tests of strains selected to show up discrepancies. Each method performed better than the others in some tests. Reproducibility of zone measurements was better with Kirby–Bauer than with other methods but there were no significant differences in interpretation between the methods.

Optimum inoculum in the ICS and comparative methods is 'not quite confluent growth'. The ICS and Kirby–Bauer methods of standardizing inoculum are laborious and must be rigidly followed, particularly in the Kirby-Bauer method, because it is impossible to judge subsequently whether correct standardization has been achieved; the inoculum, although fairly light, is confluent and too heavy inoculum, which will profoundly affect the result, cannot be recognized. We think this is a serious disadvantage for diagnostic laboratories (where pressure of work may sometimes lead to poor standardization) and outweighs the better reproducibility of zones when the method is performed correctly. This method is also extravagant because specially large Petri dishes have to be used to prevent overlapping zones from the comparatively high content discs.

The greater flexibility of the comparative test is an important advantage. In the trials this method was carried out on any of four different sensitivity test media. There are no criteria for interpretation of sulphonamide and fusidic acid zones by the ICS and Kirby–Bauer methods, and when a new drug needs special medium for reliable tests (e.g. trimethoprim) problems of interpretation immediately arise. The greater need for reliable controls is a potential disadvantage of the comparative method but is overcome by using swabs impregnated with a suitable dilution of the control culture (page 212). They can be prepared by a skilled member of the staff and are used to inoculate plates instead of liquid cultures, which can easily be contaminated by the inexperienced. We prefer the modification of the comparative method, first published in an early edition of this book, where the control culture is inoculated on each plate. Although this means that a zone radius rather than a diameter must be measured and the test is slightly more laborious to set up, it ensures that the control is always available for comparison, and when zones are equivalent with the control no measurement is required. This modification was tested in the trials quoted above. Anyone having to prepare discs locally would be well advised to use it because substandard discs will be easily recognized, each being tested simultaneously against test organism and control.

In conclusion, since no disc diffusion method is always accurate (tests of MIC being needed when great accuracy is required), one which is flexible, easy to perform and gives comparable results with other methods is preferred and we therefore recommend the comparative method described in detail below.

Primary tests

There are three good reasons for testing sensitivity on first isolation, instead of after subculture. First, the need for speed is met in many cases; second, the microbes tested are as fair a sample as possible of those at the site of sampling. Two strains of the same species may infect a single wound, one sensitive, the other resistant. If tests are made after subculture only the sensitive one may be found and this may be followed by an unexplained failure of antibiotic treatment. The third reason is that in a mixed culture, although the sensitivity test may have to be repeated, an unexpected important pathogen present in small numbers may be recognized by selection; for example, *Str. pyogenes* seen within a gentamicin zone or *Ps. aeruginosa* seen within an ampicillin zone.

The following objections have been raised against testing sensitivity in primary culture.

1. The inoculum cannot be standardized.
2. Results are difficult to interpret, particularly in mixed cultures.
3. Tests have to be repeated so often that a primary test is extravagant.

Answers to these objections are as follows.

Inoculum

Standardization of inoculum is of prime importance for reliability in all disc diffusion tests and it would seem that the first objection rules out primary tests. However, the optimum inoculum for the comparative test used in Britain and for the International Collaborative Study (ICS) methods is 'not quite confluent growth' which is easily recognized, making the need for a repeat test obvious. In practice, not quite confluent growth is seen in a high proportion of cultures from purulent lesions, particularly when *Staph. aureus* is present. The reliability of primary tests on urines performed in this way has been confirmed by comparing results with those done on the strains in pure culture tested in the same manner by the Kirby–Bauer and ICS methods (Waterworth and Del Piano, 1976). The inability to recognize too heavy inoculum in the Kirby–Bauer test (because the standard inoculum, although fairly light, is confluent) makes this method unsuitable for a primary test.

Mixed cultures

Provided the primary cultures are pure or only very lightly contaminated, interpretation presents no difficulty. When pus, thought to be staphylococcal, yields a mixed growth all organisms may prove to be sensitive to one or more of the drugs tested which is valuable information available to the clinician after overnight incubation. On the primary plate a penicillin sensitive organism such as *Str. pyogenes* may appear resistant to penicillin when accompanied by a penicillinase producer which enables it to grow near the disc (see Fig. 9.4). This is of clinical importance because the presence of the β-lactamase producer may lead to failure of therapy if an enzyme-sensitive penicillin is used alone. When tests cannot be interpreted (due to overgrowth by a resistant organism, too heavy or too light inoculum) they must be repeated, but only one culture plate will have been lost and some valuable information will have been gained from most of these cultures.

Extravagance

Primary tests on all specimens would indeed be most uneconomical, both in time and in materials. Such tests are indicated regularly only in acute pyogenic conditions, when the need for speed is balanced against the likelihood of a single pathogen or predominating pathogen being present. Attempts to select urine specimens for primary sensitivity testing are unreliable. Little is lost by not performing them routinely, as sensitivity test results are often predictable and treatment will, in many cases, have commenced before results are known.

Definition of sensitivity and resistance

When sensitivity tests are carried out by a diffusion method it is not possible to give precise figures for the sensitivity of a given organism to a given antibiotic, but bacteria can be divided info three groups: sensitive, intermediate and resistant.

Sensitive: strains amenable to treatment in ordinary dosage.

Intermediate: strains amenable to treatment when large doses are used or when the drug is concentrated at the site of infection – e.g. in the urinary tract or by local application; combination with another agent may be synergistic.

Resistant: strains unaffected by high concentration and therefore unlikely to respond to any dosage of the antibiotic.

For clinical purposes the term 'sensitive' must be related not only to the MIC for the organism but also to the concentration of antibiotic obtainable *in vivo*. In most acute infections it can be assumed that if the average blood level exceeds the MIC by a safety factor of 2 or 4 the infection will respond to treatment.

In the comparative method to be described, grading is achieved by testing in parallel unknown organisms with a sensitive control and comparing their inhibition zones.

Comparative disc method

Antibiotic-impregnated discs can be obtained commercially, and have superseded home-made discs. Those from reputable firms are subject to stringent quality control, and will give reliable and repeatable results in the comparative method. The choice of disc content is critical, even with a properly controlled method. The zone size must allow decreased sensitivity to be easily detected, without producing a false indication of sensitivity or resistance. If the content is too high, there will be little change of zone over a wide range of difference in MIC. Unless strains are highly resistant they will appear sensitive, despite the actual MIC being above the clinically relevant level. When the content is too low, the zone will be small and a slightly heavy inoculum will make the organism appear resistant. Indiscriminate use of high or very low content discs can give grossly misleading results. Table 9.1 indicates suitable contents for the comparative disc method. Two strengths are recommended for some drugs because

Table 9.1　Suitable disc contents (μg)

Antibiotic	Organisms from sites other than urine	Organisms from urine
Amikacin	10	10
Ampicillin/amoxycillin	10*	25
Azlocillin	75	75
Cefotaxime	30	30
Ceftazidime	30	30
Cefuroxime	30	30
Cephaloridine	5	30
Chloramphenicol	10	–
Clindamycin	2	–
Erythromycin	10	–
Fusidic acid	10	–
Gentamicin	10	10
Kanamycin/Neomycin	30	30
Methicillin	5†	5
Metronidazole	5	–
Mezlocillin	75	75
Nalidixic acid	–	30
Netilmicin	10	10
Nitrofurantoin	–	50
Penicillin	2‡§	2
Piperacillin	75	75
Polymyxin B	300‡	300
Spectinomycin	10	–
Sulphafurazole	100	100
Tetracycline	10	30
Ticarcillin	75	75
Tobramycin	10	10
Trimethoprim	1.25	5
Vancomycin	30	30

*For *Haemophilus* spp. 2 μg.
†Strip containing 25 μg also available.
‡Units.
§0.03, 0.25 and 1 unit for *N. gonorrhoeae*; 0.25 unit for *Str. pneumoniae*.

their high concentration in urine makes treatment of urinary infection possible when the organism in any other site would be regarded as of intermediate sensitivity or even resistant.

Because sensitivity in the report indicates a drug suitable for treatment in particular circumstances it is possible to report *Esch. coli* isolated from blood as of intermediate sensitivity to, say, ampicillin when the same strain isolated from the patient's urine will be reported sensitive. This seems illogical but it is inevitable if the report is to be both rapid and reliable in indicating appropriate treatment. It happens only with penicillins and cephalosporins which are concentrated in the urine and are sufficiently harmless to be given in exceptionally large doses when the need arises; the term 'intermediate' reminds the clinician that a high dose will be needed.

Discs may be stored at 4°C, observing the manufacturer's expiry date. When removed from the refrigerator for use, the vials should be kept unopened for sufficient time to avoid condensation. Metronidazole is light sensitive, and discs must be kept in a dark bottle (Jones and Scott, 1977). Discs can be applied using a needle or forceps, and each must be pressed into position; even diffusion will occur only when the disc is in complete contact with the medium. The discs must be sufficiently widely spaced (2 cm) to prevent overlapping of the zones. Dispensers are now available (Oxoid Ltd) which provide a convenient means of storing discs in cartridges, and ensuring even and rapid delivery onto the medium (see page 216). Paper strips instead of discs are also available (see page 217).

Medium

Many drugs are affected by various constituents of laboratory media. The most important examples are sulphonamides and trimethoprim, which act by inhibiting folate metabolism. If the medium used for these tests contains end products of folate metabolism (e.g. thymidine), sensitive organisms will be able to bypass the actions of these drugs. On such media inhibition zones are not simply reduced in size, but also colonies, often much smaller than normal, will grow right up to the disc. Media containing small amounts of such substances can be rendered suitable for use by the addition of lysed horse blood.

Other ingredients which may affect some antibiotics are salt, which may reduce the activity of some (e.g. aminoglycosides) and enhance that of others (e.g. fusidic acid); carbohydrates, which may enhance the action of nitrofurantoin and ampicillin in some diffusion tests; and some minerals such as calcium, magnesium and iron (e.g. tetracycline and gentamicin). Many ingredients such as peptone, yeast extract, tryptone and the agar used for solidifying the medium vary in their mineral content, not only between different manufacturers but also even between different batches from the same source (Bovallius and Zacharias, 1971). For further information about the need for uniformity in sensitivity test media, see Waterworth (1978).

The results of sensitivity tests are both more reliable and easier to interpret if a specially defined medium is used. For the Kirby–Bauer method, Mueller–Hinton agar is essential; however, for the comparative method there are several choices of media. Oxoid Diagnostic Sensitivity Agar (to which 5% lysed horse blood must be added for tests with sulphonamides and trimethoprim) and Oxoid Iso-sensitest Agar (which is free of sulphonamide inhibitors) are suitable for most purposes. For testing sensitivity to *Haemophilus influenzae*, plates are 'choco-lated', or Mueller–Hinton agar plus 5% lysed horse blood is used. Wilkins–Chalgren agar plus 5% lysed horse blood is suitable for fastidious anaerobes.

The medium should be poured into flat-bottomed dishes on a flat horizontal surface, to a depth of 3–4 mm (20 ml in an 8.5 cm Petri dish). An increase in depth of 1 mm will not significantly affect the results but very thin plates are unsatisfactory.

The antibiotics most affected by pH are tetracyclines, which give large zones on acid medium, and the aminoglycosides, which are most active in alkaline medium. Many other drugs are affected to some extent; for example, the cephalosporins, the macrolides (erythromycin group) and lincomycin are favoured by alkalinity whereas methicillin, cloxacillin and fusidic acid perform better in acid medium. Conditions for sensitivity tests should resemble as nearly as possible conditions in the patient's tissues. The buffering action of blood is beneficial in nullifying the effect of minor changes. The pH of sensitivity test media containing no blood must be carefully adjusted and conditions such as incubation with added CO_2 which may alter pH should be borne in mind.

Inoculum

All zones of inhibition are affected by the size of the inoculum, and whenever pure cultures are tested adjustment of the inoculum is essential. When this is too heavy, zones are always reduced in size and the edges become indistinct, but with sulphonamides the zone will completely disappear even though the organism may be fully sensitive. The inoculum which gives the most consistent results is that which gives dense but not confluent growth (once growth is confluent it is impossible to judge how heavy it is); it is essential that it is evenly distributed over the whole area. Small variations in the weight of growth are unlikely to invalidate the results but the use of uncontrolled and inadequately spread inocula is one of the main sources of error in these tests. For the preparation of inoculum, see page 216.

Choice of drugs to test

Suggestions for suitable drugs to be tested against various bacteria and specimens are given in Table 9.2. The number of tests can be reduced by including as a routine only one representative of closely related drugs amongst which cross-resistance always occurs. Only one tetracycline need be tested; methicillin should represent all penicillinase-resistant penicillins and cephalosporins against staphylococci (see page 219); kanamycin will serve for neomycin, clindamycin for lincomycin, cephaloridine for first-generation cephalosporins (but see page 219), and either polymyxin or

Table 9.2 A suggested choice of drugs for sensitivity test

	Primary culture		Secondary tests on subcultures				
	Pus	Urine	Staphylo-cocci	Strepto-cocci	Haemo-philus	Coliforms	Pseudo-monas
Penicillin	+		+	+			
Methicillin*	+		+				
Ampicillin		+			+	+	
Ticarcillin							+
Azlocillin							+
Cephaloridine		+				+	
Cefuroxime	+	+				+	
Ceftazidime							+
Erythromycin	+		+	+	+		
Fusidic acid			+				
Tetracycline	+		+	+	+	+	
Chloramphenicol			(+)†	(+)†	+		
Kanamycin/ neomycin			(+)‡				
Gentamicin	+	+	+			+	+
Polymyxin B						(+)‡	+
Trimethoprim	+	+			+	+	
Sulphonamide	+	+			+	+	
Nalidixic acid§		+				+	
Nitrofurantoin§		+				+	

() = not recommended for all specimens.
*See page 219 concerning this drug.
†Ocular/aural use.
‡Topical/aural use.
§Applicable to urinary isolates only.

colistin will serve for both. Only one sulphonamide need be tested and sulphafurazole is satisfactory; some confusion arises because *Ps. aeruginosa* may appear resistant to this but sensitive to Sulphatriad used on some discs; this is due to the greater activity of sulphadiazine (included in Sulphatriad) against this species, but this is not thought to be clinically significant. New variants of well established drugs are constantly being produced. However, a difference between members of the same class in an *in vitro* test is not necessarily reflected in its *in vivo* performance. Pharmacological factors such as penetration to the site of infection or reduced toxicity are more important than small differences in bacterial sensitivity.

Tests with hexamine mandelate (Mandelamine) are both unnecessary and misleading. This drug acts because formalin is released in acid urine; all organisms are sensitive to formalin but if they split urea (e.g. *Proteus* spp.) they render the urine too alkaline for it to be liberated.

Maintenance and choice of control cultures

Control cultures are essential and should always be included with any method. In general, difference in species between the control and test strains does not matter provided both grow at approximately the same rate; an exception is *Ps. aeruginosa* (see page 220).

Control organisms should be maintained on agar slopes kept in the dark at room temperature. A broth culture is made at the beginning of each week and further subcultures in broth daily from this. The agar slopes are subcultured monthly. No attempt should be made to purify a contaminated control culture by picking a single colony because of the risk of variation. When the slope is contaminated the control should be revived from a lyophilized preparation.

When plates are to be inoculated with swabs, a more convenient method of maintaining controls, less liable to contamination, is to impregnate sterile 7.5 cm swabs in bulk and store these in screw-capped glass or plastic jars (Felmingham and Stokes, 1972). About 20 drops of overnight broth culture in 20 ml broth, well mixed, will impregnate and be quickly absorbed by about 90 Q-tip swabs (obtainable from EL KAY Laboratories) and will give a suitable inoculum when one swab is used per plate. They can be stored for up to 1 week at 4°C. *Ps. aeruginosa* will continue to grow at 4°C, and should be used within 5 days.

The control must be an organism known to respond to treatment with normal doses of the drug, and the choice depends on the site of the infection and the concentration of drug attainable there. Drugs which are excreted by the kidneys produce high concentrations in the urine and more resistant organisms are likely to respond to treatment. In these circumstances a high content disc and a more resistant control organism can be used. It must be remembered, however, that when coliforms or enterococci are isolated from specimens other than urine, they must be compared with the fully sensitive control. This is particularly important with ampicillin and the cephalosporins because, although urinary infections with these organisms respond well to low doses, coliforms and enterococci are really only moderately sensitive to these drugs and the report must make it clear that higher dosage will be required for infections in other parts of the body (see page 209). For most practical purposes, the Oxford staphylococcus (NCTC 6571) can be used as the sensitive control for all drugs except polymyxins and metronidazole. *Esch. coli* (NCTC 10418) should be used for all tests with polymyxins and for all drugs with organisms from the urine. An anerobic control is essential for tests of metronidazole sensitivity because no aerobes are sensitive. Control of diffusion tests for anaerobes is more difficult than for aerobes because the rate of growth of anaerobic species is more variable. Two controls have been widely used in Britain. *Cl. perfringens* (NCTC 11229) is sensitive to penicillin and has a growth rate comparable with the Oxford staphylococcus. For control of tests on non-sporing anaerobes, *Bact. fragilis* (NCTC 9343), which grows more slowly, has been employed, but it is penicillin resistant and cannot be used for tests with this drug. Both species are resistant to aminoglycosides but this does not greatly matter since almost all anaerobes are resistant and these agents are not used for infections caused by them. When testing metronidazole sensitivity, culture of the control on each plate is desirable because a poor degree of anaerobiosis in a slightly leaking jar alters the size of inhibition zones and may make sensitive anaerobes appear resistant; the control will then also appear resistant and the error will be discovered (Milne *et al.*, 1978). Swabs are prepared as described above by impregnating them with a tenfold dilution in broth of a well mixed cooked meat broth culture not more than a week old (in a screw-capped bottle with well fitting cap). This is kept in the dark on the bench at room temperature (20–26°C). Each swab is placed in transport medium before refrigeration (see also page 309).

Methods for primary tests

A separate plate for sensitivity tests is set up when the cultures for identification have been made, before the swab is placed in cooked-meat broth or on any antibiotic-containing medium. Blood agar must be employed for primary tests since the organism isolated may be fastidious, and the blood should be added to medium specially prepared for sensitivity tests (see above). This is essential for sulphonamide and trimethoprim tests and important for other tests also. The disc content recommended is related to the medium employed and may be inappropriate for other media. For example, tetracycline discs will show smaller zones and false resistance may be reported if the blood agar base recommended here for diagnostic cultures is also employed for sensitivity tests.

The swab, loopful of pus or loopful of *uncentrifuged* urine is seeded heavily and evenly in a band across the middle third of the plate, in the manner described below (see 'Urine'). The control is applied on either side of the test organism, either by inoculating one small loopful of overnight broth culture and spreading with a dry sterile swab or by using one pre-impregnated swab per plate (Figs. 9.1 and 9.2). Using flamed forceps or a needle, up to four antibiotic-impregnated discs are placed on the gap between the inoculated areas. Discs should be lightly pressed onto the agar, ensuring that they touch the edge of the central inoculated area and are about 1 cm from the edge of the plate.

The control and test material must be inoculated within about 15 minutes. A delay of not more than 2 hours may be allowed before the discs are applied when this is more convenient.

When tests need repeating because, for example, the primary growth of

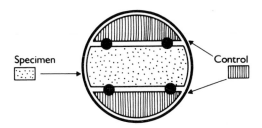

Specimen   Control

Fig. 9.1 Primary sensitivity test.

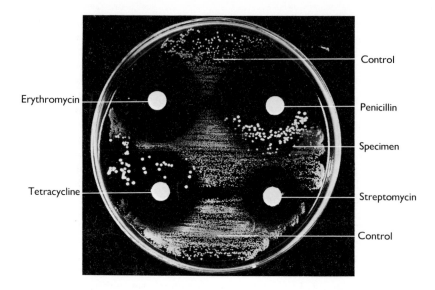

Fig. 9.2 Sensitive control (Oxford staphylococcus) spread over the top and bottom thirds of the plate. Specimen of pus from an abscess spread over the middle third. The specimen yielded two staphylococci: one sensitive to all drugs (i.e. zones equivalent to control) and a smaller number of a penicillinase-producing staphylococcus also resistant to tetracycline.

an important pathogen is too scanty, or it has been overgrown by another resistant organism or is itself resistant to all four drugs, the same method can again be employed. The inoculum of the test organism must be adjusted to match the control (see 'Secondary tests', below).

Pus swabs and liquid pus
Sensitivity test cultures are normally incubated aerobically but when anaerobes are likely to be present (e.g. septic abortion pelvic or abdominal abscess) it may save time to do anaerobic sensitivity tests as well. Since by the method described below anaerobic incubation does not invalidate results on facultative aerobes, one (anaerobic) test plate only can be employed. Methicillin may be included in primary tests on blood agar when staphylococci are expected, provided the culture is incubated at 30°C (see page 219).

Urine
There is little to be gained from routinely doing primary sensitivity tests on urines. The majority of patients with symptoms of uncomplicated urinary tract infection are treated with antibiotics before the outcome of culture and sensitivity tests are known. Sensible choice of antimicrobial agent based on local sensitivity patterns will ensure a high success rate for therapy. When a primary test is requested, an optimal inoculum of

infected urine can almost always be achieved by placing a loopful (5 mm external diameter, held vertically) of *uncentrifuged* well mixed urine on a plate of sensitivity test medium. The inoculum is spread evenly using a dry sterile swab. Swabs dipped directly into the urine will usually give too heavy an inoculum.

Results are interpreted as for tests with pure cultures, but when zones are significantly smaller than the control, particularly if the inoculum is heavier, tests must be repeated. It is also important to assess the significance of the growth before reporting sensitivity tests. Reporting the sensitivies of commensals may lead to unnecessary treatment in the first place or to a change in established therapy, possibly detrimental to the patient.

If large square dishes are used or if the cultures are spread using a rotator* (Pearson and Whitehead, 1974), six antimicrobials can be tested on each: suitable drugs for routine use are given in Table 9.2. The drugs listed are necessarily a personal choice, reflecting the likely sensitivity pattern in our practice and the current local antibiotic stock-list. Further discs are kept available (see Table 9.1) for use on organisms resistant to first-line antibiotics or where different antibiotics are in clinical use for specific reasons. The extra time taken to apply the control cultures to each plate can be greatly reduced if preimpregnated swabs prepared in bulk are used (page 212), and it is compensated for by the ease with which zones can be compared. Discs can be speedily and efficiently placed on a rotary inoculated plate using either a manual inoculator (Oxoid Hand Dispenser System) or a semi-automatic machine (Oxoid Discamat) (Fig. 9.3). Using cartridges, sets of discs can be prepared on a removable head to cater, for example, for Gram-positive organisms or Gram-negative organisms.

Secondary tests on pure cultures

Inoculum

Even when the diagnostic culture appears to yield a pure growth it is seldom desirable to test a single colony in case there is variation in sensitivity, and part of several colonies should be taken. It is not usually possible to achieve a satisfactory inoculum (semiconfluent growth, see page 210) by transferring solid growth directly to the plate; a suspension, approximately equivalent in density to an overnight broth culture, can be made by emulsifying the colonies in a small volume of broth or peptone water. A small loopful (2–4 mm diameter) of this or of an overnight broth culture is transferred to the centre of the plate and spread as evenly as possible with a dry sterile swab. When colonies are very small or not easily emulsifiable it may be possible to achieve an optimal inoculum by picking one or two and after seeding them centrally on the plate spreading with a swab, but broth should also be inoculated so that tests can be repeated

*Obtainable from Denley Ltd. Rotation speed 150 r.p.m.

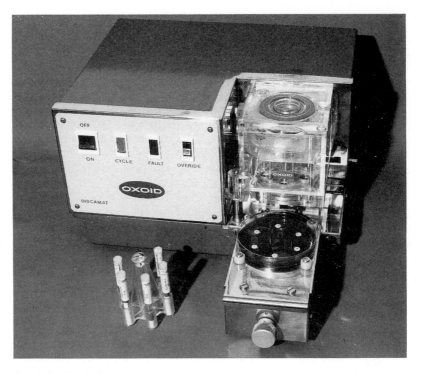

Fig. 9.3 Oxoid Discamat – an antibiotic – impregnated disc dispenser.

when necessary from a liquid culture next day. Plates are inoculated as described for the primary test.

Interpretation of results

Zones of inhibition of the test organism are compared with those of the appropriate control organism, and when there is any doubt as to their relative size, they are measured with calipers or by laying a millimetre rule across the dish. Provided the inoculum is optimal and the control zones are 8–15 mm radius, results are reported as follows.

Sensitive: zone radius equal, wider, or not more than 3 mm smaller than the control.

Intermediate: zone more than 3 mm radius but smaller than the control by more than 3 mm.

Resistant: zone of 2 mm radius or less.

This method of interpretation is not valid for some tests with penicillinase-producing staphylococci nor for tests with polymyxin (colistin). They are interpreted as described below.

The paper strip method

When a number of organisms have to be tested against only one or two drugs, blotting paper strips are more convenient to use than discs. Suitably

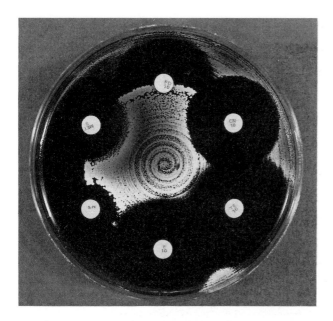

Fig. 9.4 Primary sensitivity test of staphylococcal pus incubated at 30°C overnight. Preimpregnated control swab inoculated peripherally. P 2 = 2 units penicillin; MET 5 = 5 µg methicillin; FD 10 = 10 µg fusidic acid; CN 10 = 10 µg gentamicin; TE 10 = 10 µg tetracycline; E 10 = 10 µg erythromycin. Note the penicillinase production around the penicillin disc.

diluted cultures are streaked across the plate; eight strains (seven tests and a control) can be accommodated on one plate, and an impregnated strip is placed at right angles across the inocula.

Several drugs are now commercially available in this form (Mast Laboratories). The method is valuable for testing staphylococci with methicillin (see below).

Tests presenting special difficulty
Penicillinase-producing staphylococci

The penicillin-inhibition zone of a sensitive organism may be reduced if it is mixed with a penicillinase producer (see Fig. 9.5). If sufficient penicillinase is formed and the logistics of its production and the growth of the organisms are favourable, satellitism of the sensitive organism round colonies of the penicillinase producer will be seen.

If a penicillinase producer fails to form enough of the enzyme to neutralize the penicillin close to the disc, it will show an inhibition zone. It can, however, be recognized because the colonies at the edge of the zone are large and well developed and there is no gradual fading away of growth towards the disc (see Figs. 9.2 and 9.4). They are easy to recognize in contrast to the fading edge of the control zone when test and control are cultured on the same plate. These strains are therefore reported as resistant.

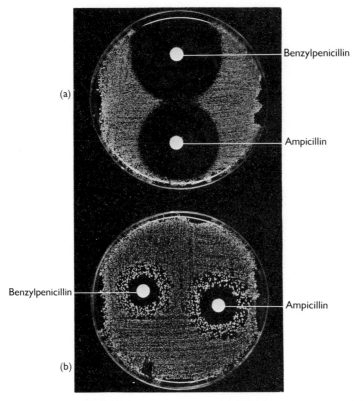

Fig. 9.5 Cultures showing the effect of a penicillinase-producing staphylococcus on inhibition zones to penicillin of a sensitive staphylococcus mixed with it. (a) Sensitive strain alone showing wide zones. (b) (same strength discs) Sensitive staphylococcus plus penicillinase producer showing (1) small zone with well defined edge typical of a penicillinase producer, and (2) zone of sensitive strain smaller than in (a).

Methicillin-resistant staphylococci

Methicillin-resistant staphylococci will often appear fully sensitive when tested in the ordinary way. Many of these organisms grow more slowly in the presence of methicillin and growth will appear within the zone only when incubation is continued for 48 hours. This difficulty can be overcome either by incubating the culture at 30°C (Annear, 1968) or by using 5% salt agar (Barber, 1964) when most of the culture will appear resistant overnight. The interpretation of sensitivity tests to other drugs is not adversely affected by incubation at 30°C.

Although there is cross-resistance between methicillin and all other penicillinase-resistant penicillins both clinically and when tested by a dilution method, many resistant strains appear sensitive when tested against cloxacillin or flucloxacillin discs (Hewitt *et al.*, 1969; Garrod and Waterworth, 1971). Methicillin only should be used in diffusion tests but it should be made clear in the report that results apply equally to the other drugs.

Estimation of minimal inhibitory concentration (MIC) of these peni-cillins is not straightforward because very small numbers of resistant cells are common and a test in liquid medium is therefore very inoculum dependent. Moreover, there is no way of knowing whether the patient's defences will overcome the small number of resistant survivors or whether they will take over during treatment, rendering the penicillin useless. It is safest to test MIC in liquid culture using a heavy inoculum. A strain sensi-tive to this test should be possible to eliminate by treatment. MIC titration on solid medium with a heavy inoculum will reveal the true state of affairs and small numbers of resistant colonies can be ignored when it is thought reasonable to do so; for example, when the penicillin is to be used in com-bination with another drug which will kill the survivors, or when the penicillin is to be used locally in the treatment of burns (Lowbury et al., 1977).

Cephalosporin
Cephaloridine can be used to represent the older cehalosporins (e.g. ceph-radine or cephalexin) in disc diffusion tests. However, the more recent β-lactamase-stable cephalosporins should be tested individually. Cephalo-ridine is only moderately resistant to staphylococcal penicillinase. As there is cross-resistance between methicillin and cephalosporins, sensitivity to the latter can be assumed from tests with the former. The disc method is misleading for testing staphylococci to cephalosporins, and should not be used (Blowers et al., 1973).

Co-trimoxazole
This is a mixture of sulphamethoxazole and trimethoprim, and discs containing both drugs in a ratio of 20 : 1 are widely used for sensitivity tests; such discs may be misleading. When both drugs are present it is impossible to know whether the organism is sensitive to both or only to one of them. Each drug should therefore be tested separately, and if sulphonamide is already being tested one extra disc containing trimetho-prim alone is needed. An organism should be reported sensitive to co-trimoxazole only when some sensitivity is shown to both drugs (see also page 228). Disc diffusion methods are more susceptible to differences in inoculum than are dilution methods, and this is particularly important in tests of these folate inhibitors (see page 209). Quality control trials in Britain in which more than 300 laboratories participate have demons-trated an unacceptably high rate of errors in some of these tests. Urinary pathogens which grow well on the thymidine-poor medium required can be reliably tested provided inoculum does not exceed 'not quite confluent growth'. Streptococci grow poorly on sensitivity test medium, even when blood is added. Moreover, streptococci, staphylococci and N. gonor-rhoeae often show intermediate sensitivity to sulphonamide, which makes them more difficult to test. Consequently, care is required when interpret-ing the results of testing folate inhibitors against Gram-positive organisms by disc diffusion. Should it be clinically necessary to use these compounds to treat such infections, determination of MIC is to be preferred (see page 222).

Polymyxin and colistin

Polymyxins diffuse very poorly in agar and the measurements above cannot be applied. The *Esch. coli* control gives a zone radius of 3–4 mm and this can easily be reduced by too heavy an inoculum. Most Gram-negative bacilli are sensitive, notable exceptions being members of the proteus/providencia groups and *Serratia* species.

Ps. aeruginosa

The sensitivity of this species to gentamicin is much affected by the magnesium content of the medium; when this is low the organism will appear unduly sensitive (Garrod and Waterworth, 1969).

A further difficulty arises because this organism is only moderately sensitive to both gentamicin and ticarcillin, often the drugs of choice, and zones will be smaller than those of either the *Esch. coli* or the staphylococcal control. It will therefore be difficult to detect moderate increases in resistance to these drugs.

Both these difficulties can be overcome by using a strain of the same species of known sensitivity (NCTC 10662) as a control for tests with this organism and when the zone is not significantly reduced, as judged by comparison with the control, the organism can be reported sensitive (Garrod and Waterworth, 1971). Preimpregnated swabs can be prepared for convenience as described for the *Esch. coli* control (page 212).

Swarming organisms

These invade inhibition zones even when the organism is sensitive. The zone edge should be measured as for other organisms and swarming should be disregarded. In mixed cultures when no colonies forming a zone can be seen the test must be repeated (see also page 227).

N. gonorrhoeae

Isolates of *N. gonorrhoeae* fall into one of three groups with respect to penicillin sensitivity. Sensitive organisms will require an MIC equal to or less than 0.06 mg/l (0.1 unit/ml). Moderately resistant strains require an MIC greater than 0.06 mg/l but usually less than 0.2 mg/l (0.34 units/ml), and they are β-lactamase negative. The third group consists of the β-lactamase-producing strains. A three-disc sensitivity test is recommended for routine purposes. Using the comparative technique, discs containing 1.0, 0.25 and 0.03 unit penicillin are employed, with a sensitive control strain of *N. gonorrhoeae* for comparison (see page 213). Strains showing comparable zones to the control for all discs, or a reduced zone size to the 0.03 unit disc only, are reported as sensitive. Organisms showing full or reduced sensitivity to the 1.0 unit disc only are reported as moderately resistant, unless found to be β-lactamase producing. All strains showing reduced zones to any disc should be tested for β-lactamase production (see page 310).

Str. pneumoniae

Isolates of *Str. pneumoniae* with reduced susceptibility to penicillin will not be recognized using a 1 unit disc. Sensitivity to penicillin should therefore be evaluated using discs containing either 0.25 unit penicillin or 1 μg oxacillin.

Anaerobes

Aminoglycoside antibiotics are partly inactivated by anaerobiosis; therefore the control must also be incubated anaerobically. Disc diffusion tests are not as satisfactory for anaerobes as they are for aerobes. Nevertheless, disc tests by the method described will often serve as a guide to treatment of infection by anaerobes which grow overnight. Primary tests of pus from pelvic sepsis, where anaerobes are very common, will give a quicker result if the culture is incubated anaerobically. Results for facultative anaerobes will not be invalidated and an additional aerobic test is not essential, but note the effect of added CO_2 which tends to acidify the medium and may affect the zone size. When metronidazole is included, the anaerobic control *Cl. perfringens* (NCTC 11229) or *Bact. fragilis* (NCTC 9343) will be required (but see page 212).

Fungi

Media used for bacterial sensitivity tests inactivate 5-fluorocytosine; therefore special medium must be employed. Yeast nitrogen base (Difco) with 0.15% asparagine and 1% dextrose as supplements is suitable. Discs containing 1 μg give a large zone with a sensitive *Candida* and are preferred to the 10 μg disc. When the zone for the test strain is smaller than that of a sensitive control tested in parallel, the MIC should be determined by a reference laboratory.

Technical faults (see also 'Inoculum', page 215)

Zones are sometimes found to be oval or eccentric. There are three common causes for this. If the disc is dropped on the medium and then shifted to a different position, sufficient antibiotic will be absorbed at the first site of contact to inhibit growth. If the medium 'sweats' on incubation, antibiotic may be carried in the surface moisture. If the discs are placed too near the edge of the plate, i.e. less than 1 cm from it, the zones may be eccentric, due to sideways diffusion of the antibiotic which is prevented from further radial diffusion when it reaches the edge of the plate.

If the culture is accidentally left on the bench for an hour or two after the discs have been placed on it, the zones will be large because the antibiotic will have had time to diffuse before growth began. Provided that the control and the test material were seeded before the discs were placed in position, this does not greatly matter because when the result is read the test zone is compared with the control zone and both are similarly affected. Delay between seeding the test organism and the control may, however, lead to reduction in zone size of whichever was seeded first. This is most likely to happen in the paper strip method when all the cultures to be tested are not ready at the same time.

Determination of minimal inhibitory concentration (MIC)

Although the rapid test already described is a sufficient guide to treatment in the majority of infections, a more accurate estimate is sometimes desirable particularly when a patient needs prolonged treatment with an antibiotic which may be toxic. Numerous methods of measuring the MIC have been devised; they fall into two classes. Zones of inhibition can be measured by diffusion through agar under standard conditions, or growth of the organism can be assessed in a series of doubling dilutions of antibiotic in liquid or solid media. Dilution methods are usually preferred because zones are often ill-defined and difficult to read.

An organism of known sensitivity, usually the Oxford staphylococcus, should always be titrated in parallel with an unknown organism. When reporting, the MIC for both test and control organisms should be stated so that a comparison can be made. A statement of MIC without some standard of comparison and without details of the method employed has very little meaning.

Factors, other than antibiotic concentration, which affect the end point are as follows.

Inoculum

Individual bacterial cells are not constant in their antibiotic sensitivity. Irregularity in reponse is much more marked with some drugs than with others. For example, sensitive staphylococci titrated against benzylpenicillin will show only a small rise in MIC when the inoculum is increased one-thousandfold; the end point with methicillin, however, varies widely with inoculum. A strain may appear fully sensitive when tested with a small inoculum, but when tested with a very heavy inoculum the MIC may rise to a level unattainable when normal doses are given. Tests in liquid medium with very large inocula are misleading because when even a single bacterial cell out of hundreds of millions is uninhibited growth will be seen. Under these conditions in the patient the drug may succeed because very small numbers of uninhibited cocci would find it difficult to withstand the normal tissue defences and it is unlikely they would be able to flourish *in vivo*.

When β-lactamase-producing organisms are tested against β-lactamase-susceptible antibiotics, the MIC is greatly influenced by the inoculum. This is particularly noticeable when the organism produces large amounts of extracellular enzyme. The use of heavy inocula of such organisms will introduce preformed β-lactamase into the test system, reducing the activity of the antibiotic and enabling growth to begin.

Inoculum may also be affected by adherence of organisms to the wall of the tube, above the meniscus, during inoculation. The organisms will not be exposed to antimicrobial action, and will be resuspended in the broth during mixing prior to subculture. Adherence is most marked with plastic tubes.

Dilution tests of sulphonamides are also very susceptible to inoculum size. Inoculum effect is much less important in tests on solid medium because very small numbers of survivors of a heavy inoculum can be seen and ignored. Moreover, when large numbers of strains are to be tested, a multiple inoculator can be employed. This method is therefore preferred.

Composition of the medium

For non-fastidious organisms either Iso-sensitest or Mueller-Hinton medium is suitable. These should be supplemented with 5% lysed horse blood for tests involving sulphonamides or trimethoprim, on solid media. Serum (5–10%) or blood may be added to broth media for fastidious organisms. Considerations of the protein-binding properties of an antibiotic are probably unnecessary, provided that suitable control organisms are always used to ensure that the test conditions are optimal.

Incubation time

Tests should be read at about 12–18 hours. Further incubation will allow growth to appear in higher concentrations, partly because slightly inhibited bacteria will begin to grow and also because many antibiotics are unstable in low concentration at 37°C; as they are destroyed, bacteria previously inhibited will flourish. In the patient, doses will be repeated and the drug level maintained so that this effect will not be seen. Strains which acquire resistance sometimes grow more slowly in the presence of the drug than normally; for example, erythromycin resistant staphylococci. Attempts to read results more quickly than 12 hours are liable to lead to error when such strains are encountered (Waterworth, 1976).

Growth phase

Penicillin and many other antibiotics are most active against rapidly dividing bacteria. Anything which reduces the rate of cell division will render the organisms less sensitive. For example, penicillin is relatively harmless to sensitive bacteria at low temperatures. Appropriate dilutions of an overnight liquid culture should therefore be employed in order to standardize inoculum and minimize differences due to testing during different phases of growth.

Broth dilution methods

The range of dilutions to be tested can usually be limited in the light of the paper disc method result. When no disc test has been made, it should run from a concentration higher than can be maintained in the blood to a concentration lower than that which is known to inhibit the control strain. When the organism to be tested was recovered from urine the range must be increased to include the high concentrations obtainable in urine.

Antibiotics used for making stock solutions are best obtained pure from the manufacturers for laboratory use only. Capsules and tablets often contain material other than antibiotic, which will affect the result. Solutions prepared for parenteral treatment when available are satisfactory, with the exception of chloramphenicol and clindamycin phosphate (see page 210) because they are only activated after *in vivo* hydrolysis. For details of the solubility of various drugs, see Garrod *et al.* (1981).

Tube titration method
Materials:

Sterile graduated 10 ml pipette
Sterile graduated 1 ml pipettes
Sterile capped 3 × 1.25 cm tubes or small screw-capped bottles
Pasteur pipettes
Overnight broth culture of test organism
Overnight broth culture of control organism
Antibiotic solution of known concentration
Broth or serum broth (see page 223)

The method to be described for preparation of a row of doubling dilutions of an antibiotic, has proved to be economical in time and materials. It is unnecessary to prepare a set of master dilutions, thus avoiding a possible source of error. Stock solutions of antibiotics are prepared at concentrations of 10, 100 and 1000 mg/l and kept frozen at −20°C, ready for use. Penicillins and cephalosporins should be freshly prepared.

A suitable control, usually the Oxford staphylococcus, is tested in parallel and an antibiotic-free tube is included to check the viability of test organism and control.

Procedure
Prepare two rows of sterile capped 7.5 × 1.3 cm tubes in a rack. (Each tube will contain 1 volume, usually 2 ml, of the appropriate antibiotic dilution.) Prepare in a sterile 30 ml (Universal) screw-capped bottle 4 volumes of broth containing the concentration of antibiotic required for the first tube in each row. (This antibiotic dilution is prepared from the appropriate stock solution.) Mix the contents of the Universal bottle, using a pipette, and transfer 1 volume to the first tube in each row. Using a fresh pipette, add 2 volumes of broth to the remaining 2 volumes in the Universal, mix and add 1 volume to the second tube in each row. Repeat this process until all but the last tubes are filled. Place 1 volume of antibiotic-free broth in each last tube. Inoculate one row with one drop of an overnight culture of the test organism per tube diluted approximately 1 : 100 and the other row with a similar dilution of overnight culture of the control organism. This gives a concentration of about 10^5 organisms per ml and is comparable with the inoculum recommended for the disc diffusion test. Incubate all tubes for 18–24 hours at 37°C.

Results
Sensitivity is expressed as the lowest concentration which inhibited growth, judged by lack of opacity in the tube. The sensitivity of the control is also reported. This is important because it enables comparison to be made between titrations performed in different laboratories. After further incubation, growth may be seen in tubes in which it was originally inhibited, it is disregarded (see page 223).

When deciding on the range of antibiotic dilutions to be used in this test it is strongly recommended that twofold dilutions are always based on 1. Thus the range will be 1, 2, 4, 8, etc. when doubling and 0.5, 0.25, etc. when halving the dilutions. This facilitates comparison between the results from other laboratories and between resistant and sensitive strains of the same organism.

This estimation of MIC can be extended to find the minimal bactericidal concentration (MBC) by explanting on solid medium from tubes showing no opacity after overnight incubation in the manner described on page 229. A highly bactericidal drug such as penicillin or an aminoglycoside will yield little, if any, growth from the clear tube containing the least drug. A bacteriostatic drug, such as a tetracycline, is likely to yield heavy or moderate growth from all clear tubes.

Plate dilution method
The preparation of agar media containing accurate concentrations of anti-biotics is a skilled process. Tablets containing suitable concentrations of antibiotics are available (Adatabs, Mast Laboratories) or, alternatively, Sensititre (Seward Laboratories) can be used. Dried dilutions of anti-biotics, applicable to a group of bacteria (e.g. coliforms, staphylococci, etc.), are provided in microtitre trays. The antibiotic is reconstituted when a measured, 50 microlitre drop of a dilution of an overnight broth culture of the test strain is delivered to each well of the series. A control strain is tested in parallel. The trays can be stored at room temperature. The method was assessed by Phillips *et al.* (1978).

Materials:

    Sterile graduated 1 ml pipettes
    Sterile graduated 25 ml pipette
    Screw-capped sterile bottles 30 ml (1 oz)
    Sensitivity test agar, sterile horse blood
    Sterile Petri dishes
    Overnight broth cultures of test organisms and control.

Procedure
Prepare molten sensitivity test agar at 56–60°C.

Make a range of dilutions of antibiotic in sterile distilled water twenty times stronger than the final dilution required in the medium. Label one sterile 8.5 cm Petri dish for each dilution and one for the control plate. Add 1 ml of diluent (distilled water) to the control plate and then, starting with the weakest dilution of antibiotic, transfer 1 ml of each dilution to the appropriate labelled dishes.

Using the 25 ml pipette (with its tip cut off to allow rapid delivery), transfer 19 ml of medium to each dish, mixing well. A mechanical rotator fitted with a large tray to take the dishes can be used to facilitate mixing.

When the medium has set, dry the plates in the incubator, with the lids of the dishes tilted, for from 30 minutes to 1 hour according to the humidity of the incubator. Well dried plates are essential; once dried, they can be stored at 4°C for up to 1 week (Ryan *et al.*, 1970).

Inoculate the plates using either a loop or a multiple inoculator with overnight broth culture diluted 1/100 approximately.

Include a standard sensitive control organism on each plate.

Read after overnight incubation, disregarding abnormally minute colonies and growth of one or two colonies only.

When swarming bacteria are tested by this method, the agar content should be increased by 1 per cent.

A multiple inoculator in available (Denley Ltd) which will allow up to 25 organisms to be tested per 8.5 cm plate.

Relation between disc diffusion and titration

Under standard conditions rapidly growing organisms, showing the same zone of inhibition as the Oxford staphylococcus after overnight incubation, will prove to have the same order of sensitivity when tested by titration. It does not follow, however, that one showing half as large a zone will be half as sensitive when titrated because the relation between concentration of the drug and distance from the disc is not a simple linear one.

The relation between zone size and MIC is likely to be quite different if the organism grows slowly. The zone will tend to be large because the antibiotic will have had time to diffuse further from the disc. When the lag phase of growth is prolonged for several days, this effect may be somewhat counteracted by destruction of the drug.

During titration the dose of antibiotic remains constant until it begins to degenerate. Therefore, when the drug is stable, rates of growth will not affect the result.

Spreading organisms are capable of swimming on the surface of moist medium near discs even when they are sensitive. Therefore, in the disc method, readings should be taken from the edge of growth of inhibited colonies. Parallel tests with *Proteus mirabilis* by tube titration and agar diffusion are consistent only when spreading is disregarded.

Sensitivity tests for mycobacteria

Testing the sensitivity of *Myco. tuberculosis* is potentially dangerous and most hospital laboratories in Britain isolate few strains. Experience shows that much better results are obtained when specialist laboratories undertake this work; moreover, the inevitable additional delay in transporting cultures and returning reports is not important because it is a small fraction of the time taken to test such slow-growing microbes.

Antibiotics in combination

Acute bacterial infections by single pathogens usually respond to treatment by an antibiotic which inhibits growth of the organism in laboratory tests, provided the drug is able to reach the site of infection in sufficient concentration. In certain circumstances, however, it may be necessary to give more than one antibiotic, either because two infecting microbes with different sensitivity patterns have to be dealt with or because treatment must be prolonged and there is danger of resistance developing.

Bacterial endocarditis frequently requires treatment with a combination of antibiotics, to ensure killing of the organism. Inhibition of bacterial growth will often provide temporary relief of symptoms, but relapse is inevitable unless a bactericidal antibiotic, or combination of antibiotics, is used.

The laboratory should, therefore, be prepared to test strains isolated from the blood by a method which shows bactericidal power as well as inhibition and which will demonstrate antagonism when inappropriate combination of drugs are proposed for treatment. Once treatment has started, the patient's serum should be tested against his own organism to check that the strain is killed by the concentration of the antibiotic achieved.

The synergistic action of some combinations of antibiotics against certain bacteria is well known. Synergy between penicillin and the aminoglycosides against streptococci, particularly *Str. faecalis*, is demonstrable *in vitro*. In contrast, tetracyclines and chloramphenicol are invariably antagonistic in combination with penicillin. Other combinations, such as flucloxacillin and fusidic acid, will give equivocal results. At certain concentrations antagonism is seen *in vitro*, whilst at other concentrations the combination may demonstrate synergy. Determination of the fractional inhibitory concentration (FIC) of each antibiotic in the combination, and from these results the fractional inhibitory concentration index (FICI), goes some way to resolving the problem (Japan Co-operative, 1973). The mathematical concepts of synergy are discussed further by Berenbaum (1978).

It must be stressed that *in vitro* tests are only a guide as to what may be expected to occur *in vivo*. In endocarditis, results of therapy match well with bactericidal tests of antibiotic combinations, but in other circumstances (e.g. deep-seated chronic abscesses) the response is less certain. It cannot be assumed that combinations of antibiotics theoretically synergistic will be proved to be so when used for therapy. The proportion of each drug at the site of the lesion is unknown, and the bacterial load may be overwhelmingly large. Combinations of antibiotics designed to be synergistic may, for example, induce enzyme-mediated resistance. Such a possibility has been suggested by Sanders (1983) for combinations of β-lactam antibiotics. It is therefore difficult to devise a laboratory test relevant to all conditions, and it is too much to hope that an apparently good combination will always succeed in fibrosed and avascular lesions. ·

For the demonstration of bacteriostatic synergy between two antibiotics, the best method is the 8×8 chessboard titration in liquid culture. A suitable range of dilutions of each antibiotic is prepared in broth, such that each antibiotic is present alone and in all combinations. A standardized inoculum or the organism is added to each tube prior to incubation. Details of the method, which is tedious and time consuming, will be found in Garrod *et al.* (1981). The FIC (the inhibitory concentration of drug acting in combination divided by the MIC of the drug acting alone) can be calculated. The FIC index (FICI) is the sum of the two FICs. Synergy is defined as FICI of less than 0.25.

Synergism and antagonism in disc tests

Tests of mixtures of drugs on discs are misleading and do not necessarily indicate combined action. Two single discs or strips of blotting paper, each impregnated with one of the proposed drugs, can be placed side by side or at right angles on blood agar preseeded with the pathogen. After overnight incubation the shape of the inhibition zones may indicate synergism or antagonism but cannot be relied upon to do so. None of these tests indicates the effect of combining the drugs on killing power and they are therefore insufficient as a basis for recommending treatment in endocarditis.

The synergistic action between sulphonamide and trimethoprim which are normally given as a mixture, co-trimoxazole, is frequently seen when these drugs are tested separately and the discs are placed 3 cm or less apart. This is an exception to the general rule that mixing drugs on discs is undesirable because co-trimoxazole discs will show a larger zone than either constituent separately when tested against an organism sensitive to both. Nevertheless, the increase is not very great and an organism resistant either to sulphonamide or to trimethoprim but not to both is likely to be reported sensitive to the combination. Bacteria are much more often resistant to sulphonamide than to trimethoprim and this can be recognized by testing separately for sulphonamide. Trimethoprim-resistant strains are sometimes sensitive to sulphonamide and they will not be discovered unless trimethoprim is also tested separately. Ideally, three discs should be used, each drug separately and the combination. All essential information will, however, be revealed if sulphonamide and trimethoprim are tested separately, and the combination is omitted. It can safely be assumed that when activity of whatever degree to either constituent is seen (when tested

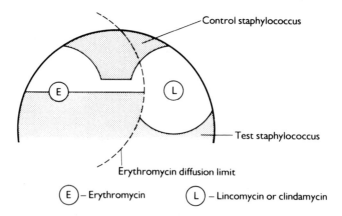

Fig. 9.6   Dissociated resistance to erythromycin.

against the disc content recommended, see Table 9.1) the combination will be active, whether synergism can be easily demonstrated or not.

Antagonism is often seen in tests on staphylococci when erythromycin and clindamycin discs are placed about 3 cm apart. Strains which, when tested alone, are erythromycin-resistant but sensitive to clindamycin are seen to be resistant to clindamycin also when erythromycin is present (Fig. 9.6). It is well known that clindamycin resembles the macrolide antibiotics too closely to be useful in combination with them, but it is not always appreciated that when clindamycin is used alone to treat staphylococcal infection by an erythromycin-resistant strain the organism will quickly become resistant to clindamycin also. When reporting the clindamycin result, a warning should therefore be given; this applies also to the closely related drug lincomycin.

Bactericidal tests

Endocarditis caused by unusual organisms may be difficult to treat. Tests of synergy between unusual combinations are therefore essential to guide therapy.

Two kinds of methods are suitable for bactericidal tests in hospital laboratories. Both kinds are qualitative. In one ('the half chessboard'), a series of dilutions of drugs are tested both singly and in combination against a heavy inoculum of the organism in liquid culture. After overnight incubation, the contents of tubes are subcultured onto solid medium and reincubated to demonstrate bactericidal activity. The method is simple to perform but has the disadvantage that only a single concentration of each drug can be tested. There is, of course, no guarantee that this concentration will be the operative strength at the site of infection. In addition, only a small proportion of the total inoculum is sampled on subculture to solid medium. The other method is a modification of Chabbert's cellophane transfer technique (Chabbert, 1957). It is easier to perform, and also allows two drugs to be tested against each other over a range of concentrations produced by diffusion through blood agar.

Combined tube dilution method (adapted from Chabbert, 1953)

A set of 10 tubes is arranged as in Fig. 9.7. Serum broth and antibiotic is added to each tube so that the volume of fluid per tube is the same and each contains the appropriate concentration of the drugs. The dilution of drugs in the tubes is that judged to be the average concentration of each at the infection site when full doses of each are given. If the volume per tube is about 2 ml, one drop of a 1 : 10 dilution of an overnight culture of the pathogen is seeded into each tube. A control tube is included which contains the same volume of medium but no antibiotic.

All the tubes are very thoroughly shaken and then subcultured immediately to sectors of two blood agar plates. The loop should be withdrawn edgewise to prevent overfilling, thus ensuring that each sector receives approximately the same volume. Duplicate seeding from each tube, using four plates, increases reliability. Tubes and plates are incubated overnight. Next day the tubes (which all appear clear except the control) are removed from the incubator, shaken thoroughly and again subcultured to blood agar. The first incubated plates are kept in the refrigerator so that overnight growth on them may be compared with that of the second subcultures which will be seen on the third day.

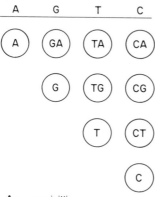

A =   ampicillin
G =   gentamicin
T =   tetracycline
C =   chloramphenicol

Fig. 9.7   Combined tube dilution test.

Example

Meningitis in an infant, cause by *Esch. coli* sensitive to all four drugs, has responded poorly to ampicillin. Can improvement be expected if tetracycline is also given?

Result

See Table 9.3.

Table 9.3   Result of combined antibiotic bactericidal test: + + = semiconfluent growth

	Blood agar culture	
Tube	Before inc.	After inc.
1. Ampicillin	+ +	±
2. Ampicillin and gentamicin	+ +	−
3. Ampicillin and tetracycline	+ +	+
4. Ampicillin and chloramphenicol	+ +	+
5. Gentamicin	+ +	−
6. Gentamicin and tetracycline	+ +	−
7. Gentamicin and chloramphenicol	+ +	−
8. Tetracycline and chloramphenicol	+ +	+
9. Tetracycline	+ +	+
10. Chloramphenicol	+ +	+

Interpretation
A mixture of tetracycline and ampicillin or of chloramphenicol and ampicillin is less lethal to this *Esch. coli* than is ampicillin alone. Tetracycline and chloramphenicol alone fail to kill large numbers of the microbe after overnight incubation. Gentamicin is the only one of these drugs which, when added to ampicillin, is likely to improve the patient's condition.

Agar diffusion method for combined sensitivity test (after M.P.E. Slack and D.B. Wheldon, personal communication)
Materials:

Sterile Petri dish
9.9 ml nutrient broth
Overnight broth culture of test organisms (opacity adjusted to McFarland Standard No. 1)
Circular sterile filter (Millipore type HC, 0.7 μm), cut to a right angle
Iso-sensitest lysed blood agar
Sensitivity disc for each antibiotic under investigation (see Table 9.1, page 208, for concentrations)

Note. Discs are used because commercially prepared impregnated strips are not obtainable for a wide range of drugs. It is easier and more reliable to use discs than to prepare strips.

Method
Add 0.1 ml of the broth culture to the 9.9 ml of nutrient broth. The resulting suspension should contain approximately 10^6 colony-forming units per ml. Pour the diluted culture into the petri dish. Using sterile forceps, place the membrane filter (marked grid side uppermost) on the surface of the broth culture, and leave for about 15 minutes to become saturated. Place two rows of antibiotic discs (one row for each antibiotic) on the lysed blood agar, to form a right angle. (A template placed under the plate helps proper alignment of the discs.) Using sterile forceps, remove the membrane filter from the broth culture, draining off excess fluid, and place it on the blood agar plate (marked grid side *downwards*) so that the cut right angle fits into the right angle formed by the two rows of discs. Incubate overnight in an atmosphere suitable for the test organism. Next day, growth will be seen on the membrane near the curved edge, with inhibition zones seen nearest the antibiotics. Transfer the membrane aseptically to a fresh lysed blood sensitivity agar plate without antibiotic discs, and reincubate. Figure 9.8 illustrates the results that may be obtained. In addition, small numbers of persisting organisms may also be revealed by this method.

Bactericidal activity of patient's serum
A test of the bactericidal activity of a patient's serum against his own infecting organism has traditionally been a part of the microbiological

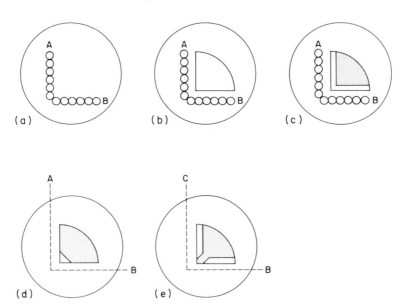

Fig. 9.8 Agar diffusion method for combined sensitivity test. (a) Lysed blood agar plate with antibiotic discs applied. (b) Membrane filter, cut as described, applied to the agar plate. (c) After incubation, growth on the membrane filter. Combination of A and B shows indifference at this stage. (d) After further incubation on an antibiotic-free plate, the growth pattern reveals synergy between A and B. (e) As (d) but the growth pattern reveals antagonism between B and C.

monitoring of endocarditis; as indicated on page 202, its value is being increasingly questioned. We still recommend this test for two reasons. First, the information is undoubtedly of use when taken in context with other parameters of the patient's response. Failure to respond clinically to the antibiotics used may well reflect an inadequate serum bactericidal activity. However, the converse is not necessarily true. Poor *in vitro* serum bactericidal power is not grounds for altering treatment when clinical response is good. Secondly, the drugs used may be potentially toxic. Serum bactericidal power measured against clinical response will guide adequate therapy and avoid excessive doses.

Serum should be tested after at least 24 hours of therapy, to achieve a stable state. Two samples should be tested: one taken 1 hour after a dose has been given, and the second immediately before a dose. (i.e. when levels of drugs will be at their lowest). Serum should be separated as soon as possible, to avoid inactivation of antibiotic in the sample.

Method
Make twofold dilutions of serum in appropriate assay medium. When there is sufficient serum it is better to test in duplicate so that the effect on two different inocula can be observed. Convenient volumes are 0.5 ml. Include a control tube without serum.

Inoculate each tube with one drop of an overnight culture of the pathogen. For staphylococci, suitable dilution for inoculation is 1 : 100. Mix each dilution well after inoculation on a vortex mixed. Explant two loopfuls from each tube onto blood agar in the manner described for the combined tube dilution test (page 229). Incubate overnight. Next day, note the inhibition titre. Mix well each tube lacking visible growth and explant again on blood agar. Keep the incubated blood agar cultures in the refrigerator for comparison and incubate the new explant plates.

In general, sterile cultures from tubes containing serum diluted 1 in 4 or greater correlate best with adequate treatment. Small numbers of organisms persisting (<0.1 per cent of initial inoculum) can usually be ignored.

Antibiotic assays

The assay of antimicrobial agents in body fluids may be necessary for the following reasons:

To ensure the maintenance of adequate therapeutic levels.
To avoid dose-related toxicity.
To adjust dosage in patients with renal or hepatic failure.
To check patient compliance.

On occasion, antibiotic levels may need to be measured in any body fluid. However, by far the majority of assays are carried out on serum samples.

Serum samples need to be collected immediately before the administration of a dose (trough level). Serum should also be taken at a time, after administration of a dose, corresponding to the highest expected level after initial distribution of the drug has occurred. The timing of this 'peak' level will depend on many factors, including the pharmacokinetics of the antimicrobial to be assayed, the route of administration and the individual's response.

Table 9.4 indicates recommended ranges for commonly assayed antimicrobial agents. These recommendations are designed to give optimal efficacy without increased risk of toxic side effects.

Table 9.4   Recommended serum levels for various antimicrobial agents

Antimicrobial agent	Trough (mg/l)	Peak (mg/l)	Time after dose (h)
Gentamicin ⎫ Tobramycin ⎭	<2.0	4–8	1
Netilmicin	<3.0	8–10	1
Amikacin	<5.0	20–30	$\frac{1}{2}$ p.i.
Vancomycin	5–10	25–35	$\frac{1}{2}$ p.i.
Chloramphenicol	5–10	15–35	1–2
Sulphamethoxazole* + trimethoprim		100 ⎫ 5 ⎭	1
5-Fluorocytosine		80	1–2

p.i. = post infusion.
*For treatment of *Pneumocystis carinii* infections.

The aminoglycoside antibiotics have a narrow margin between efficacy and safety. They are widely used in hospital practice, despite potential oto and renal toxicity. As a result, they are the most frequently assayed antimicrobial agents in the laboratory. Assay is required when renal function is impaired or treatment lasts longer than 48 hours. The frequency of assay will depend on the circumstances, but in general should not exceed 3 days.

There are many methods available for the assay of antimicrobial agents. Some methods are suitable for virtually all drugs; for example, microbiological assay and high-performance liquid chromatography (HPLC). Others have a more restricted use; for example, immunoassay for aminoglycosides and vancomycin, or colorimetry (sulphonamides).

It is beyond the scope of this book to review or detail all available methods. Further information and comprehensive methodology can be found in Reeves and Bywater (1976), Reeves *et al.* (1978) and Lorian (1986).

Methods

Microbiological assay

This assay is within the capabilities of any hospital laboratory, and with attention to detail can provide accurate results. The major disadvantage is the time taken to obtain a result. By using a rapid growing indicator organism (e.g. *Klebsiella edwardsi* NCTC 10896), zones of inhibition may be read within 4–5 hours' incubation. Results are therefore usually obtainable within the 8 hour dose period commonly employed, enabling the clinician to be informed and the dose adjusted when necessary.

Another major disadvantage of this method is a lack of specificity when antimicrobial agents other than the one for which the test is required are also present in the sample. This problem may be overcome by selective inactivation. Penicillins and cephalosporins can be inactivated with a mixture of broad spectrum β-lactamase (Genzyme Biochemicals Ltd). Alternatively, an assay strain known to be resistant to the other antimicrobial agents present may be used. To this end, every laboratory should save organisms with resistance profiles useful for this purpose.

Agar plate assay

Medium

Pour 100 ml of molten sterile DST agar (Oxoid) into a carefully levelled bioassay Petri dish (243 × 18 mm) (Nunc, Kamstrup, DK 4000, Denmark) and allow to gel. Dry thoroughly at 37°C.

Inoculum

Prepare 20 ml of a 1 : 50 dilution of an overnight broth culture of *Klebsiella edwardsi* (NCTC 10896) in sterile nutrient broth.

Method

Flood the surface of the agar plate with the inoculum, and ensure that all of the surface area is seeded. Drain the plate at a shallow acute angle, and carefully remove excess inoculum. Dry thoroughly at 37°C. Using an 8 mm cork borer, cut 30 wells in the agar in a 6 × 5 pattern (see Fig. 9.9).

Preparation of standards
A standard solution is prepared using pure antimicrobial agent of known potency. The pure substance is kept ready for use in a desiccator at 4°C. Final dilution is prepared in sterile horse or human serum which has been tested for, and found to be free of, inhibitory activity against the indicator organism.

A maximum of five standard concentrations are used. For gentamicin, tobramycin and netilmicin, standards of 1,2,4,8 and 16 mg/1 are suitable. For amikacin and streptomycin, 2.5,5,10,20 and 40 mg/1 are used. Each standard or test specimen is assayed in triplicate. One of the test specimens should comprise an external quality control of known potency.

Using a random distribution (e.g. Fig. 9.9), each well is completely filled (until the meniscus has disappeared) with standard or test solution.

After application of standards and test samples, plates are incubated at 37°C overnight. For rapid assays, seeded plates are preincubated for 1 hour at 37°C before cutting wells and applying standards and test sera. After application, further incubation at 37°C for 2½–3 hours usually produces zones of inhibition which can be measured. Zones should be read with microcalipers or an optical zone reader. Results are plotted on semi-logarithmic graph paper, relating zone of inhibition to $\log_{10}$ concentration of antibiotic. The average of the set of three readings for each standard is plotted and a straight line drawn between them. The average zone diameter of each test is then read off to give the concentration of antibiotic. Alternatively, and preferably, a computerized linear regression analysis is used. The programme will calculate the line of best fit for the standards, and determine the concentrations of the test samples from this.

The basic methodology described above is applicable to virtually all antimicrobial agents, with suitable modifications to medium formulation, and a relevant indicator organism as follows.

Choramphenicol   Oxoid DST agar is used, with *Esch. coli* (NCTC 10418) as indicator organism. Standards of 2.5, 5, 10, 20 and 40 mg/1 are recommended.

Vancomycin   Oxoid Antibiotic Medium No. 2, adjusted to pH 5.6–5.7 by the addition of 1.25 ml of 1 M HCl to 1 litre of medium after sterilization, is used. Suitable indicator organisms are *Bacillus subtilis* spores (NCTC 8236) incorporated into the agar prior to pouring, or surface seeding a *Staph. aureus* (this may be rifampicin- and/or aminoglycoside-resistant when appropriate).

Streptomycin   Oxoid Antibiotic Medium No. 2, adjusted to pH 7.9 by the addition of 5 ml M NaOH to 1 litre of medium before sterilization, is used. *Esch. coli* (NCTC 10418) is a suitable indicator organism.

1	2	3	4	5
6	7	8	9	10
11	12	13	14	15
16	17	18	19	20
21	22	23	24	25
26	27	28	29	30

Standards   (e.g. gentamicin assay)

	Well numbers
1 mg/l	1, 13, 25
2 mg/l	7, 20, 21
4 mg/l	5, 12, 23
8 mg/l	4, 15, 22
16 mg/l	3, 19, 27

Tests

a	6, 17, 28
b	2, 14, 26
c	8, 11, 30
d	9, 16, 24
e	10, 18, 29

Fig. 9.9   Random code for a 30-hole assay plate.

5-Fluorocytosine   This antifungal drug can be assayed using the following medium:

Base agar   Dissolve 2 g Oxoid No. 1 agar in 90 ml sterile distilled water and autoclave at 15 lb for 15 minutes. After cooling to 60°C, 10 ml of concentrated yeast nitrogen base glucose solution is added (prepared by dissolving 6.7 g Bacto Yeast Nitrogen Base (Difco) and 10 g glucose in 100 ml sterile distilled water, and sterilizing by filtration). The indicator organism is *Candida pseudotropicalis* (NCPF 3234), used at a 'just cloudy' concentration (approximately 1×10^6 cells/ml). The standards recommended are 6.25, 12.5, 25, 50 and 100 mg/l 5-fluorocytosine.

Alternative methods for antibiotic assay

Immunoassay

Although applicable to most antimicrobial agents, microbiological methods are relatively labour intensive, non-specific and slow. They are therefore unsuitable when large numbers of assays need to be carried out regularly. A number of immunoassay techniques are now commercially available for the assay of aminoglycoside antibiotics and (in one case) for the assay of vancomycin. These include substrate-labelled fluoro-immunoassay (Fluorostat, Ames), enzyme immunoassay (Emit, Syva) and fluorescence polarization assay (TDX, Abbott). At present the Fluorostat is a manual method, whilst the Emit and TDX are mechanized. The TDX will assay vancomycin in addition to the aminoglycosides. These machines are expensive to purchase, but in most cases the manufacturers operate schemes for laboratories to acquire the machines on permanent loan in return for a guaranteed purchase of a certain number of assay kits during the year. This arrangement makes these techniques cost-effective for laboratories with a heavy workload of assays.

Colorimetric methods

Chemical methods may be used for a number of antimicrobial agents. Of particular importance is the assay of sulphamethoxazole during treatment of *Pneumocystis carinii* infection in immunosuppressed patients. The method described is straightforward, requiring a standard spectrophotometer.

Sulphonamide assay (Modified after Bratton and Marshall, 1939)
Principle
The proteins in the serum sample are precipitated following treatment of the sample with trichloracetic acid and centrifugation. Sulphonamide present in the supernatant is diazotized, then coupled with *N*-(1-naphthyl)-ethylenediamine dihydrochloride, after removing excess nitrite with sulphamic acid. The resulting colour is read at 540 nm, giving an absorbance proportional to the amount of sulphonamide present when compared with a standard curve.

Preparation of standard solutions
Prepare a stock solution of 100 mg of the appropriate sulphonamide in 1 litre of water. A range of standards is prepared by adding 1.25, 2.5, 5.0, 7.0 and 10 ml each of stock solution to 40 ml of trichloracetic acid. The final volume is made up to 200 ml with sterile distilled water. These standards are equivalent to 25, 50, 100, 150 and 200 mg/l sulphonamide respectively. (It should be noted that these concentrations are 40 times greater than their *actual* concentrations in order to compensate for the 1 : 40 dilution of sample in the test (see below).

Test method

Pipette 3 ml of water into a 7.5 × 1.3 cm tube, add 0.1 ml of sample serum and 0.9 ml 20% w/v trichloracetic acid. Mix well, and allow to stand for a few minutes before centifuging at 3000 r.p.m. for 5 minutes.

Prepare sufficient 7.5 × 1.3 cm tubes for standards and samples. Pipette 2 ml of standard or sample or water into each tube (the water-containing tube will act as a blank). Add. 0.2 ml of sodium nitrate (1g/l) to each tube, mix and stand for 3 minutes. Add 0.2 ml of ammonium sulphamite (5 g/l) to each tube, mix and stand for 2 minutes. Add 1 ml of coupling agent (500 mg/l of *N*-(1-naphthyl)-ethylenediamine dihydrochloride) to each tube, and stand for a further 10 minutes. Set the spectrophotometer to read at 450 nm, zero on blank and read absorbance for all tubes in turn. From the standards, a graph of concentration against absorbance is plotted on arithmetic graph paper. This should produce a straight line passing through the origin. Concentrations of sulphonamide in the test samples are then read from the graph.

Note. This method estimates free drug. Some sulphonamide may be present in the sample as the acetyl derivative. However, because only free drug is active, it is probably valid to estimate only the free fraction.

High performance liquid chromatography (HPLC)

The technique of quantitative physical separation by column chromatography is applicable to virtually all antimicrobial agents. Pro-drugs (e.g. chloramphenicol succinate) and drug metabolites (e.g. desacetyl cefotaxime) can also be measured. The equipment is costly and requires a high standard of technical expertise. HPLC use is generally confined to larger laboratories with a need to perform rapid assay of chloramphenicol, or for research applications. The method is least applicable to aminoglycosides because these antibiotics require derivatization, making the procedure tedious and time consuming. It is likely that HPLC will be of increasing use for the assay of β-lactam and related antimicrobial agents.

Quality control of antimicrobial agent assays

All antimicrobial agent assays should include an external quality control to check accuracy and reproducibility. Control sera are available commercially (Lyphochek[R], Bio-Rad Laboratories Ltd) for some antibiotics, or, in certain cases, are obtainable from the appropriate pharmaceutical company on a regular basis. Laboratories should also take part in the National Quality Control Scheme (see page 22).

References

Annear, D.I. (1968) *Medical Journal of Australia* 1, 444
Barber, M. (1964) *Journal of General Microbiology* 35, 183
Bauer, A.W., Kirby, W.M.M., Sherris, J.C. and Turck, M. (1966) *American Journal of Clinical Pathology* 45, 493
Berenbaum, M.C. (1972) *Journal of Infectious Diseases* 137, 122
Blowers, R., Stokes, E.J. and Abbott, J.D. (1973) *British Medical Journal* iii, 46
Bovallius, A. and Zacharias, B. (1971) *Applied Microbiology* 22, 260
Bratton, A.C. and Marshall, E.K. (1939) *Journal of Biological Chemistry* 128, 537
Brown, D.F.J. and Kothari, D. (1978a) *Journal of Antimicrobial Chemotherapy* 4, 19
Brown, D.F.J. and Kothari, D. (1978b) *Journal of Antimicrobial Chemotherapy* 4, 27
Chabbert, Y.A. (1953) *Annales de l'Institut Pasteur* 84, 545
Chabbert, Y.A. (1957) *Annales de l'Institut Pasteur* 93, 289
Ericsson, H.M. and Sherris, J.C. (1971) *Acta Pathologica et Microbiologica Scandinavica* Section B Supplement, 217
Felmingham, D. and Stokes, E.J. (1972) *Journal of Medical Laboratory Technology* 29, 198
Garrod, L.P., Lambert, H.P. and O'Grady, F. (1981) *Antibiotic and Chemotherapy*. Churchill Livingstone, Edinburgh and London
Garrod, L.P. and Waterworth, P.M. (1969) *Journal of Clinical Pathology* 22, 534
Garrod, L.P. and Waterworth, P.M (1971) *Journal of Clinical Pathology* 24, 779
Hewitt, J.H., Coe, A.W. and Parker, M.T. (1969) *Journal of Medical Microbiology* 2, 443
Japan Co-operative Bacteriological Study Group for Cotrimoxazole (1975) *Journal of Infectious Diseases* 128, S502
Jones, P.H. and Scott, A.P. (1977) *Journal of Clinical Pathology* 30, 1028
Kucers, A. and Bennett, N. (1979) *The Use of Antibiotics*. Heinemann Medical, London.
Lorian, V. (Ed.) (1986) *Antibiotics in Laboratory Medicine*. Williams and Wilkins, Baltimore
Lowbury, E.J.L., Lilly, H.A. and Kidson, A. (1977) *British Medical Journal* i, 1054
Mellors, J.W., Coleman, D.L. and Andriole, V.T. (1986) *European Journal of Clinical Microbiology* 5, 67
Milne, S.E., Stokes, E.J. and Waterworth, P.M. (1978) *Journal of Clinical Pathology* 31, 933
Pearson, C.H. and Whitehead, J.E.M. (1974) *Journal of Clinical Pathology* 27, 430
Phillips I., Warren, C. and Waterworth, P.M. (1978) *Journal of Clinical Pathology* 31, 531
Reeves, D.S. and Bywater, M.J. (1976) In: *Selected Topics in Clinical Bacteriology*. Ed. by J. de Louvois, Baillière Tindall, London
Reeves, D.S., Phillips, J., Williams, J.D. and Wise, R. (Eds) (1978) *Laboratory Methods in Antimicrobial Chemotherapy*. Churchill Livingstone, London.
Ryan, K.J., Needham, G.M., Dunsmoor, C.L. and Sherris, J.C. (1970) *Applied Microbiology* 20, 447
Sanders, C. (1983) *Journal of Infectious Diseases* 147, 585
Simmons, N.A. (1980) In: *Antibiotics and Chemotherapy*, p. 157 Ed. by R.N. Grüneberg. MTP Press, Lancaster

Stokes, E.J. and Waterworth, P.M. (1972) *Association of Clinical Pathologists Broadsheet* No. 55 (revised)

Waterworth, P.M. (1976) *Journal of Antimicrobial Chemotherapy* **2**, 104

Waterworth, P.M. (1978) *Journal of Antimicrobial Chemotherapy* **4**, 4

Waterworth, P.M. and Del Piano, M. (1976) *Journal of Clinical Pathology* **29**, 179

Weinstein, M.P., Stratton, C.W., Ackley, A *et al.* (1985) *American Journal of Medicine* **78**, 262

10

Clinical Immunology

Antigen–antibody reactions are employed both for the identification of microbes and to demonstrate antibodies in human serum to pathogenic organisms. Specific antigen–antibody reactions are now so sensitive that very small amounts of antigen can be detected. This is a great advantage when patients have received antimicrobial treatment which makes isolation of the pathogen impossible. By demonstrating specific antigen in cerebrospinal fluid, serum or exudate a specific laboratory diagnosis can be made, often within an hour or two of receiving the specimen. A positive result is valuable in indicating appropriate treatment in meningitis, in pneumonia and in virus infections. Except in speed of result such methods are, however, inferior to culture because only antigen is identified, which may be common to more than one microbial species, and because there is no possibility of testing sensitivity of the pathogen to antimicrobials. Serological tests in routine use for the identification of pathogens have been described in Chapter 5. Those commonly made to demonstrate antibody in the patient's serum have now to be considered. This will be followed by an account of tests for demonstrating microbial antigen in specimens.

Demonstration of antibody

The value of a search for antibodies varies greatly in different clinical conditions. For example, in the diagnosis of syphilis the causative spirochaete cannot be cultivated. Antibody tests are therefore important because the reaction is usually specific, and, furthermore, the reagin antibody diminishes in treated patients. Even here, however, serological diagnosis is not entirely satisfactory, for two reasons. First, none of the serological tests for syphilis distinguishes between the treponeme causing syphilis and treponemes causing other diseases, such as yaws; further, the reagin test may be positive in a range of diseases unassociated with treponemes. Secondly, the mere presence of treponemal antibody does not in itself confirm a diagnosis of syphilis. Antibody may persist long after the successful treatment of syphilis, or may reflect previous yaws or other treponemal infections. Its presence may lead to a mistaken diagnosis of syphilis as the cause of unexplained disease when in fact the patient is suffering from a new growth or a granuloma caused by some other infection.

Serology in pyrexia of unknown origin

The specific agglutinins formed in serum as a result of bacterial infection are of greater value in excluding the infection than in making a positive diagnosis. They are found in serum long after the patient has recovered and also in the serum of a certain proportion of healthy people with no history of severe febrile illness. Infection by other microbes or severe bleeding may be followed by a rise in titre of antibodies originally formed months or even years previously, the so-called anamnestic reaction. Lack of history of previous infection does not exclude previous antibody formation because diseases such as typhoid fever, which are usually severe, can occur in a very mild and clinically unrecognizable form. Furthermore, previous vaccination, although not wholly protective, will result in antibody production which may confuse the interpretation of test results.

Agglutinins can almost always be found in the serum at the end of the second week in enteric fever. When a patient has suffered from a febrile illness for 2 weeks or more and his serum when adequately tested reveals no enteric agglutinins, this type of infection is very unlikely.

Brucellosis is often diagnosed by the presence of antibodies and a typical temperature chart. If the organism is not isolated the diagnosis remains essentially clinical because brucella agglutinins are sometimes found in serum from healthy people and their presence is therefore not diagnostic. Even when samples of serum are tested and a rising titre is demonstrated, the evidence is still not good enough to stand alone and is of the same kind as the demonstration of acid-fast bacilli in sputum, which is discussed in Chapter 1. When the patient is seen in the acute stage of the disease, blood culture should always be attempted. If performed by the method described on page 25 it is almost always successful.

With very few exceptions, which will be mentioned later, significant antibody titres are not found in the serum until infection has persisted for at least 10 days. Even if antibodies are found in high titre in the first few days they are most unlikely to have been produced in response to the present infection and it is hard to assess the significance of low titres. Therefore serological tests will not as a rule aid early diagnosis. A positive result during the second week is, however, of much greater value if in the early stages of the illness no antibodies were found, but this does not mean that serum must be tested within the first few days of every undiagnosed fever. The following procedure is satisfactory and labour saving. As soon as possible after a generalized infection has been clinically diagnosed, blood is collected for culture. About 5 ml more than is needed for culture is withdrawn and placed in a sterile screw-capped bottle or plugged tube and allowed to clot. The serum is separated and kept in the refrigerator. If in 10 days' time no diagnosis had been made a second sample of blood is taken and tested; when positive the two specimens are tested in parallel. This saves testing each of all paired samples. In many cases by the tenth day the diagnosis will have been made, in which case the original sample of serum can be discarded. Apart from the time saved in avoiding unnecessary early tests, this method is more satisfactory because, when titres are to be compared in two samples of serum, the tests should always be made on the same day by the same person, using the same reagents.

When all appropriate tests described in this chapter are negative, the possibility of invasion by other viruses, fungi, protozoa or helminths should be borne in mind. Enteroviruses can cause febrile illness lasting for several months. The symptoms caused by them are extremely variable and fever may be the only sign. There are so many serological types of these viruses that diagnosis by serology in the absence of isolation is impracticable. Therefore specimens for virus isolation should be taken at the outset when culture is most likely to succeed. Faeces and a throat swab in virus transport medium can be stored at $-70°C$ while investigations for bacterial infection proceed. Isolation of enterovirus alone is not sufficient evidence of infection because healthy people often carry them. Diagnosis must therefore be confirmed by demonstrating at least a fourfold rise in antibody titre when the isolated virus is tested against the two samples of the patient's serum already obtained for bacteriological tests.

Cytomegalovirus is another likely cause of fever without localizing signs, particularly in immunosuppression and in patients who have received many blood transfusions. In this case, diagnosis can be made by the demonstration of a rising titre of complement-fixing antibody; isolation is not essential.

Reactions of diagnostic value

There are three different types of antibody which are commonly demonstrated in patients' serum as an aid to the diagnosis of bacterial infection: agglutinins, complement-fixing antibodies and precipitins. Antibody can also be demonstrated by specific binding with microbial antigen in smears on glass slides. The attached antibody is then recognized by staining with fluorochrome conjugated antihuman globulin. In addition to these a variety of different kinds of antibody such as antitoxins, antihaemolysins, bacteriolysins, bacteriotropins and antifibrinolysins can be found. These are not, however, sufficiently constant, specific and easily demonstrable for aid in routine diagnosis; tests for them may occasionally be helpful.

Empirical antigen–antibody reactions, in which the test antigens are not derived from the causal antigen, were widely used in the past. Examples include the reagin tests employing ox-heart extract as antigen and the Weil–Felix test employing three different *Proteus* suspensions to diagnose rickettsial infection. Cold agglutinations and streptococcus MG agglutination in mycoplasmal pneumonia are a further example. By their nature, these tests lack specificity and, in some cases, sensitivity. In all these conditions, the specific microbial antigen can now be successfully employed. In Britain, where rickettsial infection is uncommon, it is more reliable and economical to confirm the diagnosis by sending serum to a reference laboratory. Tests for reagin retain their usefulness because, unlike specific tests, the titre falls rapidly with successful treatment.

A search for antibody may be needed when deep-seated staphylococcal infection is suspected (e.g. osteomyelitis of the spine). Blood culture is often positive in these patients but may not be when antimicrobial treatment has been given recently. Antibodies to several different staphylococcal antigens have been studied in an attempt to improve the diagnostic value of these tests but interpretation is difficult because many healthy people have staphylococcal antibody in their serum. However, a high titre of one or more of the staphylococcal antibodies is of some diagnostic value. Since interpretation is difficult and the tests are not often required, serum is best examined and the results assessed by a reference laboratory.

Reliability of standard techniques

Although combination between antigen and specific antibody has been studied by many workers for a number of years, many phenomena associated with the reactions are still not well understood. The tests which have been evolved for use in diagnosis are the result of much detailed investigation. It is impossible here to discuss fully the reason for each step as the tests are described, and in fact the only reason for many procedures is that they have been found to give reliable results in a large series of cases. It must be stressed, however, that if reliable results are to be obtained each step must be slavishly followed. Minor departures from the original technique may not apparently make any difference, but no difference is likely to be noticed unless a large number of sera (proved positive and negative by other means) are tested by the original and the modified method in parallel, and this is necessary whenever a modification is introduced. The factors which are known to influence the reactions are: the proportion of antigen and antibody in the mixture; the time and temperature of the reaction; the rate at which the reagents are mixed (which includes the volume of each of the fluids to be mixed and the size and shape of the vessel in which they are mixed); the presence and concentration of electrolytes; and the pH of the diluting fluids.

All glassware used for serology must be specially cleaned apart from the rest of the laboratory glassware. Saline solutions are made with pure (Analar) sodium chloride in water twice distilled in a glass still. Buffer solutions are often recommended and can be obtained in concentrated form for easy preparation. The laboratory must ensure that the distilled water in which they are diluted is of very high quality. Bottles of distilled water or saline prepared in the hospital pharmacy for therapeutic use are sometimes employed. This is undesirable because pyrogen-free solutions for parenteral use in patients may be insufficiently pure for serological tests.

Instructions sent with commercially obtained antigens should be read with care and the technique recommended should be followed or there must be a good reason for any departure from it. The antigen may not perform reliably when the conditions of the test are altered.

Newer techniques, especially those employing viral antigens, need micro methods because reagents are costly. Manual methods must be

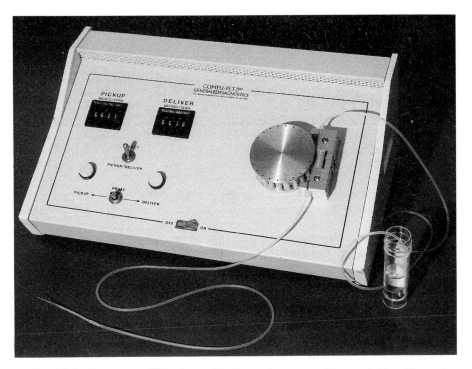

Fig. 10.1   Compu-pet 200 electronic diluter dispenser with microtubing (General Diagnostics).

performed with great dexterity if they are to be accurate when handling very small volumes, and some form of mechanical aid is essential if speed and accuracy with minimal fatigue are to be attained. The Compupet 200 electronic dispenser-diluter (General Diagnostics Warner & Co.) (Fig. 10.1) has proved to be versatile and reliable and needs very little maintenance (Cremer *et al.*, 1975). Micro methods using this machine are described but they need only minor adjustment for those having other equipment.

Specific agglutination tests

Tests for *Salmonella* agglutinations are based on the Widal test. In Britain, the test should cover not only typhoid and paratyphoid species but also other salmonellae and the *Brucella* group. The typhoid and para-typhoid organisms possess both flagellar (H) and somatic (O) antigens, and it is necessary to test for both types of corresponding antibodies.

The commonest cause of brucellosis in Britain is *Br. abortus*. Specific agglutinations will be present in the patient's serum from the second week of an acute attack. Specimens of serum should be tested against both *Br. abortus* and *Br. melitensis* suspensions because these species have antigens in common. Moreover, some biotypes of *Br. abortus* give rise to antibody which, when tested against standard suspensions, agglutinates *Br. melitensis* to a higher titre than the typical standard *Br. abortus* suspension.

Agglutination tests may show the prozone phenomenon. This is a particular problem with specimens containing brucella agglutinins, where it may extend to a high titre. This must be taken into account when screening tests are performed (see below). Paratyphoid A and C are rare in Britain, and tests for them may be omitted if the patient is known not to have been abroad or in contact with travellers.

Agglutination tests for brucellosis are no longer performed on serum from all febrile patients. They are needed when exposure to infection seems likely or when specially requested. Culture methods have improved and *Brucella* may be isolated in the absence of agglutinating antibodies. Antigens must be prepared from absolutely smooth strains, otherwise false positive agglutination will be seen. Agglutination is finely granular and micro methods have not proved satisfactory. Cross-reaction between *Br. abortus* and serum from patients infected with *Yersinia enterocolitica* type 9 will be seen because they have O antigens in common. Such sera will, however, agglutinate the H antigen of *Y. enterocolitica* (Lindberg *et al.*, 1982). Negative serum from patients clinically likely to have brucellosis but who are also culture negative should be further examined by a reference laboratory. Positive agglutination when cultures are negative should also be checked.

Method

The antigen suspensions used in the following descriptions are available from Wellcome Diagnostics. The serum is not inactivated since heating to 56°C will destroy some agglutinating antibodies.

Salm. typhi and *Salm. paratyphi*

Using U-well plastic microtitre trays and the Compu-pet diluter, make a 1 : 5 master dilution and nine rows of doubling dilutions from it for each serum to be tested as follows. Prime the tubing with saline (see page 55). Pick up 100 μl serum and dispense into a 5-ml capped container with 400 μl saline; mix by inversion of the container. Pick up 50 μl of this master dilution, and dispense with 50 μl of saline into the first well of a 96 U-well plastic microtitre tray. Pick up 50 μl from well 1, and dispense with 50 μl of saline into well 2. Continue doubling dilutions to well 7, and then discard 50 μl from well 7. Well 8 is left empty. This process is repeated using the same dilution to produce nine rows of diluted serum. Add 50 μl of saline to well 8 in each row. To each well in a single row add 5 μl of the appropriate antigen as follows:

Row 1 *Salm. paratyphi* A-H
Row 2 *Salm. paratyphi* B-H
Row 3 *Salm. paratyphi* C-H
Row 4 *Salm. typhi* H
Row 5 Non-specific *Salmonella* H

Row 6 *Salm. paratyphi* A-O
Row 7 *Salm. paratyphi* B-O
Row 8 *Salm. paratyphi* C-O
Row 9 *Salm. typhi* O

To all wells, in all rows, add 50 μl of saline. This serves to mix the constituents, and provides the final dilutions as follows:

Well	1	2	3	4	5	6	7	8
Dilution	1/20	1/40	1/80	1/160	1/320	1/640	1/1280	Control

Cover the microtitre tray and place it in a 50°C incubator for 4 hours or overnight before reading. Plates are best observed with a concave (magnifying) mirror under the plate, using transmitted light. The antibody titre is the weakest dilution to show agglutination. O agglutinations are granular, whereas H agglutinations are floccular in appearance. The suspension is unchanged in a negative well and in the saline control. The titre of the serum for each antigen is reported. This record may be important for the assessment of any future serological tests.

Br. abortus and Br. melitensis
A suitable volume for the test is 1 ml in 50 × 12 mm glass tubes. The reaction occurs best when incubated at 37°C; therefore 0.25% phenol saline is employed.

Set up two rows of 9 tubes for each serum to be tested. Make 2 volumes of a 1 : 20 dilution of serum in the first tube of each row (0.1 ml serum in 1.9 ml 0.25% phenol saline). To each of the remaining tubes add 1 volume saline. Double dilute from tube 1 to tube 8, discarding 1 volume from tube 8. Add 1 drop of *Br. abortus* concentrated antigen to each tube in row 1, and 1 drop of *Br. melitensis* antigen to each tube in row 2. Tube 9 is the antigen control. Mix by shaking, and incubate in a waterbath at 37° for 24 hours. Examine tubes macroscopically in a bright light, using a concave mirror to see the fine granular pattern in positive tubes more clearly. Negative tubes and the antigen controls are unchanged.

The titre is the weakest dilution to show macroscopic agglutination. A prozone is often observed with high titre sera.

Control positive sera are available to confirm the activity of the antigen suspensions. A rapid screening test is also available. We do not recommend it for diagnosis in individual patients but it is of value for screening large numbers of sera. At least two serum dilutions must be tested because of the likelihood of a prozone.

Antibodies in enteric fever
Salmonellae causing enteric fever stimulate the formation of three types of agglutinin which are of use in diagnosis; they are H, O and Vi. The H antibody, which is produced in response to stimulation by flagellar antigens, appears towards the end of the first week of the disease, and usually reaches the highest titre. It persists longer than the others after recovery, sometimes for many years, and its formation may again be stimulated non-specifically in subsequent febrile illnesses. Agglutination is rapid (it

can usually be seen after 2 hours' incubation) and the agglutinated bacilli form large fluffy clumps. There is no evidence that H antibody is protective or helps to combat the disease.

Formation of O antibody is stimulated by O somatic antigens. It also appears in the first week of illness and seldom rises above a titre of about 640. After recovery the titre falls and it is seldom demonstrable a year later. Production is not easily stimulated non-specifically in subsequent illness. Agglutination occurs more slowly (after 4 hours' incubation) and the clumps of bacilli are small and dense.

The Vi antigen, also somatic, is possessed by *Salm. typhi., Salm. paratyphi C* and other coliforms, including certain strains of *Esch. coli.* Typhoid and paratyphoid bacilli which possess large quantities of this antigen often give rise to severe disease. Occasionally, only Vi antibody can be demonstrated; such cases are rare, however, and there is no need to perform the Vi agglutination test in every case. The antibody is probably of value in combating infection by Vi strains (see page 249).

In the majority of patients H and O agglutinins can be easily demonstrated. Occasionally only one of the agglutinins is found, and very occasionally no specific antibody is demonstrable in enteric fever confirmed by blood culture.

Significance of results

It is impossible to lay down definite rules for the significance of various titres. The agglutination results must be judged in the light of all other findings. Their significance depends on (1) the duration of the illness at the time the specimen was taken, (2) evidence of previous infection or prophylactic inoculation and (3) the level of titres found in the sera of healthy people in the population of which the patient is a member.

In Britain, titres to the enteric group in healthy people are low, and at the end of the first week an H agglutinin titre of 1 : 80 in an uninoculated patient who has had no previous salmonella infection may be significant. An O agglutinin tire of 1 : 80 or more is good evidence of active infection, especially if it has been shown to rise to this level since the beginning of the disease. This finding has some significance even in inoculated and previously infected patients because O, unlike H, agglutinins are not maintained in the serum for long periods, neither are they often increased non-specifically. In general, diagnosis of enteric fever by agglutination tests alone is unsatisfactory, and, in previously infected patients and those who have received prophylactic typhoid inoculation, it is often impossible. Other salmonellae share H and O antigens with the enteric fever group; for example, *Salm. typhi* and *Salm. dublin* share 09. Thus, infection with non-enteric fever strains will produce specific antibody rises which may lead to errors of interpretation.

Agglutination tests for *Br. abortus* are more easily interpreted and therefore of more value in diagnosis. Although humans are not commonly inoculated against brucellosis, a kind of accidental inoculation often occurs in people whose way of life exposes them to the risk of infection, such as those who drink large quantities of raw milk and those in contact with infected animals or carcases. Provided such people are excluded, a titre of 1 : 80 or more in the second week of the disease can fairly safely be taken as evidence of infection. Later the titre rises much higher but at the end of 3 months or so no reaction may be seen. In chronic brucellosis the standard agglutination test is often negative, but antibody may be demonstrable by the antiglobulin agglutination (Coomb's) test, or by a complement fixation test employing the agglutination suspension as antigen. Since symptoms are variable these additional tests should be done on serum from patients suffering from chronic undiagnosed ill health who have been exposed to brucella either by drinking raw milk or by nature of their work. Further information will be found in the PHLS Monograph No. 14 (1980).

Other causes of enteric-like fever

When the extended Widal test is negative in the second week of an enteric-like infection, other agglutination tests may indicate the cause. The Vi agglutination test may be positive, although by this time the infection will probably have been diagnosed by blood or faeces culture; infection by a non-motile Vi-positive strain is very rare.

The Vi agglutination titre is now considered unsuitable for performance, except by reference laboratories. The test is not easy to carry out, and is seldom required in Britain.

Positive agglutination with leptospiral suspensions may enable a diagnosis of Weil's disease or canicola fever to be made. Infections which must be considered, and which are diagnosed by other means, are meningococcal and other subacute bacteraemia, rickettsial diseases, infective hepatitis, glandular fever and toxoplasmosis. In any undiagnosed febrile illness tuberculosis must be excluded; it is sometimes very difficult to diagnose in the first few weeks. Finally, although very rare in Britain, generalized fungal infections such as histoplasmosis and coccidioidosis must be considered   (see Chapter 7). Protozoa other than toxoplasma must be borne in mind, particularly in patients who have lived abroad within the last 2 years (see Chapter 8).

Complement fixation tests

Complement fixation tests have played an important part in the serological diagnosis of infections for very many years. They have been employed for all varieties of microbe, including bacteria, viruses, fungi, protozoa and helminths. The principle involves an antibody/antigen reaction in the presence of complement. The end result of this reaction is not visible to the naked eye in most circumstances. A second reaction is therefore used to provide an indicator system. The most convenient indicator is the complement-dependent lysis of sheep red blood cells sensitized by an antibody prepared against them in rabbit serum. If complement-fixing antibody is present in the patient's serum, complement will be fixed in the primary reaction, and will be unavailable to take part in the sheep red cell/antisheep red cell reaction; lysis will not therefore occur.

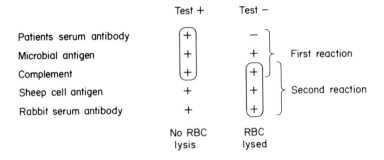

Fig. 10.2   Complement fixation test.

In the absence of antibody, complement will not be fixed, and will be available to take part in the secondary reaction, resulting in lysis of the sheep red blood cells (Fig. 10.2).

The amount of complement (usually obtained from guinea-pig serum) needs careful adjustment so that it is impossible in any one test for both reactions to occur completely. All reagents require careful preparation and standardization. Complement fixation tests are therefore demanding of technical time and expertise. Additionally, these tests are often of low specificity and low sensitivity. Advances in serological diagnostic techniques and (to a lesser extent) antigen detection techniques have considerably reduced the usefulness of the complement fixation test in the diagnostic laboratory. Complement fixation remains a useful method for research and for reference procedures, especially in virology, but has been superseded by more sensitive and less labour-intensive techniques for the diagnosis of syphilis, which was its main role in hospital laboratories. It is not a technique likely to be reliable when seldom performed. Previous editions of *Clinical Bacteriology* (Stokes and Ridgway, 1980) provide details of the technique and may be referred to by anyone wishing to perform the test.

Enzyme-linked immunosorbent assay (ELISA)

The development of enzyme-linked immunosorbent assays (ELISA) has been a major advance for the detection of both antibody and antigen in clinical specimens. The technique was originally described by Engvall and Perlmann (1971), and has undergone a rapid evolution to produce the various modifications of the system available today. The underlying principle is illustrated in Fig. 10.3. The solid phase may take the form of tubes, microtitre plates or beads, usually or polystyrene or polyvinyl. A number of enzyme detection systems are available, but those most frequently encountered in clinical practice utilize horseradish peroxidase or alkaline phosphatase. The colour change (which may be production of a colour or decolorization, depending on the system) may be observed macroscopically or read by machine. Large numbers of specimens can be conveniently processed by these methods, often requiring very small samples.

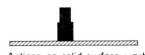

1. Antigen on solid surface, wash.

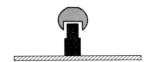

2. Add serum, antibody attaches, wash.

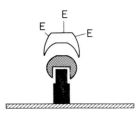

3. Add enzyme - labelled antiglobulin, wash.

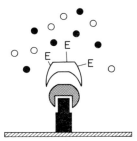

4. Add substrate, observe colour change.

Fig. 10.3 Enzyme-linked immunosorbent assay (ELISA).

Variations in the technique, such as the double antibody–sandwich ELISA, allow the detection of antigen. The tests in general have a sensitivity similar to radioimmunoassay, but do not require expensive and potentially hazardous reagents nor sophisticated counting machines.

Many ELISA systems are now available in commercial kit form, and doubtless many more will be available in the future. As with all innovative methods, it is incumbent upon the user to satisfy himself that the test has been properly evaluated in the field, and to be fully aware of the limitations of both the technique and the test kit.

Serological tests for the diagnosis of syphilis

Three kinds of antibody are present during the course of syphilis: reagin antibody, group antitreponemal antibody and specific antitreponemal antibody. The first to appear and the last to disappear is the specific antitreponemal antibody, which is recognized in most laboratories by the absorbed fluorescent treponemal antibody (FTA-ABS) test. Another test, the *Treponema pallidum* immobilization (TPI) test, is the most specific one available. However, the TPI utilizes living treponemes, maintained by passage in rabbits' testes. The test is expensive, potentially hazardous and available at only a few reference laboratories world wide; it is rarely required. A third test for specific antitreponemal antibody is the

Tr. pallidum haemagglutination (TPHA) test. Sheep, chick or turkey red blood cells, sensitized by attaching killed *Tr. pallidum* to them, will agglutinate in the presence of antibody. The test is much easier to perform and to read than the FTA-ABS test and no special microscopic equipment is required. It is less sensitive than the fluorescence test and therefore is not as reliable for the diagnosis of primary syphilis. Occasional false positive results are encountered and the diagnosis should always be confirmed by the FTA-ABS test.

The detection of specific antibody is mandatory for the diagnosis of the disease but the titre does not alter very much during treatment. A positive test does not necessarily imply that further treatment is required, neither does a continuing positive test imply that treatment already implemented is ineffective – indeed, this is to be expected.

Group antitreponemal antibody is detected by the Reiter protein complement fixation test (RPCFT). Antibody appears later in the disease than specific antibody, and some syphilitic patients do not develop it at all. The RPCFT has been superseded for diagnostic purposes by the more convenient and sensitive specific antibody tests.

The Wassermann reaction, which has in the past been the most widely practised test for diagnosis, is a complement fixation test employing non-specific lipoidal antigen derived from animal tissue. It recognizes reagin, an antibody produced in the active stages of the disease which is much more commonly found in syphilis than in other infections but is not specific for this disease. The most important false positive reactions are caused by the presence of antibody in the serum associated with other diseases. These biological false positives (BFP) are of two kinds, acute and chronic. Acute BFPs may be found following any infection associated with fever. Bacterial and viral pneumonias, vaccination with live attenuated viruses and malaria are common examples. The reagin antibody is usually of a low titre and transient (less than 6 months). It may occasionally occur in normal people for no apparent reason, and in pregnancy. Chronic BFPs are found in autoimmune-type diseases, and sensitive antilipoidal assays outside the scope of this book are employed in their diagnosis. Leprosy is the only known infection associated with a chronic BFP.

A quantitative test for reagin is needed to monitor progress since the titre of this antibody falls rapidly during successful treatment. Indeed, in the past when the Wassermann reaction alone was relied on for the diagnosis, there was a danger that treatment with penicillin for other infection might obliterate reagin before the diagnosis of syphilis could be made. This led to a late diagnosis when the disease relapsed after inadequate treatment and reagin reappeared.

There are now a large numbers of tests for reagin. The original Wassermann reaction and its modifications are less favoured than previously, partly because it does not lend itself to automation but also because other more easily performed and more sensitive tests are now available, one of the most popular being the Venereal Diseases Reference laboratory (VDRL) test. The rapid plasma reagin (RPR) card test is convenient for diagnostic purposes. The antigen is mixed with fine carbon particles, making the flocculation in a positive result easy to see. The automated reagin test (ART), which is a modification of the VDRL test, is ideal for screening blood for transfusion but even large diagnostic departments handle insufficient blood samples to justify the purchase of the costly equipment required; mechanization using an electronic diluter which can easily be employed for other purposes is more satisfactory, much less expensive and requires no special maintenance.

Although there is an increasing tendency for all veneral disease serology to be performed in reference laboratories by automated methods, hospitals with large outpatient departments of genitourinary medicine usually prefer the hospital diagnostic laboratory to undertake these tests, and indeed discussion between clinician and laboratory is as rewarding here as in other fields.

The tests which have so far proved most satisfactory for diagnosis and monitoring treatment are the rapid plasma reagin (RPR) card test, and the *Treponema pallidum* haemagglutination (TPHA) test. As a check on positive results and for diagnosis of primary infection, the absorbed fluorescent treponemal antibody (FTA-ABS) test is also needed. In each of these tests known positive and negative sera must be tested in parallel.

The above tests may be used for cerebrospinal fluid (CSF). However, it should be stressed that the cell count and protein content are more sensitive indicators of neurological involvement in syphilis. On occasion, they will be abnormal in the presence of negative serological tests on the CSF.

Methods
Control sera
Sera (either positive or negative to all these tests) which are clear and non-fatty are pooled and then distributed in aliquots sufficient for one batch of tests. These are frozen and one aliquot of each is thawed for use on the day of the test, when it is heated again at 56°C for 10 minutes. Both a weak and a strong positive control serum are needed for the FTA-ABS test. Each new pool of positive serum is tested in parallel with the previous pool.

Rapid plasma reagin (RPR) card test
This test is a flocculation test employing a modified VDRL antigen containing carbon particles. It was originally developed in 1962 for work in the field, and it can be done on either plasma or unheated serum without special laboratory equipment. It was modified by Portnoy, one of the original inventors, in 1963 for large-scale screening in the laboratory and a quantitative test was developed. The advantages of the test for laboratory use are that it can be done in small batches as the sera arrive, without inactivation, and no microscope is needed for reading. No glassware is employed, and it is at least as sensitive and specific as other reagin tests (Scrimgeour and Roslin, 1973).

Materials:
> Qualitative test kit, VDRL carbon antigen (Cambridge Biomedical Ltd).
> Quantitative test kit No. DR525 (Oxoid Ltd)
> Test cards (Oxoid Ltd)
> Dispenser/stirers, 0.05 ml (Dispenstirs, Oxoid Ltd)
> Mechanical rotator to rotate at 100 r.p.m. in 1.9 cm circle.
> Unheated patients' sera.

Positive and negative serum controls. These will be inactivated frozen aliquots (see above); the titre will be a little reduced by inactivation but will remain stable for several months.

All reagents must be allowed to reach room temperature, not be tested cold direct from the refrigerator.

Method
Instructions are included in each antigen package. The serum is dispensed with the plastic tubes, which resemble short plastic drinking straws with a flattened end. When squeezed between thumb and finger, sufficient serum can be drawn up and transferred to the appropriate, prenumbered, circle on the card; it is distributed over the area of the circle using the flattened end of the tube, which is then discarded. A drop of antigen is added, from the container and delivery needle provided, and the card is then placed on the rotator for 8 minutes, which mixes antigen and serum. The serum and antigen must not be mixed before rotation. The tests are then read in the wet state. In practice about 40 tests can be done at a time – there are 10 circles on each card; attempts to do more than this will lead to drying during rotation. While 4 cards are rotating, another 40 tests can be prepared. Covers for the cards during rotation can be obtained from the manufacturers but in Britain where the atmosphere is usually damp they are not needed. The majority of tests are easy to read. All positive tests and any where the result is in doubt are tested quantitatively.

The kit for the quantitative test contains disposable pipettes with which twofold dilutions can be made in saline on the cards. We have found the titre to be approximately twofold higher than for the quantitative VDRL in parallel tests. A prozone effect is occasionally seen, the reaction becoming more positive on dilution and then fading away, but false negative results in the screening test due to this effect are very rare (Scrimgeour and Roslin, 1973).

Treponema pallidum haemagglutination (TPHA) test
The reagents for this test are commercially prepared and provided in kits containing an absorbing diluent, lyophilized sheep cells sensitized with *Tr. pallidum* and unsensitized control cells. A reactive (positive) serum is included. The reagents cannot be obtained separately. Control and sensitized red cells are standardized and batches are not interchangeable; excess reagents must therefore be discarded. Two standard dropping pipettes for delivery of sensitized and control cells are included; a leaflet describing methods for macro-and micro-assay is provided. Since the reagents are costly, laboratories will normally use the micro method.

Microtitre trays and diluters (Takatsi loops) are needed for the micro method described in the leaflet. Alternatively, if the method is slightly modified, an electronic dispenser–diluter, Compu-pet 200 (see page 245), can be employed which is highly accurate and enables large numbers of tests to be done by one person without fatigue; for a description of this machine, see Cremer *et al.* (1975).

Since the TPHA is recommended for screening and all positive sera are further examined by other methods, a quantitative test is not essential although this can be carried out if desired. No prozone in this reaction has been recorded; therefore only one dilution need be tested. The method using the Compu-pet 200 and only one dilution is believed to be the most economical and least laborious way of performing this valuable test.

Mechanized micro method:
Materials

TPHA Test Antigen kit (FD101E, Diamed Diagnostics Ltd)
Microtitre trays with U-wells and covers
Compu-pet 200 with microtubing and pipette
3 conical flasks (100 ml) or beakers
Wash-out receptacle
Clean absorbent paper wipes

Method
Reconstitute the red cells with the reconstituting fluid provided, as directed.

Fill one flask with absorbing diluent and prime the machine by placing the non-delivering end of the microtubing in it and pressing the constant delivery switch.

When the tubing and pipette are full of diluent and free from air bubbles, make a 1 : 20 dilution of each serum (1 : 5 for CSF) to be tested and dispense them into wells of the microtitre trays as follows:

Pick up 5 μl serum, deliver 100 μl into well 1.

Pick up 10 μl of air (to separate diluent from serum dilution during dispensing).

Pick up 50 μl of the 1 : 20 dilution from well 1 and deliver 20 μl into each of the next two wells. Wash the micropipette by delivering 20 μl three times into the waste receptacle. Wipe the tip of the pipette on fresh absorbent paper and proceed to the next serum. Continue thus until all sera have been diluted and dispensed, including a positive and a negative control which should be dispensed in this order to check efficiency of wash-out.

Leave the diluted sera at room temperature for 30 minutes to complete absorption of non-specific reactive substances which they may contain.

Prime the microtubing, in the manner described above, with sensitized cells and dispense 60 μl into each well 2.

Wash the whole of the microtubing and pipette through with distilled water, prime with control unsensitized cells and deliver 60 μl into each well 3.

Mix thoroughly by tapping the tray gently. Cover and leave undisturbed at room temperature for 3–4 hours, when a preliminary reading is possible. Read finally after 18 hours at room temperature. Appearances of positive and negative tests are described in the manufacturer's leaflet.

Absorbed fluorescent treponemal antigen (FTA-ABS) test

This test has replaced the original indirect fluorescence test in which the patient's serum was diluted 1 : 200. The sorbent removes the group treponemal antibody, enabling the test for specific antibody to be performed on serum diluted 1 : 5. This greatly enchances the sensitivity of the test.

It is an indirect test in which absorbed patient's serum is applied to killed *Tr. pallidum* suspension on microscope slides. After incubation the slides are thoroughly washed in phosphate buffer to remove serum which has not bound specifically to the treponemes, and then treated with fluorescein–isothiocyanate-conjugated antihuman gamma-globulin serum. When this is washed off, only those treponemes which have been in contact with specific antibody in the patient's serum will retain the fluorescent antiserum.

The reagents are costly; therefore the test is limited to sera which are positive in at least one of the screening tests and to those from patients suspected of primary disease. Confirmation of a positive result, by repeating the test, is often desirable and is necessary in primary syphilis when the diagnosis rests on this test alone; to retest repeatedly during treatment serves no useful purpose.

Materials

Sorbent	Difco 3259–57 Bacto FTA sorbent
Antigen slide, ready coated with *Tr. pallidum*	Clinical Sciences Inc. FTA-absorbed slides (No. 1871, Diamed)
Fluorescein-conjugated antihuman gamma-globulin serum	Wellcome MF01 Fluorescent Antibodies antihuman globulin (sheep)
Phosphate-buffered saline (PBS)	Mercia Diagnostics PBS pH 7.2 for ANF test (100 ml to make 2.5 litres)
Coverslips (70 × 20 mm)	Chance Propper Ltd
Mounting fluid	Difco Bacto 2329–56 FA mounting fluid
Plastic pipettes of uniform size to drop 0.05 ml approx.	Liquipettes 127-P511-000 (ELKAY)
Coplin jars	

Moist chamber, e.g. a plastic box with well-fitting lid containing moist blotting paper.

Microscope with integral iodine quartz or mecury vapour discharge lamp. Darkground condenser or incident light system. Objective lens (with diaphragms) to magnify about × 500.

Filters. For dark-ground system, a yellow barrier filter (OGI) and a blue exciter filter (BG12 for mercury vapour lamp) will be required.

For incident light use interference filter (DS500), and blue barrier filter (LP515).

Note. An incident light system has two important optical advantages: Much less transmitted light is lost, and the system, once set up, is always in optical alignment. There is no substage condenser; both light from the source and that transmitted from the fluorescing specimen travel through the objective. A dichroic mirror separates the source of light from the transmitted light. Most major microscope manufacturers are now marketing such systems.

Titration of conjugate

The activity of commercially produced conjugate varies considerably, and a good conjugate is essential; those supplied by Nordic Pharmaceuticals, Baltimore Biological Laboratories and Wellcome Diagnostics Ltd have been found satisfactory (PHLS Monograph No. 1, 1972). The working titre of each batch should be tested as follows.

Make twofold dilutions of conjugate from 1 : 10 to 1 : 320 in phosphate-buffered saline (PBS). Test each against a strong positive, a weak positive and a negative (PBS only) control. Use slides with three test areas each (i.e. one slide for each dilution of conjugate tested).

The working dilution is half the weakest dilution which gives brilliant fluorescence with the strongly positive, and weak fluorescence with the weakly positive control. Treponemes in the negative control area should not fluoresce with the strongest (1 : 10) dilution of conjugate.

Store undiluted conjugate frozen in small aliquots. Once thawed for use, store at 4°C, preferably with 0.1% azide as a preservative; repeated freezing and thawing is harmful.

The test

Specimens of serum are inactivated at 56°C for 30 minutes before testing. Place in a rack one small (75 × 13 mm) tube for each serum to be tested and deliver into each of them 4 drops sorbent from a standard dropper. Then deliver 1 drop serum into each using a separate pipette for each serum; include strong positive, weak positive and negative serum controls (see page 253). The pipette must be held vertically and the drops allowed to form naturally, not prematurely shaken off. Mix by shaking the rack and stand it at room temperature (22°C) for 30 minutes. Then place 2 drops of the serum sorbent mixture from each tube onto a prepared area on a slide and spread gently over the area with the tip of the pipette, taking care not to scrape the slide.

Incubate in a moist chamber at 37°C for 30 minutes. Wash the slides well with PBS into a sink and then place them in PBS in a Coplin jar for 10 minutes, changing the buffer three times during this time. Blot dry carefully.

Spread 2 drops conjugated antihuman globulin serum at the optimum titre on each test area and reincubate in the moist chamber as before. Repeat the washing procedure and blot dry.

Mount the slides using the fluid and coverslips listed above. Read.

When an ordinary cardioid dark-ground condenser is used, non-fluorescent immersion oil (Gurr Products) must be placed between the condenser and the slide. An oil immersion objective is not required.

When using a dark-ground condenser system it is important that the condenser and lenses give maximum fluorescence over a small field; immunofluorescence is weaker than simple staining with a fluorescent dye (see page 146). Precise adjustment of the optical system is vital, and incident light microscopy systems are to be preferred.

Inspect the controls first.

An indirect fluorescence test, similar to the FTA-ABS but using a specific fluorescent serum conjugate reacting only with IgM human globulin, can be employed. This test is of particular use in the diagnosis of congenital syphilis. Its value in other situations, such as reinfection, is less clear as IgM class antibodies may persist after treatment.

Significance of serological reactions in the diagnosis of syphilis

Much has been written on this subject and it is impossible here to do more than indicate briefly a few important points.

Rapid plasma reagin (RPR) card test, VDRL, ART, WR, Kahn

All these test for reagin. A positive result in a syphilitic patient (diagnosed by specific tests) may indicate the need for treatment. The RPR is the most sensitive of these tests (Scrimgeour and Roslin, 1973). In secondary and active tertiary syphilis it is almost invariably positive. During therapy of early syphilis the titre is expected to fall and the test is of value in monitoring progress. A prozone may be encountered with strongly reactive sera.

None of these tests alone or combined are satisfactory for the diagnosis of syphilis. Non-specific results are comparatively common.

Reiter protein complement fixation test

A group specific treponemal antibody test, positive in syphilis and other trepanematoses shortly after the onset of symptoms. It may be positive before tests for reagin and has been a useful screening test. The more specific TPHA test is now preferred for screening.

Tr. pallidum haemagglutination (TPHA) test

A positive TPHA test in Britain is good evidence of syphilis; it will also be positive in yaws and related treponemal diseases but not in other infections. It is a sensitive screening test and becomes positive earlier than the Reiter protein CFT, which it has replaced, but is less sensitive than the FTA-ABS test. Occasional false positives are seen and the diagnosis should always be confirmed by the FTA-ABS test.

Absorbed fluorescence treponemal antibody (FTA-ABS) test

This is the most specific and most sensitive of the common diagnostic tests. The FTA-ABS may be positive early in the disease, before the reagin or TPHA tests. It is therefore important to perform this test on all cases of genital ulceration in addition to the other tests for syphilis. It is believed to detect the same antibody as the TPHA. When both tests are positive on more than one occasion, it is certain that the patient has at some time

suffered treponemal infection. However, positive results give no indication of the activity of the disease. Occasional false positives may occur,
particularly in patients with systemic lupus erythematosus. An atypical
beaded fluorescence of the treponemes is usually seen in these cases.

Treponemal immobilization (TPI) test
This is the most specific of all available tests for treponemal antibody, but
it is rarely performed (page 251).

None of the above tests will distinguish syphilis from yaws or other
related treponemal infections. Should it prove impossible to rule out
active syphilis after consideration of the patient's history and the results of
serological investigations, then antibiotic treatment is indicated.

Gonorrhoea

Gonococcal complement fixation test (GCFT)
In the past this test was routinely performed on the serum of patients
suspected of venereal disease, but this is no longer the case, partly because
culture methods (page 77) are so much improved that even in chronic
infection culture is a more reliable method of diagnosis than a serological
test and partly because it has proved very difficult to maintain a supply of
satisfactory antigen commercially.

The test does not differentiate between current and past infection, and
false positive results are a problem. Despite much active research into new
methods there is at present no satisfactory technique for the serological
diagnosis of gonococcal infection.

Serological tests for Chlamydial infections

The genus *Chlamydia* is now recognized as a major cause of disease world
wide (Ridgway, 1986). *Chlam. psittaci* is a zoonosis, causing atypical
pneumonia in man when acquired from contact with birds. More recently,
the organism has been increasingly associated with abortion in women in
contact with infected sheep.

In adults, *Chlam. trachomatis* causes conjunctivitis (including
trachoma), lymphogranuloma venereum, non-gonococcal genital infection, salpingitis and infertility. In the neonate, *Chlam. trachomatis* is a
cause of non-gonococcal ophthalmia neonatorum and of a characteristic
pneumonitis.

Diagnostic laboratories are under increasing pressure to provide a
diagnostic service for chlamydiae. The most efficient and least contro-
versial method of diagnosis is the isolation of the organism in cell culture
(Ripa and Mårdh, 1977). However, the majority of hospital diagnostic
laboratories will not have easy access to cell culture facilities. Recent
advances in monoclonal antibody technology have produced kits based on
immunofluorescence or enzyme-linked immunosorbent assay (ELISA,
see page 250) suitable for the identification of chlamydial antigen directly
from clinical material. These tests are not ideal (see page 270), requiring

some care with performance and interpretation. An attractive alternative would be the use of antibody assay tests on serum for diagnostic pupposes.

The two species of chlamydiae share a common group lipopolysaccharide antigen. Antibodies to this antigen can be detected by a complement fixation test. However, the sensitivity of this test is such that its use is restricted to the diagnosis of psittacosis and lymphogranuloma venereum. More sensitive techniques are required to detect antibody produced by the common oculogenital chlamydial infections. Wang and Grayston (1974) described a microimmunofluorescence test, directed against the major outer membrane protein, which is species and serotype specific. Although important as a research technique for epidemiological studies, the method is technically demanding and the antigen preparations required are not readily available. Certain serotypes, of *Chlam. trachomatis* cross-react widely with other serotypes, and with *Chlam, psittaci*, and the use of such a strain as a source of common antigen is the basis of the whole inclusion immunofluorescence test described by Richmond and Caul (1975). The test is group specific, and, in common with the complement fixation test, cannot differentiate between *Chlam. trachomatis* and *Chlam. psittaci* infections. Variations of the test (including ELISA techniques) are now commercially available, and will detect IgG, IgM or IgA class antibodies. However, it must be appreciated that the positive predictive power of a single antibody level determination by these tests is poor. Group chlamydial antibody is common in adults. Demonstration of rising antibody titre is therefore necessary. The detection of specific IgM class antibody in sera from neonates suspected of suffering from chlamydial pneumonitis is good confirmatory evidence of the diagnosis.

Legionnaire's disease

The demonstration of serum antibody to *Legionella pneumophila* is, at present, the most reliable way of diagnosing this disease. However, the appearance of antibodies may be delayed for up to 3 weeks; consequently, it may be necessary to examine several samples of serum. Moreover, cross-reactions with other causes of atypical pneumonia, in particular *Mycoplasma pneumoniae*, have been described. Two samples taken not less than 1 week apart should always be examined.

Rapid Microagglutination Test (RMAT)

This test has proved to be a useful method of screening sera for *L. pneumophila* antibodies. Positive results should be confirmed either by a reference laboratory or using the fluorescence antibody test described below.

Materials:

> Antigen: *L. pneumophila* suspension, supplied at working dilution for RMAT (obtainable from Division of Microbiological Reagents and Quality Control

(DMRQ) (see Appendix), Code No. BBA 50883)
Comu-pet 200 (or 20 μl dispenser pipette)
V-well microtitre trays
Phosphate-buffered saline (PBS), pH6.4

Method
Prime Compu-pet with PBS (see pages 245 and 255). For each test serum and positive control pick up 20 μl of serum and dispense 40 μl into first well. Double dilute in 20 μl aliquots out to well 8 (discarding 20 μl from this well) to give a final dilution of 1 : 256. Add 20 μl of antigen to each well. Shake for 10 seconds on a microshaker. Leave undisturbed for 10 minutes at room temperature. Centrifuge for 4 minutes at 1200 r.p.m. at 10°C. Incubate the plate at an angle of 70 degrees for 10 minutes before reading. A positive result is shown by a tight button at the base of the well. Negative wells will show a 'teardrop' streak on one side of the well. Titres greater than 4 are likely to be significant.

Fluorescence antibody test
Materials:

Antigen: Formolized yolk-sac suspension of *L. pneumophila* (obtainable from DMRQ (see Appendix), Code No. BBA 20884) distributed as 1 : 50 working dilution in phosphate-buffered saline (PBS), containing 0.8% sodium azide.*

Conjugate: Wellcome MFO1 Fluorescent Antibodies antihuman globulin (sheep).

Positive and negative control sera. Positive control obtainable from DMRQ, as for 'Antigen' above.

Microscope slides: PTFE-coated Henley-Essex with 3 mm spots No. SM010 (C.A. Henley and Co.)

Method:
Preparation of slides   Place 1 volume of antigen dilution (approximately 5 μl) on each spot on the slide and dry at 37°C for 20 minutes. (Four spots per slide will each receive one of a series of dilutions of a serum to be tested.) Fix in acetone at room temperature (22–25°C) for 15 minutes. Dry in air.

Test   Make twofold dilutions in PBS of each test serum and the positive control serum. The dilutions to be tested are 1 : 32 to 1 : 256, but this can be extended for high titre sera. Number each prepared slide and place 2 volumes of each serum dilution on the appropriate spot on a slide. Continue thus until all spots on all slides have been covered. One spot only is needed for the negative control serum. Incubate all slides in a moist box at 37°C for 30 minutes. Rinse with PBS, then wash with PBS for 15

*More clear-cut results may be obtained by calculating the working dilution for each sample of antigen in the manner described for the FTA-ABS test (page 257).

minutes with two changes of buffer. Finally rinse the slides with distilled water and dry in air.

Add 1 volume of conjugate at the working dilution to each spot. Incubate again at 37°C for 30 minutes in a moist box. Repeat washing and rinsing described above. Dry in air and mount as described for the FTA-ABS test (page 257). Examine by fluorescence microscopy at × 40 magnification.

Fluorescence may be seen with normal serum diluted up to 1 : 16. A significant positive result is a greater than fourfold rise when sera taken early and later in infection are tested in parallel. A titre of 128 or more in a single sample is significant.

Rubella antibodies

Routine screening of antenatal patients, hospital staff and post-vaccine patients for rubella antibody is now widely established. The most useful test currently employed is single radial haemolysis (SRH), which measures the long-lasting serum IgG antibody.

Single radial haemolysis (SRH) (after Grillner *et al.*, 1975)

Materials:

Agarose	(Miles Laboratories)
Complement fixation buffer tablets	(Code No. BR16: Oxoid Ltd)
Sodium azide	
Rubella haemagglutination antigen (1 ml ampoule)	(Flow Laboratories Ltd)
Complement (lyophilized)	(LIP Ltd)
Sheep red blood cells in Alsever's solution	(Tissue Culture Services)
Square plastic Petri dishes (100 × 100 mm)	(Code No. 109: Sterilin Ltd)
Moist box	
Compu-pet 200 (See page 245)	

Procedure

Dissolve 1% agarose in fresh complement fixation buffer (CFB) by autoclaving at 10 psi for 10 minutes or standing the flask in boiling water for 1 hour. When cool (50°C), add sufficient sodium azide to give a final concentration of 0.1%. Distribute in 30-ml volumes, in autoclavable screw-capped bottles, and allow to solidify. Gel prepared in this manner will store at room temperature for up to 3 months.

To prepare plates for use, melt the agarose/buffer gel by autoclaving at 10 psi for 10 minutes. Cool in a 56°C waterbath. Reconstitute the haemagglutination antigen by adding 0.5 ml of distilled water. Reconstitute the lyophilized complement with distilled water as advised (each plate will require 0.25 antigen and 1 ml complement).

Wash the sheep red blood cells at least three times in CFB, until the supernatant after centrifugation is clear. Sensitize red blood cells by the addition of 0.5 ml undiluted complement and 0.25 ml antigen to 0.1 ml of packed, washed red blood cells. Mix well, and stand at room temperature for 20 minutes. Centrifuge at 2000 r.p.m. for 5 minutes. Wash in cold (4°C) CFB, and recentrifuge at 2000 r.p.m. for a further 5 minutes. Remove the supernatant and resuspend the cells in 1 ml of cold CFB.

Add 1 ml of sensitized cells and 0.5 ml undiluted complement to 30 ml of agarose/buffer gel at 56°C, and pour immediately into the Petri plate. This is the test plate. At the same time, a control plate should be prepared, substituting CFB for the rubella antigen. It is important that the test and control plates are a matched pair. Plates thus prepared may be stored at 4°C for up to 1 week.

Test proper
On day 1 punch 3-mm diameter holes, 9 mm apart, in a pair (test and control) of SRH plates to make a 7×7 matrix on the 100×100 mm square Petri plate. This enables 46 sera and 3 controls to be tested on each pair of plates. Inactivate sera to be tested at 60°C for 20 minutes, to destroy natural complement, which may interfere with the test. Using the Compu-pet 200, pick up 20 μl of serum and deliver 10 μl into the appropriately marked wells of the test and control plates. The following controls are also included: serum known to contain no rubella antibodies (negative control); a serum known to contain rubella IgG antibodies at a concentration of 12.5 i.u./ml (low positive); and a serum known to contain rubella IgG antibodies at a concentration of 50 i.u./ml (high positive). (Control sera are available from the DMRQ – see Appendix. The PHLS Monograph No. 16 (1982) gives details of the method for standardization of control sera, allowing laboratories to prepare local control sera of matched potency to reference sera.)

Incubate the plates in a moist box at 37°C overnight.

Next day, examine them for zonal lysis. Interpret results as follows:

Test zone > zone of 12.5 i.u./ml control, and > corresponding well on control plate	Rubella antibody present Report as immune
Test zone < zone of 12.5 i.u./ml control, but > corresponding well on control plate	Low level of rubella antibody present. Immunity not guaranteed Report as 'susceptible'
No test zone, or test zone equal or < corresponding well on control plate	Rubella antibody absent Report as 'susceptible'.

The SRH has proved to be a convenient and economical screening test, and has now replaced the haemagglutination inhibition test (HAI) for this purpose (see Stokes and Ridgway, 1980). However, the SRH test does not reliably detect IgM class antibodies. It is therefore vital that a contact history is available before a report based solely on SRH results is sent out. Patients with active but subclinical rubella could be erroneously reassured as immune to rubella, because IgM class antibody was not detected. It is therefore our practice to report the presence of rubella antibodies in patients on whom we have no information as 'rubella antibodies detected; interpretation not possible owing to lack of clinical information'. SRH gives false negatives in less than 1% of sera. It is therefore recommended that negative and non-specific results by SRH are checked by a different method (see below). However, vaccination of patients reported as falsely negative is of little consequence. For the demonstration of rising titres of rubella antibody, the HAI test is to be preferred.

Rubella Monoclonal Latex Test (Rubalex, Orion Diagnostics, obtainable from Oxoid Ltd)
The recent advances in monoclonal antibody technology have permitted the re-evaluation of latex agglutination techniques using the inert carrier particles bound with specific monoclonal antibody. The Rubalex text is suitable for screening small numbers (<20) of sera for the presence of rubella-specific IgG.

Method
Pretreatment or dilution of the test serum is not required. The test is performed on a glass slide. Add one drop each of serum and antigen/latex suspension, mix, then rock the slide for 3 minutes. Agglutination at this time indicates the presence of IgG to rubella.

The method compares well with other detection techniques, but is expensive and time consuming for large numbers of sera owing to the critical incubation time. The test does not replace SRH, but provides a convenient method for checking negative and non-specific SRH reactions.

The further evaluation of sera for rubella antibodies requires facilities for the detection of IgM. A number of methods are available, including modifications of the HAI test (Luton and Ridgway, 1979), ELISA and radioimmunoassay (solid phase or antibody capture assay). These tests are best performed by reference laboratories, but details of these and other methods are given in the PHLS Monograph No. 16 (1982).

Human immunosuppressive virus (HIV) antibody

Currently, evidence of infection by HIV is sought by testing serum for antibody to the virus. The presence of antibody indicates that infection has occurred at some time in the past. Most of the antibody produced does not neutralize the virus, and antibody-positive individuals are consequently potentially infectious.

A number of commercially produced kits are available for HIV antibody testing, and all incorporate enzyme-labelled detector antibodies. Most are standard solid-phase immunoassays, with the viral antigen coated onto the solid surface. Test serum is incubated with the viral antigen. Antibody that becomes attached to the viral antigen is detected by adding an indicator system (enzyme-labelled antihuman globulin and substrate) to the final reaction mixture and observing the colour change.

Laboratories are under increasing pressure to provide a diagnostic service for this virus. Until more is known about the performance of these tests, we believe that viral reference laboratories provide the most reliable service. It is important to follow precisely the manufacturer's instructions when using these kits. False positive and false negative results do occur. A positive result has serious implications for the patient. The test should be repeated, and if necessary a further specimen obtained. The positive result must be confirmed by retesting using a different test system. At present, confirmatory tests should be carried out only by reference laboratories.

The appearance of specific antibody may only occur some months after exposure to the virus. It is thought that patients are infectious during this lag period, and they will not be detected by antibody tests. On the other hand, it is presumed that not all patients with demonstrable antibody are equally infectious. Tests for viral antigen are currently under development, and are likely to become available in the near future. Whether such tests will be primarily for use by reference laboratories or will become more widely applicable remains to be evaluated.

To date, all HIV antibody tests in the UK have incorporated antigens from the virus now designated HIV-1. It is becoming apparent that other related viruses may also occur in different parts of the world. These viruses will not be detected by the currently available antibody tests, and further developments will be necessary. Safety precautions for handling specimens are essential (see pages 10 and 302).

Toxoplasmosis

The most reliable test for demonstrating antibodies to *Toxoplasma gondii* is the Sabin–Feldman Dye test (see PHLS Monograph No. 13, 1980). The test is difficult to perform, requiring a ready source of *T. gondii*. Consequently, its use had been restricted to reference laboratories. A kit comprising latex particles coated with inactivated toxoplasma antigen has provided a useful technique for screening sera for the presence of toxoplasma-specific antibodies.

Latex Screening Test
Materials:

Latex particles coated with toxoplasma antigen (Toxoreagent, Eiken Chemical Co., obtainable from Mast Laboratories)
Buffer solution (provided in kit)
Postive control serum (provided in kit)
U-well microtitre trays
Glass test tubes (50 × 12 mm)

Method
Set up a rack of 50 × 12 mm test tubes (one for each serum sample). Add 350 μl of buffer solution to each tube, and 50 μl of serum. Add 25 μl

buffer to each required well of the microtitre plate (including control wells), and then 25 μl of serum dilution. Mix, and discard 25 μl from each well. This gives a screening dilution of 1 in 16 for the original serum. (The positive control is supplied ready diluted to 1 in 16.) A serum-free negative control should be included. Add 25 μl of well mixed latex suspension to each test and stand at room temperature for at least 12 hours.

Wells showing a tight white button are reported as 'toxoplasma screening test <1 : 16, negative'. Wells showing agglutination contain antibody >1 : 16 and are referred to the reference laboratory. Negative results on pregnant women should also be referred, as false negative tests are not unknown in this group. The test is not suitable for the investigation of congenital toxoplasmosis; therefore sera from children under 1 year of age should be referred for the Dye test. The Dye test (in which toxoplasma tachyzoites fail to stain with alkaline methylene blue in the presence of specific antibody and complement) is highly specific and sensitive.

Empirical antigen–antibody reactions

Paul–Bunnell test for glandular fever

The classic sheep-cell agglutination test, made more specific by absorption with ox red cells and guinea-pig kidney, has been replaced by a slide test employing stabilized horse red cells, obtainable from Mercia Diagnostics (Hoff and Bauer, 1965). Because of the typical changes in blood cells in glandular fever, the screening test is more conveniently carried out in the Haematology Laboratory where it can be related to the haematological findings.

Specific antibody to Epstein–Barr (EB) virus can be estimated but, unlike the Paul–Bunnell test, the result will be positive in sub-clinical infection or in other diseases caused by this virus. The empirical test therefore retains its usefulness. The test may be positive as early as the fourth day of the disease but may be negative until several weeks after the onset of symptoms. A positive test is generally taken to indicate some degree of active infection.

Clinically typical glandular fever may be Paul–Bunnell negative. A negative test for EB virus antibody will then confirm that the infection has some other cause, but a positive test does not necessarily signify infection. Serial tests showing a rising titre which falls in convalescence suggest Paul–Bunnell-negative glandular fever, but this is rare.

Cold agglutination test in mycoplasmal pneumonia

Specific *Mycoplasma pneumoniae* antigen for a complement fixation test can now be obtained, but care is needed in the interpretation of positive results because high titres are sometimes seen in serum from symptom-free contacts with no history of infection. As in other infections, a rise in titre at least fourfold in samples tested in parallel is needed before the diagnosis can be made. Since isolation of *Mycopl. pneumoniae* is uncertain even in the most experienced hands, diagnosis by serology has to be relied on.

An antibody which will agglutinate human group O red blood cells is found in the serum of about 50 per cent of patients suffering from mycoplasmal pneumonia. The agglutinin appears about the fourth day of the disease and the titre rises to become maximal early in convalescence. Cold agglutinins are also found in other conditions; for example, haemolytic anaemia, Raynaud's disease, trypanosomiasis and paroxysmal haemoglobinuria. Provided these conditions can be excluded, and particularly when a rising titre can be demonstrated, their presence is good evidence in favour of mycoplasmal pneumonia. They are not found by the method to be described in influenza, the common cold, Q fever or psittacosis. A test for them is therefore of value as a preliminary step in the serological investigation of respiratory virus infections.

Method
Take about 5–10 ml of blood by venepuncture into a sterile bottle. Allow it to clot in the 37°C incubator. Separate the serum (do not inactivate it because heating to 56°C destroys the agglutinin). Make a series of twofold dilutions in saline 1 : 10 to 1 : 160, each about 0.5 ml in volume in small test tubes. Include in the test a saline control. Add to each dilution and the control an equal volume of a freshly prepared 2% suspension of thrice-washed group O red blood cells. After shaking well, refrigerate the tubes for 2 hours or overnight, and read.

The final dilution of the series will be 1 : 20 to 1 : 320. The titre of the serum is the highest dilution which shows agglutination when viewed with the aid of a hand lens. The agglutination is reversible and will disappear on warming the fluid.

A titre of 1 : 40 or more is considered to be suggestive of mycoplasmal pneumonia provided the other conditions listed above can be excluded. An attempt should always be made to demonstrate a rise in titre by taking at least two samples of blood – one towards the end of the first week of the illness and one early in convalescence. If the patient is seen for the first time late in the disease it may be possible to demonstrate a fall in titre which is also of much greater significance than a single positive result.

Skin tests

Hypersensitivity
In chronic infective disease when no likely pathogen and no specific antibodies can be found, it may be possible to demonstrate that the patient's tissues have been invaded by the microbe suspected of causing his disease by inoculating intradermally a small quantity of antigenic material, prepared from cultures or from experimentally infected tissues. A positive reaction indicates that previous infection with the suspected microbe, or close contact with some closely related antigen, has rendered his tissues hypersensitive. Hypersensitivity usually develops about 4–8 weeks after the original microbial invasion and lasts for many years; a

positive reaction does not necessarily indicate present infection. The power to develop hypersensitivity is possessed by a very high proportion of people but not by everyone. Negative reactions to some antigens (e.g. tuberculin) make long-standing infection by the microbe very improbable, but steroid treatment often renders previously positive reactors negative. Very ill-nourished patients are also likely to give false negative reactions which become positive when nutrition improves (Lloyd, 1968; Harrison *et al.*, 1975).

The tuberculin test for evidence of tuberculous infection is one of the most useful and frequently performed. It has been described in Chapter 6. Similiar tests are made for the diagnosis of many chronic infections; examples are the Casoni test for hydatid disease, the Frei test for lymphogranuloma venereum and the coccidioidin and histoplasmin tests. Brucellin is occasionally of use in the diagnosis of brucellosis and mallein in suspected glanders. Results are usually read 48 hours after inoculation. The Casoni test antigen stimulates an immediate or a delayed reaction and a comparatively large weal is seen. Different types and preparations of antigen give different results, and instructions for reading the results are usually issued with each batch. If its activity is unknown, at least one person known to give a positive reaction and several negative controls should be inoculated for comparison with the patient's test inoculation. Advances in serological diagnostic techniques, coupled with the difficulty of obtaining standardized antigen preparations, has rendered the tests (with the exception of tuberculin) essentially obsolete.

Sensitivity tests

When small doses of diphtheria toxin or erythrogenic streptococcal toxin are injected intradermally they give rise to a local reaction, unless the person injected possesses specific neutralizing antitoxin. This is the basis of the Schick test, which shows the patient's susceptibility or immunity to diphtheria.

Schick test

Schick testing is used for two main purposes: to identify at-risk individuals during an epidemic, and to check on the immune status of health care workers. Traditionally, the main reason for testing was to avoid adverse reactions to vaccine given to previously immune people. However, modern low-dose vaccines are no more likely to produce adverse reactions in immune persons than is the Schick test itself. The role of routine Schick testing is therefore questionable.

Method

Inject intradermally 0.2 ml of diphtheria toxin (containing one Schick dose) into one forearm and 0.2 ml of toxin (inactivated by heating to 70°C for 5 minutes) into the other, to serve as a control. The following reactions may be observed.

Negative: no reaction in either arm.

Positive: no reaction in the control arm. In the test arm a flush appears after 24–36 hours, which increases to become maximal between the fourth and seventh day.

Negative + pseudo-reaction: a flush appears in both arms within 24 hours which rapidly fades. It has usually disappeared by the fourth day.

Positive + pseudo-reaction: a flush appears in both arms within 24 hours. It fades rapidly in the control arm and is replaced by the true positive reaction in the test arm which develops as described above.

A positive reaction indicates susceptibility to diphtheria. A very high proportion of negative reactors are immune.

Detection of microbial antigens in specimens

Methods for the detection of microbial antigens and specific products of metabolism in clinical material are being rapidly developed. Many methods are still applicable only to research but it is certain that in the future these techniques will find an increasing place in the diagnostic laboratory.

There are a number of sophisticated techniques for the separation and identification of components in mixtures. Examples of these include gas-liquid chromatography (GLC), high performance liquid chromatography (HPLC), mass spectrophotometry and nuclear magnetic resonance (NMR). Increasingly, these techniques are finding a role in diagnostic microbiology for the recognition of specific microbial components in specimens or cultures.

The major use of GLC in the clinical microbiology laboratory is the analysis of bacterial metabolites, particularly from anaerobic metabolism. These products include volatile and non-volatile fatty acids and alcohols. The enzymes involved are genetically stable, thus the end-points of metabolism provide a 'fingerprint' that is a useful adjunct to other identification techniques. The genus *Fusobacterium* is defined by the presence of butyric acid and the absence of iso-acids. In contrast, the species comprising the genus *Clostridium* produce differing end products. Analysis of the end product profile, along with other biochemical and morphological characteristics, will allow the speciation of organisms within the genus. The identification of *Actinomyces* can be confirmed by identification of both volatile and non-volatile fatty acids.

The results obtained by GLC are affected by the nutritional composition of the medium, specifically the ratio of carbohydrates to peptone, and also the period of incubation before end product analysis.

GLC has proved a rapid and reliable means of identifying anaerobic organisms directly in specimens of pus (Phillips *et al.*, 1976). The detection of volatile fatty acids in addition to acetic and propionic acids correlates well with the isolation of anaerobic bacteria. The analysis of short-chain fatty acids is not, however, sufficiently specific to allow identification of the genus or species directly from clinical material.

HPLC has applications in drug assay (see page 238) and in the identification and classification of micro-organisms, largely as a research or reference laboratory tool.

Counter-current immunoelectrophoresis (CIEP) provides a useful adjunct to more conventional means for the rapid diagnosis of bacterial pneumonia and meningitis, especially in treated patients. Positive results are diagnostic but a negative result, which in practice is often encountered, does not exclude infection. In countries where meningococcal infection due to strains of groups A and C is common, positive results are often encountered and the test is valuable, but in Britain most infections are caused by group B strains and no satisfactory serum is commercially available.

Routine examination of sputum by CIEP reveals that pneumococcal infection is much more common than would be expected from culture results, probably because patients are often investigated only when penicillin treatment (perhaps in inadequate dose) has been given. Unfortunately there are many types of pneumococci, not all of which can be succesfully recognized by CIEP, and specific sera are costly. The presence of *H. influenzae* type b can be recognized by its capsular antigen in specimens by this technique. The use of direct agglutination tests (see page 35) provides a more convenient technique for diagnostic purposes.

Enzyme-linked immunosorbent assay (ELISA) (see page 250) is an extremely sensitive technique for both antigen and antibody detection (Voller *et al.*, 1978). It is as good as CIEP for recognition of bacterial antigens (Beuvery *et al.*, 1979) and more versatile. The sensitivity of this technique is such that the need for expensive apparatus and the use of radioactive substances required for the most sensitive technique, radio-immunoassay (RIA), may be obviated. RIA has a number of applications, not only for antigen–antibody detection but also for antibiotic assay. Capital and running costs and the need for special conditions to work with radioactivity are disadvantages of this useful technique.

The following techniques for antigen detection in clinical material have been found to be convenient and reliable in our diagnostic laboratory.

Detection of *Chlamydia trachomatis* antigen

The appreciation of the importance of *Chlam. trachomatis* as a genito-urinary pathogen (see page 259) has resulted in a need for laboratories to provide a diagnostic service. As indicated earlier, cell culture remains the method of choice, but is not practicable unless facilities for tissue culture are readily available. Direct antigen detection kits are now commercially available. They are based on either immunofluorescence (Thomas *et al.*, 1984) or ELISA (Ridgway *et al.*, 1985), using highly specific monoclonal or polyclonal antibodies. These tests are not ideal, and there is still much to learn about the frequency and cause of false positive and false negative results. It is important that laboratories select a method that has been fully evaluated by independent laboratories. Furthermore, the use of the test must be limited to clinical specimens known to yield reliable results (Mumtaz *et al.*, 1986). None of the currently available tests has been properly evaluated for samples outside the urethra and cervix or from acute inclusion conjunctivitis. They are therefore not suitable for rectal specimens, external auditory meatus swabs, joint fluids or conjunctival specimens from cases of trachoma.

The choice between immunofluorescence or ELISA tests depends not only on available expertise but also on the expected workload. Immuno-fluorescence techniques are rapid, and allow evaluation of the quality of specimen (*Chlamydia* are intracellular and cells must be present in specimens). However, they are technically very demanding, requiring an experienced operator. Large numbers of specimens are very tedious to examine, restricting specimen throughput. ELISA, on the other hand, is expensive for small numbers of samples, and the specimen quality cannot be assessed. For larger numbers of samples, the tests can be mechanized. The predictive value of a positive result with either test compared to cell culture is low. Caution is therefore necessary when reporting positive results. In contrast, the tests have high negative predictive values in all populations studied. Their use primarily as screening tests is therefore to be encouraged. Because non-viable antigen may persist, antigen detection tests are inappropriate for post-treatment follow-up.

The test described below has been well evaluated within the constraints outlined above, and is suitable for use by laboratories experienced in immunofluorescent techniques.

Collection of specimens

The quality of specimen is critical for detecting *Chlam. trachomatis* antigen. Specimens from the male urethra should be obtained by inserting a cotton-wool-tipped wire swab 4 cm into the urethra. The swab is rotated and withdrawn. From the cervix, a cotton-wool-tipped wooden swab is used to sample the squamo-columnar junction, having first lightly cleaned the cervical area with sterile gauze. Specimens from the conjuctiva of adults and neonates are obtained by firmly rubbing a cotton-wool-tipped swab along the everted lower tarsal conjuctiva, having first removed excess exudate.

Materials:

>*Chlamydia trachomatis* direct specimen test (Microtrak, Syva Co.);
>Kit contains: FITC-conjugated *Chlam. trachomatis* antibody (lyophilized)
>>Reconstitution diluent
>>Positive and negative control slides
>>Mounting fluid
>Single well glass slides (Syva Co.)
>Acetone fixative
>Coverslips
>Moist box
>Fluorescence microscope system (see page 146), preferably using incident light.
(*Note*. Imagen (Boots Celltech) is a reliable alternative to the above direct specimen test.)

Procedure
Reconstitute the lyophilized specific reagent according to the manufacturer's instructions. Record the date on the bottle. Reconstituted reagent is stable for 3 months at 4°C and must not be used beyond this time. Allow cold reagent to stand at room temperature for 30 minutes before use.

Method
Firmly roll the swab across the well of the slide, ensuring that the whole swab is used. Flood the well with 0.5 ml acetone, and allow to evaporate. Apply 20 μl of reagent to the well of the fixed specimens and control slides. (*Note*: the manufacturer recommends 30 μl; we have found 20 μl to be adequate, and economic. Under no circumstances should the reagent be diluted before use.) Ensure that the whole specimen is covered by reagent. Incubate for 15 minutes at room temperature in a moist box. Aspirate excess reagent, and rinse the slide in distilled water for 10 seconds. Drain the slide, using blotting paper at the edge of the specimen area, and allow to air dry. Add 1 drop of mounting fluid, and apply the coverslip without entrapping air bubbles.

Read the slides at a magnification of × 500, examining the positive control slide first. Chlamydial elementary bodies will be seen as pinpoints of bright apple-green fluorescence against the red colour of the cells. Specimens containing no cells should be discarded as unevaluable. Particles showing yellow or white fluorescence, or being irregular or larger than the positive control particles, must be disregarded. Non-specific particles may fluoresce, but with experience the elementary bodies will be distinguished. When 5 or more such particles are seen per preparation, a positive report can be sent.

Hepatitis B antigen (HB$_s$Ag) haemagglutination test

Purified horse antibody to hepatitis B antigen is attached to tanned turkey cells to make a sensitive suspension which will agglutinate in the presence of human HB$_s$Ag. A small proportion of human sera contain agglutinins to turkey cells or horse globulins which will give a false positive reaction. These can usually be removed by treating the serum with turkey cells coated with normal horse immunoglobulin. Specific HB$_s$Ag is identified by neutralizing agglutination by treatment with specific hepatitis B antiserum, i.e. by specific haemagglutination inhibition.

The screening test eliminates all non-agglutination sera, leaving those which agglutinate specifically and those which agglutinate non-specifically for further investigation. Non-specific agglutination sera may also contain heptatitis antigen and these will need absorption in addition to the confirmatory specific haemagglutination inhibition test.

Materials:

Hepatest kit (Wellcome Diagnostics) containing buffer, test cells, control cells and positive and negative control sera. Confirmatory Hepatest kit.

U-well microtitre trays
Compu-pet 200 (page 245) electronic diluter–dispenser with microtubing and pipette (or other micro-diluter).
Mechanical rotator to rotate 100 r.p.m. in 1.9 cm circle.
Clean paper wipes.

Screening test
Prime the Compu-pet with buffer. Pick up 10 μl of inactivated patient's serum and deliver it with 90 μl buffer into well 1 of the microtitre tray. Pick up 50 μl of this 1 : 10 dilution from well 1 and deliver 20 μl each to wells 2 and 3, marked test and control. Discard the extra 10 μl, wash the pipette by discharging buffer thrice and wiping its tip. Continue thus until all sera are diluted and dispensed. Add 20 μl of test or controls cells (reconstituted as directed) to the appropriate wells. Cover the tray and mix thoroughly on the rotator (see safety precautions below). Incubate at room temperature (20–25°C) for 30 minutes.

Clumps of agglutinated cells are dispersed over the whole area of the well; when they are not agglutinated they appear as a button or ring in the centre of the well. When only the test well is agglutinated, proceed to titrate the serum. When both wells show agglutination the titration and confirmatory tests must be performed.

Titration
Prepare 1 : 10 dilution as above and deliver into well 1. Pick up 20 μl of dilute serum and dispense with 20 μl of buffer to well 2. Double dilute thus to well 6 and discard the final fraction. Repeat with the same serum from well 1 to provide test and control rows. Add 20 μl of either test or control cells to all wells of each row. Cover and mix on the rotator. Incubate at room temperature for 30 minutes. The highest dilution to show agglutination is the titre. A titre fourfold greater than the control is significant.

The titration confirms a positive test. False positive sera which do not agglutinate the control cells (third line in Table 10.1) show only a low titre and it would be unnecessarily extravagant to identify the agglutinin on all

Table 10.1   Confirmatory test for hepatitis B antigen

1	2	3	Wells containing patient's absorbed serum diluted
Horse antiserum	Normal horse serum	Normal horse serum	
Test cells	Test cells	Control cells	
−	+	−	True positive
−	−	−	True negative
+	+	−	False positive
+	+	+	Non-specific agglutination*
−	+	+	Probable positive with non-specific agglutination

+ = agglutination.
*Retest after reabsorption.

positive sera. Titres should not be reported, as they bear no relation to the severity of infection or the length of carriage of the antigen. The test detects surface protein antigen, not infective virus particles.

Confirmatory test

This test should be performed only when both control and test wells give a positive screening result. The kit contains the following:

Cells for absorption (to be reconstituted as directed)
Horse antiserum to hepatitis B surface antigen
Normal horse serum

Method

Pick up 0.1 ml serum and 0.3 ml reconstituted cells for absorption and transfer to a 7.5 × 1.3 cm test tube. Incubate at room temperature for 30 minutes. Centrifuge and remove the supernatant, which respresents a 1 : 4 serum dilution. Dilute the supernatant to give a concentration 8 times greater than the titre determined above. (If the titre was 32 or less, use the 1 : 4 dilution). Add 20 μl of this dilution of serum to each of 3 wells of the microtitre tray. Add 20 μl horse antiserum to well 1 and 20 μl normal horse serum to wells 2 and 3. Add 20 μl of test cells (from the Hepatest kit) to wells 1 and 2, and 20 μl of control cells to well 3. Cover the tray and mix on the rotator. Incubate at room temperature for 30–60 minutes. Interpretation of the results is seen in Table 10.1.

Safety precautions

The above procedures involve the handling of potentially high-risk sera. The tests should always be performed in a properly designed and maintained safety cabinet. All dilutions are discarded into hypochlorite solution (1000 parts per million available chlorine). The microtitre pipette should be soaked in hypochlorite overnight after filling and the work surface is wiped over with hypochlorite after use. Microtitre trays must be sealed with transparent adhesive tape before mixing, to prevent aerosols, and they should be discarded into an autoclavable container for destruction before removal from the laboratory.

Respiratory syncytial virus (RSV) fluorescence test

Respiratory syncytial virus (RSV) is a major cause of respiratory infection in children, causing bronchiolitis. The virus is very labile, with demanding growth requirements in tissue culture. Traditional methods are either slow to demonstrate the virus or unsuccessful. The use of specific immuno-fluorescence microscopy allows the demonstration of viral antigen in desquamated throat cells.

Materials:

FITC-conjugated RSV monoclonal antibody (Boots Celltech)
Phosphate buffered saline pH 6.4 (Oxoid Ltd)

Acetone fixative
Clean glass slides and coverslips
Mounting fluid
Fluorescence microscope system (see page 146) preferably using incident light.

Method

Collect a cell-rich nasopharyngeal aspirate, using a mucus trap. Add 2 ml of sterile phosphate-buffered saline (PBS). Break up cell clumps using a sterile plastic pipette. Repeat this step twice more, until a total of 6 ml PBS has been added. Centrifuge at 1000 r.p.m. for 10 minutes. Remove the supernatant (it may be used to inoculate tissue culture if required). Resuspend the deposit in 2 drops of PBS. Place two 20 μl drops of cell suspension on a glass slide and air dry (any remaining cell suspension may be added to the supernatant for tissue culture). Fix the smear with acetone at room temperature for 10 minutes. Stain with 20 μl of FITC-conjugated RSV antibody. Incubate at 37°C for 15 minutes in a moist box. Rinse in PBS for 10 minutes. Air dry and mount in glycerol mountant, applying a coverslip without entrapping air bubbles. Examine at $\times 200$ and $\times 400$ magnification. Infected cells show apple-green speckled fluorescence. Uninfected cells appear red (as a result of Evans blue counterstain in the reagent). A positive control (obtainable from the suppliers, or a known positive) should be tested with each new batch of reagent.

Rotavirus Latex Screening Test

This test detects rotavirus in faecal specimens. Latex particles coated with antibody to pooled human rotavirus serotypes are used. Other viral causes of gastroenteritis (e.g. coronaviruses or adenoviruses) will not be excluded by this method. The examination of the specimen by electron microscopy will be required to recognise these viruses.

Materials:

Rotavirus antigen detection kit (Rotascreen, Mercia Diagnostics Ltd); kit contains:
   Test latex reagent
   Control latex reagent
   Prediluted positive control
   Concentrated extraction buffer
   Test slides
Wooden applicator sticks
Plastic screw-cap containers (Universal)

Method

All reagents should be at room temperature before use. Dilute buffer (1 : 4) with distilled water, allowing 10 ml of working strength for each sample to be tested. Measure 10 ml of diluted buffer into a screw-capped universal container, and add approximately 1 g of faeces. Shake vigorously for 5 seconds and then stand for 5 minutes. Shake for a further

5 seconds before centrifuging at 1000 r.p.m. for 10 minutes. Place two 50-μl drops of supernatant on adjacent areas of test slide. Add 50 μl of test latex suspension to one sample drop, and 50 μl of control latex suspension to the other drop. Mix each with a wooden applicator stick, and gently rock the slide for 2 minutes. Observe for agglutination, visible to the naked eye. A positive result is indicated by agglutination in the test only, within the 2-minute period. Absence of agglutination indicates a negative result. If agglutination occurs in both control and test, the result is not evaluable.

References

Beuvery, E.C., van Rossum, F., Lauwers, S. and Coignau, H. (1979) *Lancet* i, 208

Cremer, A.W., Mellars, B. and Stokes, E.J. (1975) *Journal of Clinical Pathology* **28**, 37

Engvall, E. and Perlmann, P.J. (1971) *Immunochemistry* **8**, 871

Grillner, L., Lindberg, I.M. and Strannegard, O. (1975) *Journal of Clinical Microbiology* **1**, 491

Harrison, B.D.W., Tugwell, P. and Fawcett, I.W. (1975) *Lancet* i, 421

Hoff, G. and Bauer, S. (1965) *Journal of the American Medical Association* **194**, 351

Lindberg, A.A., Haeggiman, S., Karlson, K., Carlson, H.E. and Mair, N.S. (1982) *Journal of Hygiene Cambridge* **88**, 295

Lloyd, A.V.C. (1968) *British Medical Journal* iii, 529

Luton, P. and Ridgway, G.L. (1979) *Journal of Clinical Pathology* **32**, 931

Mumtaz, G., Ridgway, G.L. and Oriel, J.D. (1986) *Lancet* ii, 1156

Phillips, K.D., Tearle, P.V. and Willis, A.T. (1976) *Journal of Clinical Pathology* **29**, 248

PHLS Monograph No. 1 (1972) Laboratory Diagnosis of Venereal Diseases. HM Stationery Office, London

PHLS Monograph No. 13 (1980) *The Laboratory Diagnosis of Toxoplasmosis.* HM Stationery Office, London

PHLS Monograph No. 14 (1980) *Benchbook on Brucella.* HM Stationery Office, London

PHLS Monograph No. 16 (1982) *Laboratory Investigation of Rubella.* HM Stationery Office, London

Portnoy, J. (1963) *American Journal of Clinical Pathology* **40**, 473

Richmond, S.J. and Caul, E.O. (1975) *Journal of Clinical Microbiology* **1**, 345

Ridgway, G.L. (1986). *Postgraduate Medical Journal* **62**, 249

Ridgway, G.L., Oriel, J.D., Mumtaz, G. and Mellars, B.J. (1985) *Journal of Clinical Pathology* **39**, 232

Ripa, K.T. and Mårdh, P.A. (1977) *Journal of Clinical Microbiology* **6**, 328

Scrimgeour, G. and Roslin, P. (1973) *British Journal of Venereal Diseases* **49**, 342

Stokes, E.J. and Ridgway, G.L. (1980) *Clinical Bacteriology*, 5th edn. Edward Arnold, London

Thomas, B.J., Evans, R.T., Hawkins, D.A. and Taylor-Robinson, D. (1984) *Journal of Clinical Pathology* **37**, 812

Voller, A., Bartlett, A. and Bidwell, D.E. (1978) *Journal of Clinical Pathology* **31**, 507

Wang, S.P. and Grayston, J.T. (1974) *Journal of Infectious Diseases* **130**, 388

11

Hospital Epidemiology

Hospitals, where large numbers of sick people are brought together, have always been dangerous places. The potential risk of acquiring harmful microbes is as great as it ever was and no one should be admitted unless treatment is needed which cannot be safely undertaken elsewhere. Therapy which holds out hope of life to those who would previously have died has made prevention of infection more difficult because many of these patients must stay for long periods (or repeated short periods) in hospital and their ability to withstand infection by microbes foreign to them, and even to their own commensals, is often much impaired. There is no way a patient can be rendered microbe-free and attempts to do so ensure that his commensals, if they cause infection, will be antibiotic-resistant.

Fortunately, knowledge of the mode of infection and method of preventing it have advanced also. When clinician, clinical microbiologist and nursing staff work together and appreciate the need for perpetual vigilance, there is every hope that the good results which can be expected from treatment will not be nullified by infection. Without constant vigilance, therapeutic efforts, however expert and costly, will fail in a proportion of patients and some will suffer more harm than good from their hospital treatment.

The clinical microbiologist plays a leading role in prevention because specimens from the patients of all clinicians are processed in the laboratory and he is in a better position than others to discover the onset of hospital acquired infection and to investigate its extent and source. He is commonly the infection control officer. It is generally agreed that a large general hospital needs, in addition, a whole-time member of the nursing staff who must be sufficiently senior to advise her colleagues in wards and departments about aseptic techniques, to help implement decisions of the infection control committee and to collect specimens from potential carriers of hospital pathogens. This is a key appointment. An infection control nurse who understands modes of spread of microbes and has the personality needed to investigate sources of infection and advise staff in all departments – medical, domestic and administrative, as well as nursing – contributes greatly to the protection of hospital patients.

It is not appropriate here to describe in detail aseptic techniques and methods of investigating episodes of infection. The reader is referred to

277

Table 11.1   Potential hospital pathogens

Condition of people at risk *	Microbes liable to infect
1. Previously healthy young adults (not undergoing surgery) Hospital staff	*Str. pyogenes* *(Salm. typhi)* (Hepatitis B virus) (Human immunodeficiency virus, HIV) (Lassa fever virus)
2. Previously healthy adults undergoing surgery or obstetric care	*Staph. aureus* [†] *Streptococcus* group B *Cl. perfringens* *Cl. difficile* Commensal potential pathogens[†]: *Esch. coli, Klebsiella* spp. Microbes from 1 (above)

3. Patients with lowered resistance caused by age (geriatric, infant) or debilitating disease (e.g. cancer, chronic infection)	*Salmonella* spp.
	Shigella spp.
	Proteus, Providencia and *Enterobacter* spp.
	Environmental bacteria:
	    Pseudomonas, Serratia spp.,
	    Legionella spp.
	Fungi
	Microbes from 1 and 2 (above)

4. Patients with impaired immunity: congenital, acquired or induced by therapy.	Commensal microbes not categorized as human pathogens Microbes from 1, 2 and 3 (above)

() = risk mainly to staff; spread to other patients unlikely.
* It is assumed that normal aseptic and hygienic measures are skilfully employed.
† Especially strains resistant to commonly used antimicrobials. See text.

Lowbury *et al.* (1975) to Maurer (1985) and to Wilson, Miles and Parker (1983) for further information. We think it useful, however, to indicate sources and investigations likely to be profitable when infection caused by the more common hospital pathogens is encountered and to offer answers to commonly posed questions in this field. One problem inevitably faced is that recommendations have to be made which interfere with the optimum treatment of patients. These tend to be opposed by clinicians, whose first aim is the welfare of their own individual patients, whereas the clinical microbiologist is concerned with the welfare of the whole patient community. This potential source of friction is most easily overcome when the clinical microbiologist is familiar with the wards and has built up confidence in his ability to advise before there has been any threat of an epidemic (see Chapter 1).

The microbes which cause hospital-acquired infection can be categorized according to the condition of patients they are likely to infect (Table 11.1).

Potential hospital pathogens

Str. pyogenes

This species has great epidemic potential: a few cocci only are needed to initiate infection. The reasons why it is no longer a major cause of hospital infection are:

1. All strains are sensitive to penicillin and other β-lactam antibiotics.

2. Carrier rates in hospital are low because the population, both patients and staff, are exposed to these antibiotics which are present in small quantities in the environment.

Nevertheless, this streptococcus can cause death within hours and must be borne in mind. Patients admitted with streptococcal-infected excema, impetigo and tonsillitis (and, rarely, nasal carriers) are likely to disseminate the organism widely. They should not be allowed to come into contact with patients in categories 2, 3 and 4 (Table 11.1). Patients with streptococcal-infected excema should be isolated until the streptococcus is eliminated.

Salm. typhi

Salm. typhi is the most infective of all enteric pathogens, but, provided the patient is not incontinent (and the infection is more likely to cause constipation) nor a urinary excreter, infection is unlikely to spread. People at risk are those nursing incontinent or helpless patients and laboratory staff handling positive specimens. When typhoid is suspected it is worthwhile to check that all members of staff potentially at risk are familiar with the safety precautions devised to protect them and other patients. The infected patients are isolated to prevent others being exposed to contamination. To spread infection the pathogen must accidentally be swallowed. For control of epidemic diarrhoea, see page 291.

Patients in category 3 are more susceptible than others to infection. Because their physiological defence mechanisms are impaired, smaller numbers of *Salmonella* and *Shigella* will cause infection. Moreover, they need greater nursing care and therefore the chance of transfer of bacteria is increased. Those attending patients being nursed in source isolation should not also undertake the care of patients in categories 3 and 4 (see page 280).

Hepatitis B and human immunosuppressive virus (HIV)

These two viruses are considered together because their mode of infection and measures for control are similar.

Patients who have received repeated blood transfusions, especially those on haemodialysis and haemophiliacs, and those having injections with inadequately sterilized equipment, such as drug addicts and the extensively tattooed, are likely to be carriers. Sexually promiscuous people, especially homosexuals with numerous partners, are particularly at risk of HIV infection and hepatitis. The infection cannot be transmitted by carriers except by contact with their blood, other patients are not therefore at risk except through faulty sterilization of needles, syringes or surgical instruments. Infected hepatitis patients should be isolated for the first week of the illness. Patients suffering from AIDS may need isolation for their own protection because they are abnormally susceptible (category 4). All blood sent to laboratories should be in additional sealed plastic containers with a warning biohazard label in case of spillage en route. However, samples of blood from any patient, whether or not they are known to constitute a risk, must be handled as if infected, because virus may be present in blood in large numbers before diagnosis is possible and patients other than those obviously at risk may be infected.

Blood and serum must never be mouth pipetted. Staff separating serum must either ensure that blood or serum does not come in contact with their skin or they must wear protective gloves which either are disposable or must be disinfected. Hand washing after completing this work and when leaving a serology laboratory is essential.

The risk of acquiring hepatitis or HIV infection outside special units dealing with high-risk patients is not great. In clinical laboratories, treating blood and blood products in the manner which applies to other infected fluids is a sufficient precaution and has led to a very low incidence of hepatitis in British microbiology laboratories, perhaps no greater than in the general population (Grist, 1979). The risk to staff in contact with blood in a haemodialysis unit in which some patients were infected with HIV, and in which normal precautions against hepatitis virus were taken, was investigated. No evidence of transfer of virus was found (Goldman *et al.*, 1986).

For further information, see the guidelines by the Health Services Advisory Committee (1985) and by the Advisory Committee on Dangerous Pathogens (1986).

Lassa fever virus

This infection from West Africa, suffered by those in contact with cotton-rats (which carry the virus), may be diagnosed after admission to European or American hospitals. The risk to patients and staff is comparatively great because virus is present, not only in blood but also in the upper repiratory tract. Foreigners, who have no acquired immunity, are often extremely ill, incontinent and may need a tracheostomy. Close and frequent contact with them by nursing staff is essential. Because of the severity of infection, lack of specific treatment and high mortality, extreme precautions (as for smallpox) have been taken, but this is probably not necessary. High-level source isolation (barrier) nursing proved sufficient in a hospital in Sierra Leone, where a seriously ill British nurse with incontinence and tracheostomy was treated, without evidence of transfer of virus to the staff attending her (Fisher-Hoch *et al.*, 1985). Moreover, those foreigners infected in Africa have been hospital staff. There has been no epidemic among Europeans or Americans living in the endemic area. Normal aseptic precautions, carefully performed, should be sufficient to protect staff who may handle specimens before Lassa fever is suspected, but, because the consequences of accidental infection are so serious, once the diagnosis is suspected, laboratory investigations are reduced to a minimum and essential tests are carried out in reference laboratories with facilities for handling dangerous pathogens (category A, ACDP Guidelines, 1984).

Staph. aureus

In the 1960s, serious world-wide infection with epidemic strains of *Staph. aureus* was brought to an end by the introduction of methicillin and the isoxazolyl penicillins. Since 1980, strains resistant to these penicillins and many other antibiotics have increased and again we are faced with world-wide hospital-acquired staphylococcal epidemics.

All strains of methicillin-resistant *Staph. aureus* (MRSA) are potentially dangerous to hospital patients but some are comparatively easy to control. Epidemic methicillin-resistant strains (EMRSA), however, have caused serious infection in hospitals of many countries and, once established, are difficult, if not impossible, to eliminate. Methicillin resistance is chromosomal, not plasmid borne; it is therefore long lasting, and spontaneous reversal to sensitivity is unlikely. A constant watch for its appearance and draconian measures from the outset when infection is discovered are required.

In Britain, the Division of Hospital Infection of the Public Health Laboratory Service will identify epidemic strains. They are resistant also to penicillin, cephalosporins, trimethoprim, erythromycin and clindamycin. About 80 per cent at present are resistant to gentamicin and many are resistant to chloramphenicol. Resistance to fusidic acid, rifampicin and neomycin is rare and they are always, so far, sensitive to vancomycin. Phage typing sometimes identifies the strain as group III 85 but usually it is non-typable with standard phages and susceptible to additional phages 88A and 932.

A combined working party of the Hospital Infection Society and the British Society for Antimicrobial Chemotherapy has issued guidelines for the control of epidemic strains. For details of procedures to be adopted when such a strain is suspected, readers are referred to their Report (1986). Patients who are particularly vulnerable to staphylococcal infection, apart from those in categories 3 and 4, are those undergoing cardiac, neurological or orthopaedic surgery and patients in dermatology departments. They should on no account be exposed to the risk of EMRSA infection.

Streptococcus group B

Infection with this streptococcus is included, not because it has great epidemic potential but because it infects neonates born in hospital and is therefore technically a cause of hospital infection. The source of the organism is almost always the mother's vagina, not the hospital environment. However, spread from baby to baby in newborn nurseries can occur when aseptic technique is ineffective. Infected infants suffer septicaemia and menigitis. Diagnosis and treatment with penicillin are urgent. Routine swabbing of the mother's vagina is not recommended because carrier rates are variable and mothers who are carriers often give birth to healthy infants who suffer no damage. Premature infants of low birth weight are most liable to infection, which may occur *in utero*. We recommend routine swabbing of all infants admitted to neonatal special care units to screen for *Streptococcus* group B and other potential pathogens as described in Chapter 3 (page 51). The external auditory meatus is the most likely site to find *Streptococcus* group B (Ferrieri *et al.*, 1977).

Cl. perfringens

This anaerobe inhabits the human colon. Because it is a spore bearer and capable of long survival, it is also found in the human environment, particularly in hospital dust. In the wards the concentration of people is high and the risk of contamination from faecal bacteria is greater than normal. Anaerobic spore bearers do not initiate infection easily, but can cause death from gas-gangrene very rapidly. In order to test virulence in animals, it is necessary to produce a small area of necrosis to ensure suitable conditions for growth. Inoculation of virulent *Cl. perfringens* into healthy tissue often fails to cause infection. There is therefore no risk of epidemic spread and staff are not at risk. Even patients undergoing colonic operations very seldom suffer gas-gangrene, although the organism may be present in their wounds.

Those at risk are patients with traumatic wounds contaminated with dust, in whom there is impaired blood supply to the injured area or in whom surgical attention has been delayed and dead tissue has reduced the Eh in the wound to enable the anaerobe to flourish. Elderly patients having mid-thigh amputation for ischaemia or gangrene, whose skin in the operation area is liable to be contaminated with spores, are also at risk because blood supply to the wound is subnormal. *Cl. perfringens* is penicillin sensiive and prophylactic treatment is essential for these patients.

Cl. difficile (see also pages 75 and 132)

This spore-bearing anaerobe is an important cause of diarrhoea in those treated with antimicrobials. It is a commensal of the colon. Carrier rates in adult populations are low and therefore the environment is not normally contaminated. Most infections are caused by the patient's commensal strain. However, epidemics do occasionally occur in patients in categories 3 and 4, especially in geriatric wards where antibiotic treatment is frequently needed and patients may be incontinent. Under these circumstances it is likely to be difficult (and costly) to control (Bender *et al.*, 1986).

Paediatric wards, where sick infants may need hospital care and antibiotic treatment for comparatively long periods, are also at risk of epidemic spread. Carrier rates in infants are higher than in adults and spores may spread to the environment.

Commensal potential pathogens

1. Bact. fragilis (see also page 133)

This non-sporing anaerobe is the most common cause of acute appendicitis. It is incapable of surviving long outside the body and does not spread to other patients. Some strains establish themselves easily in wounds provided that conditions are suitable for anaerobic growth. Wound infection commonly follows operations in which the colon or vagina are opened. Many strains produce β-lactamase and are resistant to some other drugs. Metronidazole is the antimicrobial of choice for the necessary short-term prophylaxis.

2. Coliforms and enterococci

These aerobic intestinal commensals are usually harmless to healthy people but will infect the urinary tract after catheterization, and *Esch. coli* is the most common cause of spontaneous acute urinary tract infection. They are also found in small numbers in the healthy vagina. If they are allowed to contaminate wounds, infection may follow.

They contaminate skin near the anus, and the skin of the hands after defaecation, but are not able to establish themselves as skin commensals. Some strains will, however, establish themselves in the nares. Coliforms survive for long periods in moisture but small numbers only will survive drying. Prevention of infection by antimicrobial treatment is unsuccessful because the patient's normally sensitive commensals will rapidly be exchanged for resistant strains acquired from the hospital environment. Enterococci, *Enterobacter* and *Klebsiella* are more resistant than most bacteria to a wide range of antimicrobials. *Ps. aeruginosa* is an opportunist and flourishes only in hospital-treated patients. It is the most naturally resistant of the intestinal commensals. Antimicrobials specially developed for use against it are often required. Although carrier rates in healthy people are low, it survives better than other coliforms in the environment. Prophylaxis against coliforms, except for short periods in special circumstances, will usually fail because of the emergence of strains resistant to the prophylactic agent.

Str. faecalis and other enterococci resist drying but are much less common in dust than are staphylococci because faecal contamination is comparatively easily controlled. They have little epidemic potential and are usually found in company with other intestinal commensals. They can cause endocarditis, in susceptible patients, especially following procedures on the bowel.

Epidemic infection is most likely to be caused by *Klebsiella* or *Ps. aeruginosa*, which can easily be transferred from patient to patient on hands or equipment and will multiply at room temperature in fluids needed for treatment. They are commonly found colonizing tracheostomy sites and in the sputum of patients receiving antibiotics. Infection is likely to be caused, by spread from these sites, to those with wounds, with indwelling catheters or with pressure sores.

When infection spreads from patient to patient in intensive care units it may be necessary to close the unit until all infected and contaminated patients are discharged and the unit and all equipment can be thoroughly cleaned and, where possible, sterilized. Staff should be checked for nasal and faecal carriage of the epidemic strain, and on reopening non-carriers must practise normal aseptic technique meticulously.

It is important to distinguish between contamination and infection. Isolation of the same antibiotic-resistant *Klebsiella* or *Ps. aeruginosa* from the tracheostomy wound or pressure sore of more than one patient in a ward does not necessarily signify epidemic infection. It indicates the need to type apparently similar strains to confirm patient-to-patient spread and to look for evidence of infection in these patients. A check to make sure that staff understand, and are carrying out, prevention of cross-infection techniques is indicated. Samples for culture should be sent from all wounds and the staff should be requested to sample immediately any new lesion.

Other intestinal commensals which seldom infect previously healthy people will infect those in categories 3 and 4. *Proteus, Providencia* and *Enterobacter* are able to multiply during antimicrobial treatment because they are naturally comparatively resistant. Strains encountered in hospital are likely to have acquired high resistance to all the commonly employed antibacterial drugs. Patients who remain in hospital for a week or more and need antibacterial treatment are very likely to acquire them. For this reason, investigations needed preoperatively are best carried out before admission. It is difficult to prevent wound infection by hospital strains which have become part of the patient's commensal flora.

Normally harmless coliform bacteria present in dust and contaminating wash basins and baths can also infect patients in category 4. *Pseudomonas*, other than *Ps. aeruginosa*, and *Serratia* are likely causes. Some strains grow better at room than at body temperature. When blood cultures are negative in a patient with impaired resistance, intravenous therapy and signs of infection, it is worth incubating an additional subculture at room temperature.

3. Other commensal potential pathogens

Staph. epidermidis is often resistant to many antimicrobials, including methicillin. It is widespread on skin, nasal mucosa and in the hospital environment. However, its epidemic potential is low and, except in patients in category 4, it seldom infects. Methicillin-resistant *Staph. epidermidis* has caused epidemic endocarditis in patients with cardiac prostheses (van den Broek *et al.*, 1985). *Staph. saprophyticus* is a common cause of cystitis in young women but is not a common commensal and is seldom methicillin resistant (Pead *et al.*, 1985). It is not important in hospital epidemiology. Differentiation between these two species is required when infection by coagulase negative staphylococci is discovered.

Legionella pneumophila (see also page 135)

Treatment including erythromycin, which is active against *L. pneumophila*, should be given for respiratory infection in the elderly and in those with impaired resistance, until some other cause for the infection is established. Untreated infection has a high mortality. When diagnosed, the source of infection must be vigorously investigated because other people are likely to be at risk. The disease is not highly infectious and spread from patient to patient has not been recorded. Inhalation of aerosols from humidifiers in air-conditioning systems and domestic water supplies in which the organism is growing is the usual source of infection (Leading Article, 1981, 1983). Contamination of hospital air-conditioning or water systems is particularly likely to cause an epidemic because of the large number of patients in category 3 who will exposed to infection. Prevention depends on a high standard of engineering maintenance, and liaison between the clinical microbiologist and the hospital engineers is vital. For methods of examining the environment, see Edelstein (1981).

Fungi (see Chapter 7)

Candida albicans is much the most likely fungus to cause hospital infection because it is a common commensal in the mouth, colon and vagina and is resistant to antibacterial antibiotics. Its epidemic potential is low and, provided techniques to prevent cross-infection are skilfully applied, epidemic spread is unlikely.

Patients in category 4 are liable to be infected by fungi and bacteria from the environment normally considered to be harmless; these must not lightly be dismissed as contaminants. They may grow very slowly at body temperature. When microbes are seen in smears of specimens and fail to grow within 48 hours, prolonged incubation is required. Success may be attained by culture on non-enriched medium at room temperature.

The role of antimicrobial drugs

Bacteria most likely to cause hospital infection and epidemics are usually highly resistant to antimicrobials. The tendency to believe that treatment of individual patients while in hospital with the newest broad-spectrum antibiotic will prevent wound infection dies hard. The disadvantages of such treatment to the patient are often overlooked. Broad-spectrum antimicrobials often have unpleasant side effects, which, although not dangerous, depress the patient's well-being at a time when he needs all his natural resources for recovery. They will also alter profoundly his normal bacterial flora, which is likely to be sensitive to most antimicrobials, and leave him with only those which can withstand the treatment. Among them will be small numbers acquired from his new hospital environment, which will now be able to flourish. Much needs to be discovered about the relationship between host and commensal, but resident bacteria are likely to do more good than harm and should be preserved. The fact that bacteria with multiple antibiotic resistance are uncommon outside hospitals means that they are not biologically dominant. Without the aid of antibiotics to depress resident bacteria they are unable to establish themselves.

Operation wounds

Surgical skill is more important in preventing sepsis than is antimicrobial treatment, but prophylaxis is needed in some circumstances. Local application of antiseptic will prevent infection but is useless in treatment once it is established. It does not often cause side effects and does not interfere with resident microbes.

Hexachlorophane powder (containing 0.3% hexachlorophane) is highly successful at preventing staphylococcal infection of the umbilicus in the newborn. The wound, which is equivalent to a 'clean' operation wound, is kept dry – which prevents spread of bacteria from the surrounding area into the wound. Unlike liquid preparations, resistant Gram-negative bacilli cannot grow in it.

Povidone-iodine has also been used successfully to prevent infection of abdominal wounds which may be contaminated with small numbers of bacteria in operations which necessitate opening an abdominal viscus (Stokes *et al.*, 1977).

When systemic treatment is considered necessary it should be aimed at specific pathogens; for example, penicillin for *Cl. perfringens* in mid-thigh amputations, metronidazole for *Bact. fragilis* in acute appendicitis. The treatment should be timed to cover the period of maximum risk. The aim is to prevent small numbers of pathogens which contaminate the wound from becoming established. Experimentally this is achieved when treatment is given within 4 hours of contamination (Miles *et al.*, 1957). When given later than this, it has little effect. Keighley *et al.*, (1979) confirmed the effectiveness of early, brief prophylaxis in abdominal operations.

It follows that prophylaxis should be started at the time of operation, and, unless there is further manipulation and danger of contamination, it need not be continued for longer than 24–48 hours. The shorter the time, the less interference with resident bacteria and the less likely there will be unpleasant side effects.

Choice of drug depends on the site of operation and the pathogens known to be in the hospital environment at the time. The laboratory should be able to provide updated information on hospital pathogens. There is no drug, or combination of drugs, which can be guaranteed active against all wound contaminants.

Traumatic wounds

Although traumatic wounds may appear dirty on arrival, the chance that pathogenic microbes have entered the wound is slight. Road dust is much less dangerous than hospital dust (Fig. 11.1). The danger is from staphylococci, if the patient or those helping him are carriers, and from *Cl. perfringens* and other pathogenic spore bearers which are found in road dust. The spore bearers are all sensitive to penicillin, and staphyloccoci outside hospitals are very unlikely to be methicillin resistant. Moreover, small numbers entering the wound will not be likely to infect if surgical debridement and local treatment are performed shortly after injury. Provided contamination from the hospital is avoided, wounds

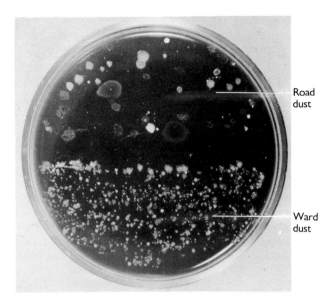

Road
dust

Ward
dust

Fig. 11.1 Comparison of growth from road dust and ward dust (blood agar incubated overnight at 37°C). The swab from the road was obviously dirty, that from the ward apparently clean.

without penetration of an abdominal viscus should heal very rapidly and short-term prophylactic penicillin should suffice.

Immunodeficient patients

Prompt treatment when sepsis develops is better than prophylaxis in these patients. They are likely to have spent long periods attending, or in, hospital and to have received antimicrobial treatment. As a result, their resident bacteria are likely to include multiple resistant hospital pathogens (see Table 11.1). To have any chance of preventing infection, broad-spectrum therapy with potentially toxic antimicrobials would be required. Prophylaxis is never 100 per cent effective and the prophylactic drugs would be useless for treatment of infection when it appeared. Moreover, some patients will escape infection without prophylaxis and their well-being is not improved by unnecessary prophylactic treatment. Contamination of the environment by multiple resistant pathogens is well known to be increased in wards where patients regularly receive prophylactic antibiotic treatment.

Febrile neutropenic patients undergoing treatment for cancer or those recovering from organ transplants need treatment immediately infection is suspected. They are at risk, not only from environmental bacteria but also from their own commensals. Laboratory diagnosis is often unavoidably delayed, treatment is urgent and has to be empirical. The numerous trials of therapy for these patients, some of them yielding conflicting results, have been summarized by Young (1986). The consensus is that a β-lactam drug combined with an aminoglycoside is most likely to succeed and is better than a single, most recent broad-spectrum antibiotic.

Investigation of hospital wound infection
Causes of breakdown in aseptic technique

Assuming that a 'no touch' dressing technique is theoretically being employed, there are five likely causes of breaddown in the technique.

1. *Rapid inspection*. The practice of taking dressings down prior to a ward round is, in general, to be deprecated. However, when dressings are extensive (e.g. plastic operations) it may be difficult to avoid. Covering the exposed wound with a loose sterile dressing, or cling-film applied aseptically, is a useful compromise but requires careful supervision.

The wound may be safely palpated if the fingers are protected with a sterile glove or by using a thick, dry, gauze swab. Sterile forceps and swabs (minimum basic equipment) should automatically be provided for those asked to inspect wounds.

2. *Shortage of forceps* is usually easily remedied. Three pairs of forceps are desirable for doing each dressing, but only two pairs are really essential for most dressings. When two pairs only are available, one of them is used to remove the inner dirty dressings and is then retained and used with the other pair to apply the clean dressing. The inner dressing is contaminated from the wound; it does not greatly matter if a few bacteria reach the clean dressing from the forceps which have removed the previous dressing. It is much safer to retain the contaminated forceps to help handle the clean dressing than to use only one pair of clean forceps and a hand.

3. *'Cleaning' operation wounds*. Accident wounds must be cleaned thoroughly. If particles of foreign matter and dead tissue remain, infection is inevitable; *sterile* antiseptic lotions are employed for this purpose. An operation wound, however, should not be cleaned with antiseptic; local antibacterial treatment may be prescribed but antiseptic lotions should be used only at the specific request of the surgeon, never routinely. Purulent discharge may need to be wiped away with a dry swab. Antiseptics sufficiently harmless to be applied to wounds are not self-sterilizing. When treatment is necessary a small quantity of *sterilized* antiseptic is applied. When a dressing is stuck to the wound it should be wetted with the smallest possible amount of sterile saline. Moisture will carry bacteria from one area to another and flooding the wound area, even with antiseptic, may carry harmful bacteria into the wound, particularly *Pseudomonas* and *Klebsiella* which are comparatively resistant to antiseptics.

4. *Frequent dressings*. It is often insufficiently appreciated that each time the dressings are removed the wound is exposed to the risk of infection, and, further, that if the wound is already infected its exposure involves dissemination of some of the pathogenic organisms into the air of the ward. Therefore, dressings should not be done unless it is absolutely necessary.

5. *Hurried dressings*. Many dressings combined with a shortage of staff means that they cannot be completed during the time that the ward is closed for dressings. If they are done at any other time the risk of infection is increased. When a dressing is done in a hurry by one person the technique is likely to be imperfect. These conditions in a surgical ward lead to a vicious circle, because more wound infections occur which lead to more dressings and so on.

Investigation and control of hospital infection

When hospital infection is suspected, the investigations required and steps to be taken to prevent spread to other patients vary with the nature of the infection. Table 11.2 lists the measures usually required when infection by any of the pathogens listed is suspected. It is a preliminary guide – each case must be individually judged; only those microbes dealt with in this chapter are included. For a comprehensive account, *Microbial Disease* by Tyrrell and his colleagues (1979) is recommended; also *Control of Communicable Disease in Man* (Benenson, 1985) an official report of the American Public Health Association approved by public health

Table 11.2 Control measures usually required

Pathogen	Isolation			Investigations		
	Strict	Standard	FU	Biohazard label	Carriers	Environ- ment
Str. pyogenes	(+)	+	–	–	+	(–)
Staph. aureus:						
MRSA	(–)	+	–	–	+	+
EMRSA	(+)	+	–	–	+	+
Staph. epidermidis	–	(+)	–	–	+	+
Salm. typhi	–	–	+	+	+	(K)
Salmonella spp.	–	–	+	–	+	K
Shigella spp.	–	–	+	–	+	K
Cl. perfringens	–	–	–	–	–	–
Cl. difficile	–	(+.)	–	–	+	–
Bact. fragilis	–	–	–	–	–	–
Coliforms:						
Klebsiella spp., *Proteus* spp., *Providencia* spp., *Enterobacter* spp., *Serratia* spp., *Pseudomonas* spp.	–	(+)	(+)	–	(+)	W
Legionella	–	–	–	–	+	
Lassa fever	+	–	–	+	–	–
Hepatitis B	–	–	–	+	(–)	–
HIV plus AIDS	p	–	–	+	(–)	–
HIV serum only	–	–	–	+	(–)	–

EMRSA = epidemic methicillin-resistant *Staph. aureus*; FU = faeces and urine; MRSA = methicillin-resistant *Staph. aureus*; W = wet sites; p = for patient's protection; K = kitchens.

authorities in Britain. Strict isolation is for highly infective microbes which spread easily, and is seldom needed. The measures recommended for the prevention of spread of dysentery (page 294) and of urinary infection (see below) will be needed for isolation category 'FU' (faeces and urine) but not for standard isolation.

Many preventive methods are tedious for those carrying them out. No recommendation should be lightly made, and it is for the clinical microbiologist to ensure that the control procedures recommended are essential and that the senior clinician in charge of the patient has been consulted. The infection control nurse ensures that the reasons for the procedures are understood and that they can be followed with as little interference with medical or surgical treatment as possible.

Urinary tract infection

Hospital-acquired infection of the urinary tract is very common. It begins as cystitis but may spread to the kidney or blood stream – catheter fever. As would be expected, the proportion of antibiotic-resistant strains is high and the pathogens are different from those causing spontaneously occuring cystitis outside hospital. Infection often follows catheterization, especially when the catheter must be retained. Epidemics in urological wards begin from one patient, perhaps with symptomless cystitis, who needs frequent catheterizaton or has a retained catheter. The pathogen, usually a coliform, is easily carried on the hands of staff to other patients who need similar attention. It can be cultivated from the environment, particularly wet areas, and coliforms more resistant than most to drying, such as *Pseudomonas* and *Klebsiella*, are found in dust. Closed drainage and strict aseptic precautions, including the use of disposable gloves, is much more important in control than is antibiotic treatment. Indeed, prophylactic treatment without prevention of spread leads to a higher rate of infection with even more resistant microbes. Antibiotics should be given to treat established symptomatic infection for as short a time as possible. It may be reasonable to give prophylactic treatment to cover operative procedures but not in the postoperative period (Casewell *et al.*, 1981).

Staph. aureus (see also page 281)

Carriage of methicillin-resistant *Staph. aureus* (MRSA) among members of hospital staff in close contact with patients requires treatment because bacteria from the nose disseminate more easily into the environment than from other carrier sites in healthy people. Carriage on healthy skin is almost always accompanied by nasal carriage and is sometimes dependent on it.

Clearance and prevention of recolonization needs prolonged treatment, including attention to personal environment, and this should be made clear from the outset. Lack of success, we think, is more often due to lack of sufficient time and diligence in treatment than to ineffectiveness of antimicrobials. The schedule outlined below was almost always successful

(Stokes *et al.*, 1965). It is based on the known time of survival of staphylococci in the environment. Now that epidemic strains are more resistant, different antimicrobials may be needed but the principles of treatment remain the same.

Method

1. Apply antiseptic nasal cream to the anterior nares four times daily: on waking, on going to bed and twice during the day immediately before going on duty. Continue this for 4 weeks.

2. Use antiseptic soap both at home and at work.

3. During the first week after starting nasal treatment, wash hair in 1% cetrimide and as soon as possible after this wash all knitted woollens in 1% cetrimide (do not rinse it all out) and send often-worn heavy garments and blankets to be cleaned. Have clean bed linen immediately after hairwashing. The cleaning programme should be complete by the end of the third week of nasal treatment.

4. After treatment has started, boil face-flannels, loofahs and powder puffs. Discard all old face powder and puffs which cannot be boiled.

All treated carriers should be followed up by culturing a nasal swab at least 3 days after the last application of cream and again 2 weeks or more, with no further treatment, after the first swab.

Epidemic diarrhoea in hospital

The patients and staff of hospitals are occasionally afflicted with epidemic diarrhoea and vomiting. Bacterial food poisoning is the most likely cause and the microbiologist is called upon to find the source of infection and to recommend measures for its control.

In Britain the organisms which commonly give rise to these symptoms are salmonellae, dysentery bacilli, *Cl. perfringens*, enterotoxin-producing strains of *Staph. aureus, B. cereus* and *Campylobacter*.

Investigation

The first step is to collect samples of faeces and vomit for culture. Then a very careful history is taken, noting especially the following points:

1. The number of people affected and the time of onset of symptoms.

2. The items of food and drink consumed by all the patients at the last meal attended by all of them.

The answers to the first question indicate the type of food poisoning. When it is caused by a bacterial toxin the onset will be abrupt, within a few hours of eating the food, and symptoms will appear in all those affected within about 12 hours. When it is caused by infection with *Shigella, Salmonella* or *Campylobacter* the incubation period will be longer, from 12 hours to 2 days, and the distribution of the time of onset of symptoms will be much more scattered. When a few people only are affected, it is as well to check carefully that they all have similar symptoms. When five or six people from the same department happen to fall ill at approximately the same time an epidemic may be wrongly suspected.

Answers to the second question usually indicate fairly clearly which dish was contaminated. It must be something consumed by all the people affected. When a number of people are symptom free, in spite of having eaten the suspected food, there are two possible explanations. Either the food was solid or semi-solid and the toxin or bacteria were not evenly distributed in it, or only a part of it was contaminated; for example, milk from an infected container might be poured into one or two jugs out of several consumed at the meal.

Any food having the following characteristics is a particularly likely source of infection.

1. Food which has been much handled in preparation.

2. Food composed of animal protein such as eggs (particularly dried egg), home-cured ham, sausage meat, minced meat and brawn.

3. Food, either cooked or uncooked, which has been prepared and allowed to stand for several hours before it is served.

Cooking often fails to kill food poisoning bacteria. Penetration of heat through a large pie in a domestic oven is not rapid, and although the temperature of the outside may be 100°C the inside can be less than 60°C. *Staph. aureus*, *Shigella* and *Salmonella* are not particularly sensitive to heat. Egg dishes, for example, are seldom heated sufficiently to kill the salmonellae which may be found in them.

Food is seldom *originally* contaminated with sufficient pathogens to cause infection. If the few pathogens originally present survive preparation and the food is not consumed immediately, they may multiply. Reheating before serving may kill them but bacterial toxins produced during growth will often survive.

Of the common causes of food poisoning, *Staph. aureus*, *Cl. perfringens* and *B. cereus* are toxin producers, and *Salmonella*, *Shigella* and *Campylobacter* are enteropathogens. *Staph. aureus* and *Shigella* are likely to contaminate food from a human carrier (or carriers) during preparation. *Salmonella* may also enter by this route, but they are widespread animal pathogens and food (eggs and meat) may already be contaminated by them. They are spread by rodents and flies in unhygienic kitchens.

The spore bearers *Cl. perfringens* and *B. cereus* are present in dust of all human habitation and inevitably enter food in small numbers, which are harmless unless they are allowed to grow and form toxin which some strains produce. Gram-stained smears of the food are likely to show large numbers of Gram-positive bacilli, usually without spores, when either of these species is the culprit. Enterotoxin production can be confirmed by sending strains isolated from remains of food consumed by those with symptoms, and from their faeces, to a reference laboratory.

Campylobacter food poisoning usually results from eating under-cooked frozen poultry. The organism can be isolated from the livers of apparently healthy birds. The incubation period is probably 2–10 days (Leading Article, 1978).

It is well known that freezing preserves rather than kills most bacteria. If pathogens have had a chance to multiply in food before it is frozen, food poisoning will result when it is consumed. Even if it is thoroughly heated, toxins in it may give rise to symptoms. Every effort should be made to culture the remains of the suspected food because a positive result may narrow the field considerably in the subsequent search for the source of infection.

The possibility that the diarrhoea may be related to antimicrobial treatment and that *Cl. difficile* may be transferred between patients must also be considered (page 282).

Measures for control
In the kitchen
Immediate measures are aimed at preventing multiplication of bacteria in the food. When several hours' delay between cooking and eating is unavoidable the food should be rapidly cooled and then refrigerated until its final preparation. In hospital kitchens, mixers, slicers, chopping boards and other equipment should be heat disinfected at least once daily. Facilities for hand washing after visiting the toilet should be inspected and improved when necessary.

In outbreaks of food poisoning caused by salmonella and dysentery organisms, carriers in the kitchen staff must be sought. When *Staph. aureus* has been isolated from the food, and from the faeces or vomit of the patients, an attempt can be made to find a nasal carrier of the same phage type among the kitchen staff. If there are no facilities for phage typing, or if the staphylococcus was killed in cooking and the diagnosis remains clinical, no good purpose is served by swabbing the kitchen staff. About half of them will probably be found to be carrying *Staph. aureus* in the nose and, without differentiation between enterotoxin-producers and others, isolation of carriers is impracticable. Further cases are prevented by keeping the food cool after preparation so that the staphylococci do not get a chance to grow and produce their toxin. Cooks with colds should be encouraged to report sick and remain off duty until cured, because frequent use of the handkerchief in the kitchen by a carrier is dangerous. Instruction of the staff in the need for frequent hand washing and the provision of antibacterial soap and plenty of clean towels will also help to lessen the risk. Cooks with septic hand lesions should not be allowed on duty. Standards of hygiene required in hospital kitchens and suggestions for maintaining them will be found in *Control of Hospital Infection* by Lowbury *et al.*, (1975), and booklets are available from the Catering and Dietetic Department of the DHSS.

Two methods are available for searching for carriers of the intestinal pathogens – serological tests and faeces culture. In an outbreak of salmonella food poisoning, when the kitchen staff have not received prophylactic TAB inoculation, a search for salmonella antibodies in their serum may lead to the discovery of a chronic intermittent carrier who would otherwise have escaped notice. The sera can be tested against the epidemic strain. A positive agglutination test does not prove that an individual is a carrier; it merely shows the need for repeated stool cultures.

Dysentery carriers do not necessarily show antibodies to the bacilli, and the method of choice for investigation is rectal swab or faeces cultures.

Kitchen staff are usually co-operative if the reason for the tests is explained to them and if they are warned from the outset that more than one specimen from each person will probably be necessary.

In the wards
Staphylococcal food poisoning is an intoxication, not an infection, and therefore no precautions against the spread of infection are necessary.

The principles of nursing patients with intestinal infections are described by Tyrrell *et al.*, (1979). A few practical difficulties may be worth mentioning here.

When there are only one or two infected patients in a general medical ward a special nurse is often appointed to look after them. This appears to be very desirable but in practice when the patients need frequent attention and when the nursing staff work in three shifts it means that six nurses are necessary if there is to be no overlap of duties, because at any time one of the infected patients may need attention while his nurse is having a meal. It is clearly impracticable to appoint six nurses to look after one or two patients. A nurse is unlikely to spread infection unless she contaminates her hands from the infected patients' excreta and then touches something which enters another patient's mouth. She may also infect herself, and staff should be asked to report any diarrhoea immediately. Disposable gloves should be worn to attend incontinent patients. Cross-infection is unlikely if it is agreed that the available staff, on each shift, are divided into two groups. Those who attend the isolated patient do not enter ward kitchens, help feed other patients or give them treatment by mouth. All other duties can be undertaken by them. Those *not* attending the isolated patients should avoid giving bedpans to *any* patient as far as possible, and wash and dry their hands meticulously after leaving the sluice if they have to do so.

Sampling the patient and his environment

1. *Nose and throat swabs*. When large numbers of contacts are swabbed it is difficult to avoid an occasional sterile specimen, which has to be repeated. If arrangements are made for the contacts to attend the laboratory for swabbing, the number of unsatisfactory specimens can be reduced because there is minimal delay between sampling and culturing. Nasal swabs need to be moistened in peptone water, broth or sterile saline before sampling.

2. *Skin*. A moistened swab is rubbed vigorously over the chosen site. The back of the wrist is a suitable area when looking for staphylococcal skin carriers. It is less likely than the hand to be contaminated with bacteria from extraneous sources. The swab is seeded over at least half a culture plate. It is unnecessary to spread the inoculum.

Since *Staph. aureus* produces phosphatase more rapidly than other staphylococci, phenolphthalein phosphate agar (Barber and Kuper, 1951) can be employed to detect them more easily in mixed culture. Phosphatase releases phenolphthalein and, when exposed to alkaline vapour (by dropping about 5 drops of concentrated ammonia into the lid of an overnight culture plate), the colonies of phosphatase producers turn bright pink. Only pink colonies need therefore be tested for coagulase production. They can be detected among similar colonies even when covered by spreading proteus; for method of preparation, see page 315. For other selective media for *Staph. aureus*, see page 92.

The skin of a surgeon or his assistants is best sampled at the end of a long operation by swabbing the hands or pressing the inner surface of carefully removed gloves on blood or phenolphthalein phosphate agar.

3. *Floors, furniture, baths, washing bowls, etc.* A moistened swab is rubbed over a wide area of the surface and then seeded on blood agar or appropriate selective medium. It is wise to streak out the pool of inoculum because even clean-looking surfaces often yield a heavy growth.

4. *Textiles.* Linen, cotton and other smooth materials are most suitably sampled by the press plate method. The part of the material to be sampled is pressed against the surface of a culture plate. The remainder is folded thickly behind it to protect it from contamination by the hand.

Woollens are conveniently sampled either by shaking them over an exposed plate or by using the edge of the plate to brush the fabric so that particles from it will land on the surface of the medium.

5. *Unsterile equipment* such as plaster shears, bandage scissors, safety pins, sandbags and mackintosh sheets are sampled as described for furniture but there is no need to streak out the inoculum from small articles.

6. *'Sterile' instruments and dressings* (see page 300). The nurse, theatre sister or dresser is asked to prepare the instrument or dressing exactly as if it were to be used on the patient. Then the operating end of the instrument is dipped into bottles containing broth and cooked meat broth. Using scissors and forceps, dry-sterilized in the laboratory, portions of dressings are cut off and cultured in broth and cooked meat broth. After 4 days' incubation the cultures are seeded on blood agar plates which are incubated in the appropriate atmospheres.

This is a very sensitive method. If one viable organism enters the broth during sampling it will grow, so the method gives little indication of the weight of contamination. Growth of aerobic spore beares, micrococci and other microbes normally considered harmless is not necessarily a serious matter. The majority of cultures carefully made in this way should be sterile but growth of a single species in say 10 per cent of bottles, if no pathogen is recovered, is not evidence of faulty technique. Most surgical techniques are not sterile in the strictest sense; they are aimed at excluding all known pathogens and reducing as far as possible the number of all other microbes which enter the wound.

7. *'Sterile' lotions* (see page 300). If the solution is not antiseptic a large volume of it can be sampled by delivering about 10 ml with a sterile pipette into an equal volume of double-strength peptone water. Two such cultures

are made, one for incubation at 37°C and one at room temperature. Some antiseptic solutions, for example those containing mercuric salts, can be rendered harmless to bacteria before culture by the addition of a neutralizing chemical. Antiseptics and disinfectants are best tested for contamination by the Kelsey/Maurer in-use test (see Maurer, 1985). For most purposes, the activity of the solution is neutralized with nutrient broth. One ml of the disinfectant is placed in 9 ml broth. Using a 50 dropper, 10 drops of this 1 : 10 dilutions are placed on each of two well-dried nutrient agar plates. One plate is incubated at room temperature (20–25°C) for 1 week, and the other at 37°C for 3 days. Five or more colonies on one or both plates indicate unsatisfactory disinfection.

8. *Air*. Two kinds of bacteria-carrying particles are found in air – small ones which remain suspended for long periods, and large ones which fall to the ground within about an hour in a still atmosphere. Infections caused by bacteria which gain entry via the respiratory system can be transferred by the inhalation of either large or small particles. If the risk of infection by this route is to be satisfactorily investigated, a slit sampler or rotary air sampler is required (see Report, 1983). The small particles, since they remain suspended, are unimportant in wound infection. The large ones can be collected by allowing them to fall on the surface of exposed blood agar.

To find the risk of aerial contamination of a wound in the theatre it is reasonable to expose blood agar plates in pairs at various sites for the duration of the longest operation likely to be performed. At least one pair of plates should be prepared sterile on the outside so that they may be exposed near the operation site.

Sterile Petri dishes without covers are placed in a sterile box. The lid of the box is lifted and blood agar is poured into them with minimal exposure. The lid is then closed and time is allowed for the medium to set. When the surgeon is ready to make the incision the box is opened and he takes out the sterile blood agar plates and places them conveniently near the wound. At the end of sampling they are handed to the microbiologist, who covers them with sterile lids in the usual way.

One plate of each pair is incubated in air, the other anaerobically. After 24 hours' incubation the number of colonies on the aerobic plates is counted. Contamination of the air is expressed as the number of colonies per minute of exposure. One colony of each type found on the anaerobic plates is streaked on blood agar to be incubated aerobically and then, without flaming the loop, onto blood agar for anaerobic culture. Those which grow on the anaerobic but not on the aerobic subculture are anaerobes and need further investigation. Known pathogens likely to appear are *Staph. aureus*, streptococci, coliforms and *Cl. perfringens*.

To obtain a good idea of the risk of infection from the air it is necessary to repeat the sampling on several occasions because the result depends on a number of variable factors, the most important of them being: (1) the number of people in the threatre; (2) the amount of movement, particularly of the patient and his coverings and of people entering and leaving the theatre; (3) the number of operations previously done in the theatre;

(4) the direction and strength of the wind and (5) the humidity of the atmosphere.

Autoclave sterilization

Sterilization of materials by steam under pressure is effective, quick and cheap, but its effectiveness depends on the proper handling and maintenance of the autoclave, which needs frequent testing and supervision. Although an old-fashioned boiler will not kill all spores and leaves instruments wet, all vegetative bacteria (i.e. all those which commonly cause hospital infection) and tubercle bacilli are killed after 2 minutes' boiling. Disinfection of instruments by this simple method is safer than 'sterilization' in a badly maintained and inefficient autoclave.

For preference, instruments and dressings should be sterilized centrally prewrapped. They should emerge dry and must not be exposed to the risk of contamination after sterilization. In hospitals this is most readily achieved by at least two high-vacuum autoclaves, operated or supervised by skilled staff, situated in central sterile supply department (CSSD). Two is the minimum number to allow for servicing. Theatre autoclaves for the sterilization of theatre instruments which need not be prewrapped can be of the cheaper downward displacement type. Wards should receive presterilized dressings and instruments from the CSSD because it is uneconomical to install ward autoclaves and usually impossible to maintain and operate them efficiently.

Tests of efficient sterilization
Hospital Technical Memorandum (HTM) No. 10

HTM No. 10 describes tests which must be carried out regularly from the commissioning of an autoclave and hot air sterilizer in order to ensure their efficiency. The microbiologist, the CSSD manager or the hospital engineer must ensure that these tests are carried out regularly and that records are available for inspection. The key to successful operation is the master temperature recording (MTR). This is a graphical chart produced when the autoclave is properly commissioned against a multi-lead thermocouple recorder. The MTR should be displayed near the autoclave, and all subsequent cycle charts should be checked against it. Autoclave dials are not sufficiently accurate to be used to assess whether sterile conditions have been obtained. When a cycle chart is not identical to the MTR, sterility cannot be guaranteed, and the autoclave should be taken out of use until the fault is repaired and the machine recommissioned. HTM 10 lists the daily, weekly, monthly and annual tests that should be performed, as part of a planned maintenance policy. With the exception of the Bowie and Dick test, which indicates air removal the tests described below are secondary to the thermocouple test, and comparison of cycle charts against the MTR. It is important to appreciate that the **cycle** time is made up of a **heating** period, a **holding** period (consisting of the **sterilization** time, plus a **safety** period of half the sterilization time) and a **cooling** period.

Downward displacement autoclaves
Air is partly evacuated either by pump or by steam ejector and steam flows in through the top of the chamber, displacing the remaining air which flows out through the chamber drain at the bottom. In this type of auto-clave, packing is extremely important because the flow of steam must not be impeded either by overloading the chamber or by packing too tightly. Waterproof materials, even when interleaved, are very difficult to sterilize by this method.

The cycle is prolonged because removal of air from the load is slow and subsequent drying is slow; in a large machine it may take more than an hour. Articles most exposed to heat in the load may be damaged if those least exposed are to be properly sterilized. These machines are therefore suitable only for sterilization of instruments where no penetration of textiles is required. They are simple to use and efficient for this purpose. They are also employed for sterilizing bottled fluids.

Tests   Browne's tubes, which change colour from red to green on exposure to heat for an appropriate time, are suitable for routine testing provided the type 1 tube (black spot) is used and that the tubes are stored in a cool place, not above 21°C (70°F). Autoclave tape which becomes striped on heating will check that articles have been through the machine but not that they have been efficiently sterilized.

High-vacuum autoclaves
These more costly machines overcome the difficulty of penetration of steam into the load and of drying, by employing much more efficient evacuation of air using high-vacuum pumps before steam flows in, and by rapid evacuation of steam after sterilization. A higher temperature is reached but the articles escape damage as the cycle is much shorter – about 15 minutes with a large machine. These are the best machines so far made for the sterilization of dressings and wrapped instruments.

Tests   The chamber may leak or the pumps be inefficient and these must be checked by daily inspection of a chart on which temperature and pressure during each cycle are automatically recorded and compared with the MTR. Browne's tubes type 2 (yellow spot) can be employed within loads, but when temperatures are high (135–137°C) the holding time must not be more than 3 minutes. After this time the capsules may change colour in dry heat, which is not a fair test as bacterial spores are not suscep-tible to dry heat for a short time at this temperature. A test of steam pene-tration within a load has been devised by Bowie and Dick employing autoclave tape; it is reliable when properly carried out.

Bowie–Dick test
Materials
Huckaback towels 90 × 60 cm to form a pile 25 × 27.5 cm high when

folded. Paper, firm but not waterproof. Autoclave tape, 3M brand No. 1222, sufficient to form a diagonal cross when stuck on the paper.

Method
The towels are washed when new or soiled, or are hung up for at least 1 hour before each test. The paper with tape on it is placed in the middle of the pile and the whole is held in whatever container is employed for dressings. It is then placed in the empty autoclave which is run for its normal cycle. When penetration is satisfactory the stripes will be uniformly darkened. The holding time must not exceed 3½ minutes at 134–137°C because the tape will change colour in dry heat. The tape must be stored in a cool place and must not be left in the warm autoclave room before testing. The test should be done in an empty autoclave at the beginning of the day after a preliminary warm-up cycle, because conditions are least favourable in this type of autoclave when there is only one pack and a large volume of air has to be evacuated from the chamber (Bowie *et al.*, 1963).

Likely faults
A common and obvious fault is wet dressings. This is often due to poor-quality steam supply, which is the province of the hospital engineer. It is also likely to happen if the jacket is not prewarmed so that there is condensation on the inside of the chamber when steam flows into the cold machine. It can also be caused by condensation on metal articles, jugs, bowls, etc., if they are sterilized with the dressings. This can often be avoided if they are packed inverted so that water cannot accumulate in them. It may be necessary to pack them separately. This is a very serious fault when dressings are packed in paper or linen because bacteria will be carried in moisture from the surroundings to the inside of the pack and the dressings will be contaminated after sterilization. More detailed information on this complex subject is given in *Control of Hospital Infection* by Lowbury *et al.* (1975).

Monitoring sterile products

There are commonly two places where sterile products are prepared within the hospital. One is the central sterile supply department (CSSD) which supplies sterile dressings and instruments, the other is the pharmacy which supplies sterile lotions and medicaments. The clinical microbiologist may be called on by either of these to monitor the efficacy of sterilization and he must be prepared to offer advice when a fault is suspected.

The CSSD sterilizes by autoclave, oven or other physical methods and the product is not exposed until it is to be used. The autoclaves and ovens are supervised by the CSSD director; daily records are kept by him and the only likely problem within this department is lack of staff or space in the sterilizers to cope with the work demanded of it. There may be a subsection which deals with equipment which cannot be heat treated, such as respirators and infant incubators. This equipment may be disinfected by a combination of formaldehyde vapour and gentle heat (80°C). Penetration is ensured by treating while a respirator is in action. Sterilization is not attempted and not required, the aim being to kill all vegetative bacteria, including tubercle bacilli (and most viruses), likely to be passed from one patient to the next by contact with the equipment.

When cross-infection is suspected from contaminated dressings, instruments or equipment, inspection of records of performance will usually show that sterilizers are perfoming efficiently. Automatic recorders should then be checked. No useful purpose is served by testing the sterility of samples of dressings or instruments. A positive result is more likely to indicate a fault in the sampling method than a fault in the autoclave or oven showing impeccable records. (Methods of testing are described on page 295, for use in hospitals with no CSSD when a gross fault in procedure is suspected.) Contamination of 'sterile' materials from a CSSD may be either because they have not been through the sterilizers or because they have been contaminated subsequently. Careful and tactful enquiry from the people *actually handling the materials at the time when the fault is believed to have occurred* will usually bring irregularities to light. The patient himself is often helpful; he may remember in detail what happened and his account must be taken seriously even when it seems improbable. The CSSD should be kept scrupulously clean and tidy, dust must not be allowed to contaminate the outside of sterilized packets, but routine bacteriological tests of a clean and well organized department are a waste of laboratory expertise.

Hospital pharmacies which prepare sterile products for use on patients are regularly inspected in Britain and evidence of some form of monitoring is demanded by the inspectors. Products which are to be sterilized are prepared in 'clean' areas; 'aseptic' areas are provided for the preparation of material which will not withstand sterilization. Hospital pharmacies do not prepare materials for prolonged storage; therefore a few contaminating bacteria do not have an opportunity to grow to dangerous numbers.

Records of performance of pharmacy autoclaves must be kept and automatic recorders must be checked regularly. 'Aseptic' areas are often plenum ventilated or have within them plenum ventilated cabinets; this equipment must be properly maintained and the air flow monitored. An 'aseptic' area must be kept clean and free from visible dust but it is not sterile. The inspectors have good reason to require evidence that the equipment in these rooms is properly maintained and performing as expected. When it is first installed it is worthwhile to incubate culture medium exposed in the sterile area to exclude an unexpected source of extraneous contamination. The benefit of *routine* monitoring by culture is unproven and in our view unlikely to be useful. Testing the sterilized products, rather than the sterilizing equipment, is as useless here as in the CSSD. Testing aseptically prepared medicaments calls for premises at least as aseptic as those in the pharmacy, which most laboratories do not possess. Moreover, bacterial inhibitors are often present and must be neutralized. This is highly specialized work and best carried out centrally in a laboratory set up for the purpose.

Culture of blood for transfusion

Blood for transfusion is sometimes sent for culture when a patient has suffered an unexplained reaction. Patients are not likely to suffer unless a bacterium, introduced into the blood at some stage, has had an opportunity to grow. Symptoms are usually caused by toxins preformed during growth rather than by infection with the organism. Toxin formation is likely when the contaminating organism grows well at 4°C, and may happen if the transfusion is given slowly and sufficient time elapses for growth to occur after the bottle is removed from the refrigerator. Since many bacteria which multiply at 4°C are incapable of growth at 37°C, routine methods have to be modified.

Procedure
Make two smears for Gram and Leishman stains. Seed three blood agar slopes (in screw-capped bottles to prevent evaporation), and incubate one at 37°C, one at room temperature in the dark and one at 4°C. Deliver about 2 ml of the blood into each of three bottles containing peptone water and incubate one with each of the blood agar slopes.

Examine the cultures daily. If no growth is visible when they have been incubated for the same length of time that elapsed between the collection of blood from the donor and the transfusion, they may be discarded. Growth may be difficult to see in the liquid cultures; they should therefore be subcultured on blood agar and Gram-stained before a negative report is sent.

The bacteria which have most often been found as the cause of this rare accident are coliform bacilli capable of growth at low temperatures (see ACP Broadsheet, 1974).

Termination of isolation

Fumigation by sealing the room and releasing formalin vapour is no longer considered to be necessary except in very dangerous infections such as lassa fever, when it is best carried out by the Public Health Department who have the training and equipment to do it properly.

After isolation procedures, terminal cleaning is carried out. This is normally done by an orderly wearing a gown who cleans the whole room and furniture very thoroughly, first with disinfectant (e.g. 1% Sudol), and then he removes the disinfectant in the same order of cleaning so that each area treated is exposed for an adequate time. Vigorous cleaning during application is very important; the disinfectant will not penetrate layers of dust. The room can be reoccupied without delay. Plastic-covered pillows and mattresses can be treated similarly; otherwise they should be heat treated with bedding and clothing. A short disinfecting cycle is sufficient since, in general, spores can be ignored; *B. anthracis* is the only spore bearer likely to cause transmissible infection.

Prevention of laboratory infection

The recognition that hepatitis B virus can cause fatal laboratory infection and that the danger of catching smallpox is now greater in laboratories handling virus than anywhere else in the world has concentrated attention on laboratory infection and its prevention. There is at present no standard practice and no compulsory notification of infection. Hospital laboratories normally only handle pathogens belonging to category B (Report, 1975), among which the most dangerous likely to be encountered in Britain are *Salm. typhi* and *Myco. tuberculosis*. Medical pathogens of category A are all viruses, and when the diagnosis is suspected the appropriate designated laboratory must be notified by telephone immediately and their instructions followed.

Tuberculosis has long been recognized as a hazard in microbiology laboratories, and rules for handling material suspected of infection are included in Chapter 6. Safety cabinets improperly installed and maintained can increase the danger. Recommendations for their construction and maintenance will be found in PHLS Monograph No. 6 (1974).

Hazards of particular techniques and safety measures are mentioned where they occur in the text. A brief list of safety rules of general application is listed below.

1. Mouth pipetting must be forbidden in all laboratories, including serology rooms.

2. Eating and smoking must be forbidden in the laboratories.

3. Protective clothing must be worn when handling all specimens and cultures.

4. Hands and exposed forearms must be washed after work at a safety cabinet and always before leaving the laboratory.

5. Discard jars must be placed conveniently on the bench to enable workers to place the tips of pipettes under the disinfectant before removing the teat. Jars must be emptied and disinfectant renewed before each day's work.

6. Discard buckets must be waterproof and withstand autoclaving. Discarded cultures and specimens must either be autoclaved in the laboratory or be placed in waterproof bags for incineration. They are the responsibility of laboratory staff until rendered safe for handling.

7. A senior member of the staff must be designated safety officer and be responsible for training junior and ancillary staff. He must have a deputy.

8. Any accident or spillage must be reported forthwith to the safety officer or his deputy and a record of it made.

9. Basic safety rules should be displayed and a written copy given to each member of the staff, who should sign a register confirming that he has read and understood the instructions.

10. Telephone numbers of designated laboratories which handle category A pathogens (see above) must be kept up to date and are best displayed for rapid emergency use.

References

Advisory Committee on Dangerous Pathogens (1984) *Categorisation of Pathogens According to Hazard and Categories of Containment*. HM Stationery Office, London

Advisory Committee on Dangerous Pathogens (1986) Revised Guidelines. HM Stationery Office, London (obtainable from DHSS)

Association of Clinical Pathologists, Broadsheet No. 54 (1974) By G.H. Tovey and W.A. Gillespie.

Barber, M. and Kuper, S.W.A. (1951) *Journal of Pathology and Bacteriology* 63, 65

Bender, B.S., Bennett, R., Langhon, B.E., Greenough, W.B. III *et al.* (1986) *Lancet* ii, 11

Benenson, A.S. (Ed.) (1985) *Control of Communicable Disease in Man*. American Public Health Association, Washington DC

Bowie, J.H., Kelsey, J.C. and Thompson, G.R. (1963) *Lancet* i, 586

Casewell, M.W., Pugh, S. and Dalto, M.T. (1981) *Journal of Hospital Infection* 2, 55

Edelstein, P.H. (1981) *Journal of Clinical Microbiology* 14, 298

Ferrieri, P., Cleary, P.P. and Seeds, A.E. (1977) *Journal of Medical Microbiology* 10, 103

Fisher-Hoch, S.P., Craven, R.B., Forthall, D.N. *et al.* (1985) *Lancet* ii, 1227

Goldman, M., Liesnard, C., Vanherveghem, J.L. *et al.* (1986) *British Medical Journal* 293 161

Grist, N.R. (1979). *British Medical Journal* 1, 192

Health Services Advisory Committee (1985) *Safety in Health Service laboratories – Hepatitis B* HM Stationery Office, London

Hospital Technical Memorandum No. 10 (1980) H.M. Stationery Office, London

Keighley, M.R.B., Arabi, Y., Alexander-Williams, J., Youngs, D. and Burdon, D.W. (1979) *Lancet* i, 894

Leading Article (1978) *Lancet* ii, 135

Leading Article (1981) *Lancet* ii, 381

Leading Article (1983) *British Medical Journal* 287, 443

Lowbury, E.J.L., Ayliffe, G.A.J., Geddes, A.M. and Williams, J.D. (1975) *Control of Hospital Infection*. Chapman and Hall, London

Maurer, I.M. (1985) *Hospital Hygiene*, 3rd edn. Edward Arnorld, London

Miles, A.A., Miles, E.M. and Burke, J.F. (1957) *British Journal of Experimental Pathology* 38, 79

Pead, L., Maskell, R. and Morris, J. (1985) *British Medical Journal* 291, 1157

Public Health Laboratory Service Monograph No. 6 (1974). *The Prevention of Laboratory Acquired Infection* Collins C.H., Hartley, E.G. and Pilsworth R. HM Stationery Office, London

Report of Working Party on the Laboratory Use of Dangerous Pathogens (1975) Cmnd 6054. DHSS, London

Report (1983) *Ventilation of Operating Theatres*. Inter-Authority Engineering Group No. 10. DHSS, London

Report (1986) Guidelines for the control of epidemic resistant *Staph.aureus Journal of Hospital Infection* 7, 193

Stokes, E.J., Hall, B.M., Richards, J.D.M. and Riley, D.J. (1965) *Lancet* i, 197

Stokes, E.J., Howard, E., Peters, J.L., Hackworthy, C.A., Milne, S.E. and Witherow, R.O. (1977) *World Journal of Surgery* 1, 777

Tyrrell, D.A.J., Phillips, I., Goodwind, C.S. and Blowers, R. (1979) *Microbial Disease*. Edward Arnold, London van den Broek, P.J., Lampe, A.S., Berbee, G.A.M. *et al.* (1985) *British Medical Journal* **291**, 949

Wilson, G.S., Miles, A.A. and Parker, M.T. (Eds.) (1983) In: *Topley and Wilson's Principles of Bacteriology, Virology and Immunity*, 7th edn. Edward Arnorld, London

Young, L.S. (1986) *New England Journal of Medicine* **315**, 580

12

Media Preparation and Other Techniques

Media preparation

Diagnostic laboratories seldom have time to test media routinely. They have to rely on quality control practised by commercial firms on their products. It has been shown by the culture of simulated specimens sent by UKEQAS (see page 22 and Appendix) that isolation of intestinal pathogens is more successful when commercially prepared powdered medium (for final preparation in laboratory) is employed. Occasionally a batch of medium below par may be supplied, but generally standards are higher than could be achieved by making media locally.

Final preparation from several commercially prepared ingredients which are mixed and poured into Petri dishes, or otherwise distributed, in the laboratory, needs supervision and monitoring. The most frequent error is failure to mix ingredients thoroughly. Inversion of containers several times will mix; swilling around, especially of a large nearly full bottle (to avoid wetting the cap or causing bubbles) is unlikely to be effective. Bottles should not be completely filled. For example, a 3 litre bottle should not contain more than 2 litres, to allow room for mixing. This fault leads to variation between plates or individual bottles and is likely to escape notice unless especially investigated. Failure to isolate pathogens from simulated specimens sent by UKEQAS should immediately lead to a check of media preparation within the laboratory.

Another likely error is to use glassware which has previously contained growth inhibitors. These are difficult to remove completely and even traces of them may prevent growth of small numbers of pathogens on primary isolation. Disposable containers can be used or glass containers of a particular shape or size can be reserved for media or solutions containing inhibitors. Tubing should be disposable. When mechanical methods are used and tubing is required, it is important to pour nutrient and enriched medium first, and selective medium, which contains inhibitors, later. For those who wish to check their media, or to investigate the potential of a new medium, suitable methods are described in *Clinical Bacteriology* (Stokes and Ridgway, 1980); see also the Miles and Misra method of making viable counts (1938).

Anaerobic culture technique

There are a number of satisfactory methods of maintaining anaerobic conditions in liquid cultures. Reducing agents in common use are strips of sheet-iron, minced meat (which contains reducing fatty acids) and thioglycollic acid. If primary anaerobic cultures of material from mixed infections are made in liquid media only, the proportion of the different species present will not be revealed. A few organisms of a quickly growing species such as *Cl. perfringens* may assume a predominance in the culture quite out of proportion to its numbers in the specimen. In order to judge which, if any, of the anaerobes found is likely to be the causal organism, primary seeding on solid medium is essential. This necessitates incubation in a container from which all free oxygen has been removed.

There is a considerable choice of equipment for maintaining anaerobiosis of plate cultures. Anaerobe cabinets can be purchased in which all manipulation is carried out in an oxygen-free atmosphere. There are modifications of the classic McIntosh and Fildes jar in which air is evacuated and replaced with hydrogen. Polycarbonate and stainless steel jars have a catalyst in the lid and commercially produced sachets to which water is added to generate hydrogen and carbon dioxide for each jar, no vacuum pump or gas cylinders being required. (They are obtainable from Oxoid or Becton Dickinson (polycarbonate) or Don Whitley (stainless steel).) These sachets cannot be used in the standard McIntosh and Fildes jar without danger of explosion because the catalyst is not suitable, but they can be employed in a modification of it (Burt and Phillips, 1977). The disadvantage of these jars is that anaerobiosis is not attained for several hours. Highly fastidious anaerobes will succumb to this length of exposure to oxygen.

An inexpensive method, suitable for laboratories without an anerobic cabinet, is a McIntosh and Fildes jar with cold catalyst, which achieves rapid anaerobiosis. A vacuum pump and a cylinder containing a mixture of hydrogen, nitrogen and 10% CO_2 will also be needed. To attain a micro-aerophilic atmosphere (page 307) and for greater versatility, two cylinders are required – one containing the hydrogen/nitrogen mixture, the other CO_2. The choice of method depends on the amount and nature of the anaerobic work undertaken. The medically important anaerobes are able to withstand short periods of exposure to air (Rosenblatt *et al.*, 1973; Watt *et al.*, 1974).

Anaerobic indicators

An indicator is essential to check on each occasion that strict anaerobiosis has been achieved; there are three kinds, chemical, physical and biological. It is important to be able to recognize a faulty jar before incubation and this can be done either by a rapid colour change of a chemical indicator or by noting the rapid development of a vacuum when an active catalyst induces rapid combination of hydrogen and oxygen. Chemical indicator strips can be purchased in sachets; one is opened and exposed in each (transparent) polycarbonate jar immediately before closure. Metal McIntosh and Fildes jars have a side arm to which an indicator tube can be attached. These have not been popular because the side arm tends to leak and commercially produced indicators have proved unsatisfactory. The side arm can be sealed off. Jars which are not transparent must be tested by noting the *rapid* development of 620 cm Hg vacuum within 5–10 minutes measured by attaching a manometer to each before it is passed for incubation.

An additional biological test which will reveal a very small, slow leak should be included in each jar. A culture of a strict aerobe which will not grow anaerobically or a strict anaerobe can be employed. The most convenient of these is *Ps. aeruginosa* cultured on Simmons citrate agar. It will not grow on this medium under strictly anaerobic conditions, and an added advantage is that traces of growth are easily detected by a colour change in the medium (Gargan and Phillips, 1978).

A hiss of inrushing air on opening the jar combined with slight discoloration of the blood agar is evidence of an air-tight jar and some change in atmosphere, but both these signs can be present when some oxygen remains and must not therefore be taken as evidence of anaerobiosis.

The catalyst is inactivated by moisture, sulphur and arsine. Hydogen sulphide given off from cultures will gradually inactivate it. Arsine inactivation is caused by traces of arsine in the hydrogen; it can be removed, when necessary, by passing the gas through 10% silver nitrate solution.

Incubation in air plus 5–10% CO_2

When a large number of cultures are required to be incubated in an atmosphere of 10% CO_2, the use of a CO_2 incubator is convenient. Accurate control of gas, humidity and temperature is achieved. A number of models are available, and in our experience Assab incubators are reliable.

When no CO_2 incubator is available a McIntosh and Fildes jar without a capsule (which need not be quite air-tight) can be employed. The jar is evacuated to 640 mm Hg and CO_2 is allowed to run in until the evacuation, as read on the manometer, is reduced by 7.6 cm approximately. Assuming atmospheric pressure to be 76 cm this is equivalent to 10 per cent.

A lighted candle placed in a jar which is then closed will reduce the oxygen and increase the carbon dioxide content of the jar. An unknown amount of fumes, possibly toxic, will also be released from the candle and there will be a small amount of carbon deposits. Undoubtedly CO_2-dependent bacteria will grow in a candle jar, which must be used for their culture when there is no better alternative.

Microaerophilic atmosphere

The oxygen requirements of bacteria can be studied in shake agar cultures, enriched with Fildes extract and serum when necessary. The molten medium in a test tube is cooled to 45°C seeded with liquid culture and well shaken; after incubation in air, microaerophilic organisms usually grow most profusely 1–2 cm below the surface. The amount of oxygen in the jar for plate cultures can be adjusted to suit the requirements of any particular organism. Most microaerophilic organisms grow well in a McIntosh and Fildes jar without a capsule if two-thirds of the air is evacuated (to about 25 cm); CO_2 is run in to give a concentration of 5% and the remaining space is filled with hydrogen or nitrogen. For an atmosphere suitable for the growth of *Campylobacter* species, commercially prepared sachets are available from Becton Dickinson.

Preservation of bacteria

It is often impossible in a diagnostic laboratory to pursue detailed investigation of interesting bacteria immediately they are isolated. Strains temporarily put aside may be lost because they need frequent subculture, which is neglected, or because after many generations they become contaminated or lose their original characteristics. In most laboratories a small collection of stock cultures is kept, comprising standard strains for antibiotic sensitivity tests and assay and a selection of the less common pathogens for use in media testing when freshly isolated strains are not available. Some species will remain viable up to a year without subculture under suitable conditions. For delicate species and longer preservation, drying is required. For further information, see PHLS Monograph No. 7 (1974).

Preservation without drying

Bacteria such as coliforms and staphylococci which grow readily will survive for several months in semi-solid (0.5–1%) nutrient agar. A loopful of young culture is stabbed into the agar, which is incubated overnight and then stored at room temperature (18–21°C) in the dark. Members of the salmonella group survive well, for a year or more, on Dorset's egg slope cultures in screw-capped bottles kept in the dark at room temperature. Shigellae keep better on nutrient agar of rather poor nutritive quality. Organisms which grow less well need more frequent attention. Streptococci will survive for at least a month in blood broth seeded with a young culture incubated overnight and then refrigerated. They survive nearly as well on blood agar slopes which are kept in the dark at room temperature and can more easily be checked for contamination. *Corynebacterium diphtheriae* is difficult to maintain, most strains need weekly subculture on Loeffler's medium; after incubation for 48 hours they are kept in the dark at room temperature. *Neisseria meningitidis* and *N. gonorrhoeae* are notoriously difficult to preserve. They need continuous incubation and subculture on alternate days in an atmosphere containing 5% CO_2. When they are well established subcultures can be reduced to once in 4 days and additional CO_2 may be discontinued. Most strains can be stored successfully for some weeks by making a heavy emulsion in 10% glycerol broth which is then frozen at $-20°C$. Anaerobes survive well in sealed cooked meat broth cultures. Clostridia will remain viable thus for many months if the tubes are kept at room temperature in the dark. Anaerobic streptococci and *Bacteroides* survive for several months in similar cultures if they are kept in the incubator. *Myco. tuberculosis* will survive on Dorset's egg medium for about 6 months if the medium remains moist and the culture remains in the incubator.

When an unknown organism is isolated which grows poorly on blood agar it should be subcultured on alternate days and incubated in the atmosphere of original growth to maintain viability during investigation; when each subculture is made the remaining growth is reincubated. The characterisitcs of the strain will remain more constant if subcultures are made from the pool of inoculum rather than from single colonies.

Most bacteria and viruses survive well suspended in broth or growth medium and frozen at $-70°C$. A special low temperature refrigerator or a supply of solid CO_2 or liquid nitrogen to maintain this temperature is required.

Preservation by drying

Even the most delicate bacteria can be preserved for long periods by rapidly drying serum broth cultures or suspensions in a vacuum. The aparatus required is expensive and not available in all diagnostic laboratories. A simple drying method in a gelatin ascorbic acid medium (Stamp, 1947) is successful for all but the most delicate bacteria. It is suitable for the stock strains and for preserving other organisms which, after identification by the usual methods, may be required later for detailed investigation.

Maintenance of control strains for antibiotic sensitivity tests and assay (see also page 211)

The standard Oxford H staphylococcus (NCTC 6571) will retain its sensitivity to antibiotics for many years if maintained in the following manner. Three preparations are made: one lyophilized or frozen at $-70°C$; one in a nutrient agar stab, which after 48 hours' incubation is stored in the dark at room temperature ($18-21°C$); and one broth culture which is subcultured daily. The agar stab is subcultured monthly.

At the beginning of each week a fresh broth culture is made from the stab for daily subculture during that week. If the stab is contaminated the strain is recovered from the dried preparation. On no account is it plated out and recovered from a single colony, because this entails the risk of picking a variant and so altering the properties of the strain. *Esch. coli* (NCTC 10418) and *Ps. aeruginosa* (NCTC 10662) are similarly maintained. *Klebs. edwardsi* (NCTC 10896), kept for rapid assay of aminoglycosides, is maintained as a suspension frozen at $-70°C$ (see page 234).

Three cooked meat broth cultures of the *Cl. perfringens* control (NCTC 11229) are prepared. One is lyophilized or frozen at $-70°C$ as described for the other controls; one is kept on the bench at room temperature (20–25°C), unopened; and the third is used to prepare swabs in transport medium for convenient inoculation (see next page). Each time a new batch of swabs is prepared (i.e. weekly or when needed), it is tested for purity by subculture to blood agar and another cooked meat is inoculated. The opened culture is then discarded. The second cooked meat culture remains unopened until the one in current use is contaminated or until it has been repeatedly subcultured for 3 months, when it is renewed from this unopened bottle. A further subculture is then made to replace it because no cooked meat culture is retained after it has been opened. If both bench cultures should become contaminated the strain is revived from the dried or frozen culture. The control *Bact. fragilis* (NCTC 9343) is maintained in the same manner.

A penicillin-sensitive strain of *N. gonorrhoeae* is also kept for comparison with β-lactam-negative strains which may show reduced sensitivity. It is subcultured daily on sensitivity test agar from the pool of inoculum and incubated until growth appears on the subsequent subculture.

Demonstration of β-lactamase production

The recognition of β-lactamase-producing strains of *N. gonorrhoeae* and *H. influenzae* and their clinical importance has resulted in a need for rapid methods to detect the presence of this enzyme in cultures. Three methods have proved satisfactory in our hands.

The method of Hodge *et al.* (1978) requires no special reagents but is not rapid. A penicillin-sensitive *Staph. aureus* is seeded uniformly over the surface of a sensitivity test blood agar plate. A known β-lactamase-producing control strain is streaked across the diameter of the plate. The test organism is then streaked across the diameter at right angles to the control to form a cross. A 10 unit penicillin disc is placed in the middle of the plate where test and control strains meet. After incubation at 37°C for a minimum of 6 hours, a β-lactamase-producing strain will distort the zone of inhibition by the pencillin to give a clover leaf effect.

A novel chromogenic cephalosporin, nitrocefin (Oxoid SR 112), is hydrolysed by β-lactamases to produce a red colour. A 0.5 mg/ml solution of this antibiotic is prepared in potassium phosphate buffer, pH 7.0. For the test, control and test organisms are each suspended in 0.5 ml physiological saline and 50 μl of the cephalosporin is added. A colour change to red is observed over the next 2 minutes in the presence of beta-β-lactamase (Skinner and Wise, 1977).

The third method utilizes commercially prepared paper strips (Mast) soaked in benzylpenicillin and a suitable indicator. Organisms are scraped off a culture plate with a wire loop and rubbed onto the test paper. Hydrolysis of the penicillin alters the pH and produces a colour change on the paper. A positive and negative control must be tested on each occasion, these need not be the same species as the test organisms for any of these methods.

Transport media

Transport medium for pathogens other than gonococci

Transport medium should be used for all pus swabs and for other swabs which may be delayed en route to the laboratory. Although the medium is as non-nutritive as possible, some species are capable of growth in it, notably coliforms including *Pseudomonas*. Therefore, a smear should be made at the bedside for microscopical examination or a separate swab without transport medium should be sent. Overgrowth of contaminating coliforms in the medium can then be recognized by its absence, or very scanty appearance, in the stained film. Each batch of commercially prepared medium should be Gram-stained before use because Gram-negative bacilli may be seen in it which have grown during preparation and have been killed during final sterilization. Their presence when no second swab is provided for microscopy can be very misleading. Moreover, harmful products of their metabolism may be present in the medium, a batch containing them should, therefore, be returned to the manufacturer.

Medium which will preserve anaerobes and retain the moisture of swabs comprises a 5 ml screw-capped bottle or plastic tube filled with a semi-solid non-nutrient agar containing reducing substances and an indicator. The swab is placed in it and the applicator is broken off so that the cap can be replaced. On culture the short swab stick is handled with sterile forceps. The indicator (methylene blue) is colourless when reduced but blue when reducing agents have degenerated, indicating unsuitability for use. Swabs and medium (Transwabs) are obtainable from Medical Wire and Equipment Ltd. (MW170) for transport of *Bord. pertussis* (see page 313).

Transport medium for *N. gonorrhoeae* and *N. meningitidis*

For the preservation of *N. gonorrhoeae*, reducing medium is required to prevent oxidation, which is rapidly lethal. In addition, charcoal is needed to absorb inhibitory substances in the medium. A convenient kit comprising medium with charcoal and a swab is also obtainable from the above company, code number MW171.

Transport medium for culture of chlamydia and viruses

Although commercially prepared media are available, many laboratories prefer to make their own. These may vary according to culture methods. Those transmitting specimens for culture should seek guidance from the reference laboratory about suitable transport methods.

Media for primary isolation

Blood agar is essential for the primary isolation of pathogens in human infection; microbes from mycoplasma to fungi will grow on it. In preparing blood agar the aim is to make a medium which will support the growth of the widest variety of pathogens as possible and to aid speed of diagnosis by demonstrating typical haemolysis when this occurs. The advantage of layered plates is that nutrient agar base, poured into a Petri dish on a flat surface, ensures that the blood-containing layer on top of it is of even thickness. Haemolysis will than appear equivalent over the whole surface of the plate. Provided the dishes are flat-bottomed internally, layering is not essential. Incubation for several days is often necessary and the medium must be at least 4 mm thick or it will dry out prematurely.

The nature of the blood employed and the basic ingredients will affect haemolysis. Human blood is not recommended because of the danger of infection from virus contamination and also because anticoagulant in blood for transfusion will inhibit some fastidious pathogens. Columbia agar base (Oxoid CM331) plus 5 per cent defibrinated horse blood is employed by most laboratories in Britain, and we recommend it. When horse blood is not available, sheep blood can be used. *Haemophilus* does not lyse sheep cells. Red cells in defibrinated blood are fragile and faults in preparation, such as overheating or the presence of contaminating chemicals, are likely to be revealed by red cell lysis.

Method
Nutrient agar:

Columbia agar   44 g
Distilled water   1 l
Autoclave at 15 p.s.i. for 15 minutes (121°C)

Blood agar
Allow the blood to reach room temperature.

Liquefy nutrient agar in the steamer, and when liquid stand on the bench for 15 minutes and then place it in the 56°C waterbath.

Stand the blood for not more than 1 minute in the 56°C waterbath, and then add 5 ml per 100 ml liquid agar. Mix well and pour 20 ml per 90 mm Petri dish.

Alternatively, when large numbers of plates are to be prepared, make the Columbia agar base in Duran bottles (heat resistant, obtainable from Schott); then transfer them from the autoclave to the 56°C waterbath where they can remain as convenient. Before adding the blood, each bottle must stand on the bench for 10–15 minutes. They are swilled around to aid even cooling of the contents; when the temperature of the outside of the bottle is bearable on the back of the hand the temperature of the medium will be about 40–45°C and the warmed blood can be added.

Nalidixic acid blood agar for selection of Gardnerella

Columbia agar   22 g
Distilled water   500 ml
Autoclave at 15 p.s.i. for 15 minutes (121°C)
Cool as for blood agar, then add:

Human (date expired) transfusion blood	25 ml
Nalidixic acid solution (3000 mg/l)	2.5 ml
Polymyxin B solution (50,000 iu/ml)	1.0 ml

Mix very well and pour as for blood agar.

Nalidixic acid blood agar for selection of streptococci

Prepare nalidixic acid solution 3000 mg/l in distilled water. Add 2.5 ml of this solution to 1 litre horse blood agar immediately before pouring. Mix very well and pour as for blood agar.

Neomycin blood agar for selection of anaerobes

Prepare a solution in distilled water containing 15 g/l neomycin. Add 5 ml of this solution to 1 litre of blood agar immediately before pouring. Mix very well and pour as for blood agar.

Liquoid (sodium polyanethol sulphonate) broth for blood culture
(von Haebler and Miles, 1938)

Prepare a 5% solution of Liquoid (Southern Group Laboratory) in 0.85% saline and sterilize it in the autoclave at 15 p.s.i. for 15 minutes.

Add 10 ml of this solution to 1 litre of nutrient broth, mix well and check that the pH is 7.6. Distribute in 10 ml quantities in narrow-necked 30-ml screw-capped bottles, and sterilize as before in the autoclave. Screw the caps on tightly to prevent evaporation; they must be free from traces of inhibitory substances. (About 5 ml of patient's blood will be added to each bottle to give a final concentration of Liquoid of 0.03–0.05 g/dl.)

Diphasic medium for blood culture

Deliver 10 ml Oxoid blood agar base No. 2 liquefied into a 50-ml flat bottle. Autoclave at 15 p.s.i. (121°C) for 15 minutes and slope. When cold, add 10 ml Liquoid broth aseptically. Incubate for 3 days. Examine in a bright light and discard any bottles showing turbidity. Commercially prepared diphasic medium (50 ml) can be obtained and is preferred. We have found Vacuneda bottles of medium from Medical Wire and Equipment Ltd satisfactory.

Thioglycollate fastidious anaerobe broth (FAB) for blood culture

This is supplied by Lab M ready for use.

Charcoal blood agar for Bord. pertussis (from Regan and Lowe, 1977)

Composition

Oxoid charcoal agar CM 119
40 mg/l cephalexin
10% defbrinated horse blood

Method

Prepare charcoal agar as instructed by the manufacturer. Cool to 56°C and add cephalexin and horse blood aseptically. Mix very well before pouring into Petri dishes.

For transport and enrichment, prepare charcoal agar at half strength. Add 40 mg/l cephalexin and 10% horse blood. Mix well. Pour into sterile 5-ml (bijoux) bottles and fill to the neck. Screw caps down well, and store at 4°C; discard any which remain after 8 weeks.

Hoyle's tellurite blood agar for *C. diphtheriae* (modified)

Base agar (Oxoid CM83)	40 g
Distilled water	1 l

Autoclave at 15 p.s.i. (121°C) for 15 minutes. When sufficiently cooled, add as described for blood agar:

Lysed horse blood	25 ml
Whole defibrinated horse blood	25 ml
Potassium tellurite solution 3.5% (Oxoid SR30)	10 ml

Pour into Petri dishes. The presence of whole blood allows haemolysis to be seen.

Medium for isolation of *L. pneumophila*

Medium and special supplements for the isolation of *Legionella* species are obtainable from Oxoid. It comprises CYE agar base (CM655) and growth supplement (SR110). Final preparation in the laboratory must follow the manufacturer's instructions precisely.

VCNT blood agar for *N. gonorrhoeae* (Philips *et al.*, 1972)
Composition:

Vancomycin	3 mg/l	
Colistin	100 units/ml	
Nystatin	12.5 units/ml	} in lysed horse blood agar
Trimethoprim	5 mg/l	
10% saponin		

Method

Prepare stock solutions in sterile distilled water as follows: vancomycin 3 g/l, colistin methane sulphonate 20 000 units/ml, trimethoprim lactate 5 g/l. Sterilize a 10% solution of saponin by autoclaving at 15 p.s.i. for 15 minutes. Mix the solutions aseptically as follows: vancomycin 10 ml, colistin 50 ml, trimethoprim 10 ml and saponin 30 ml. Distribute at 10 ml amounts and store at −20°C. On the day of preparation make 1 litre Difco GC base and cool to 50°C. Reconstitute nystatin to make a suspension containing 12 500 units/ml. Add to the base 100 ml horse blood, 10 ml VCT saponin mixture and 10 ml nystatin suspension. Mix very well and pour 15–20 ml per 8.5-cm Petri dish. Use within 48 hours.

Campylobacter selective medium

Enriched and selective medium for *Campylobacter* species can be obtained from Oxoid. It comprises Campylobacter agar base (CM689) and growth supplement (SR84); to this is added 10% lysed defibrinated horse blood and antibiotics to inhibit the growth of commensals. The antibiotic mixture can also be purchased (SR117) or can be prepared within the laboratory. The required constituents are:

Vancomycin	10 mg/l
Polymyxin B	2.5 units/ml
Trimethoprim	5 mg/l

Nystatin (12.5 units/ml) can also be added but is not usually necessary for faecal specimens.

Prepare the medium as recommended by the manufacturer. Incubate inoculated plates at 42°C in an atmosphere containing 5% air, 10% carbon dioxide and 85% hydrogen or hydrogen–nitrogen mixture, without a palladium catalyst (page 74), or use a sachet prepared for the purpose (supplied by Becton Dickinson).

Phenolphthalein phosphate agar (Barber and Kuper, 1951)

Dissolve 0.5 g sodium phenolphthalein in 100 ml distilled water. Sterilize by Seitz filtration. Melt 200 ml nutrient agar, pH 7.4, cool to 50°C and add 2 ml of the solution. Mix well and pour about 2 mm deep into Petri dishes. Store the solution at 4°C.

The solution will hydrolyse after some weeks. It can be tested by removing a little and adding alkali. A pale pink colour indicates hydrolysis and the solution must be renewed. Some batches of sodium phenolphthalein phosphate are slightly hydrolysed and are unsuitable. The medium can be made selective for staphylococci by the addition of polymyxin B in a concentration of 25 units per ml. Manitol salt agar (Oxoid CM85) with added polymixin can be used as an alternative to phenolphthalein phosphate agar.

Salt medium for the selection of staphylococci (Maitland and Martyn, 1948)

Add 10% sodium chloride to Robertson's cooked meat medium. If faeces or other heavily contaminated material is incubated in this medium overnight and then plated, it will yield an almost pure growth of staphylococci when they are present.

Cetrimide agar (Brown and Lowbury, 1965)

The medium is prepared by adding C-N supplement (Oxoid SR102) to molten Pseudomonas agar base (Oxoid CM559) according to the manufacturer's instructions.

Selective medium for isolation of *Myco. tuberculosis* (Mitchison *et al.*, 1973)

Materials

Middlebrook 7H10 agar (Difco)
Glycerol
Bacto-Middlebrook OADC enrichment (Difco)
Antibiotic solutions: Polymyxin   100 000 units/ml
                  Carbenicillin   100 000 mg/l
                  Trimethorprim 10 000 mg/l
                  Amphotericin B 2 000 mg/l

Method

Suspend 19 g of agar in 1 litre distilled water. Add 5 ml glycerol. When dissolved, distribute in 200 ml volumes and sterilize by autoclaving at 15 p.s.i. (121°C) for 10 minutes. Make 40 ml of a stock antibiotic solution by mixing together 4 ml polymyxin and 2 ml each of carbenicillin and trimethoprim and 32 ml sterile distilled water; this will keep for several months frozen. To each 200 ml molten agar cooled to 50°C add aseptically 4 ml of the antibiotic mixture and 1 ml amphotericin solution. Mix very well, distribute in 5 ml volumes in screw-capped bottles, and slope.

Kirschner medium (Marks and Thomas, 1958)

Kirschner medium base Oxoid (CM193)   1 l
Glycerol   20 ml
Horse serum plus penicillin (100 units/ml)   1 ml

To 1 litre of base medium in distilled water add 20 ml glycerol and mix well. Distribute 9 ml volumes to 30-ml (1 oz) screw-capped bottles and sterilize by autoclaving at 115°C for 10 minutes. To each bottle when cold add aseptically 1 ml sterile horse serum containing 100 units penicillin per ml.

Cl. difficile blood agar

Cl. difficile agar base (Oxoid CM601)   138 g
Distilled water   2 l

Prepare the agar as described for blood agar. When it is in the 56°C water-bath, cool further before adding:

Cefoxitin solution (10 mg/ml)   2 ml
Cycloserine solution (250 mg/ml)   5 ml
Horse blood (defibrinated)   150 ml

Mix very thoroughly and pour as described for blood agar.

The antibiotics may be obtained commercially as *Cl. difficile* supplement (Oxoid SR96).

Mycoplasma medium

Base:

Mycoplasma agar base (Oxoid CM401)	19.9 g
Yeast extract L21	20 g
Distilled water	640 ml

Autoclave at 121°C for 15 minutes.

Supplements:
All are added aseptically (after sterilization by filtration when required) to base, cooled and ready for pouring.

Horse serum	16.0 ml
Thallous acetate 1%	20.0 ml
URA (Oxoid) 10%	5.6 ml
Manganese sulphate 2%	8.4 ml
Phenol red 0.2%	3.0 ml
Penicillin 60 mg/l (stored at −20°C)	1.6 ml

The supplements may be obtained from Oxoid. Supplement G SR59 is recommended for general purposes and P SR60 enchances the growth of *Mycopl. pneumoniae* (but see page 137).

Medium for sensitivity tests

Lysed blood agar (for sulphonamide and other sensitivity tests)
    To lyse the horse blood cells, remove the serum from sedimented, defibrinated blood and replace it with sterile distilled water; mix well and store the mixture frozen solid in the refrigerator.
    Melt 100 ml of Oxoid diagnostic sensitivity test (DST) agar or Iso-sensitest agar and cool it to 50°C. Warm the frozen lysed horse red cells and some fresh whole horse blood as described for the preparation of blood agar. Add 5 ml of each to the nutrient agar, mix well and pour 20 ml per 90-mm Petri dish.
    Blood plates, left overnight to give the lysed blood time to neutralize sulphonamide inhibitors, can be 'chocolated' for tests with haemophilus by heating in an inspissator in a moist atmosphere.
    Iso-sensitest (Oxoid) agar is free of sulphonamide and trimethoprim inhibitors and can be used without blood for tests on non-fastidious organisms. Mueller–Hinton agar base (Oxoid) is used to prepared chocolated blood agar for tests on *Haemophilus* but is not suitable for testing sulphonamide or trimethoprim; it is also the base for medium for testing *N. gonorrhoeae* (page 221). Wilkins–Chalgren agar (Oxoid) is employed for testing non-sporing anaerobes.
    Medium for antibiotic assay is freshly prepared for each batch of assays, and will be found in Chapter 9 as part of the methods described.

Media for identification

Aesculin–bile medium

Add 0.1 g aesculin to 100 ml nutrient agar and autoclave at 15 p.s.i. for 15 minutes.

Dissolve 20 g Bacto dehydrated ox-gall powder (Difco) in 100 ml distilled water sterilize by steaming for 2 hours.

Sterilize 0.5% ferric citrate in distilled water by steaming for 2 hours and store both these solutions at about 2°C.

To prepare the medium melt the base (Difco) and cool to 50°C. Add 5 ml horse serum, 10 ml 0.5% ferric citrate solution and 20 ml 20% ox-gall solution. Mix well and pour into Petri dishes.

Kligler's iron agar

The agar base is obtainable in powder or tablet form from Oxoid Ltd (CM33, CM34). Instructions for making the medium are followed (see also Kligler (1918)).

Urea slope (Christensen) for identification of *Proteus* and other urease-producing bacteria (Cook, 1948)

Ingredients:

Urea agar base (Oxoid CM53)
40% urea solution (Oxoid SR20)

Prepare urea agar base according to the manufacturer's instructions.

To 95 ml prepared molten base, add 5 ml solution aseptically. Mix well and distribute, aseptically, aliquots of about 2 ml to tubes or 5-ml screw-capped bottles. Cool in a sloped position. Test for sterility by overnight incubation.

Nagler plate for identification of *Cl. perfringens* and *Cl. bifermentans*

To 20 ml molten nutrient agar at 50°C add 4 ml concentrated egg yolk emulsion (Oxoid SR47). Mix well and pour into a 90-mm Petri dish. When set, dry off the water of condensation and mark the plate into halves with a grease pencil. On one half spread a few drops of *Cl. perfrigens* antitoxin of British pharmacopoeial strength (polyvalent therapeutic antitoxin will do) and allow to dry. Seed the swab over both halves of the plate, spreading the inoculum in the same pattern on each side. Incubate in an anaerobic jar. The reaction is positive if cloudy zones are seen round colonies on the half of the medium without antitoxin and if similar colonies on the antitoxin half show no zones (page 131).

The following media mentioned in the text are obtained commercially and are prepared according to the manufacturer's instructions, when not ready for use:

Citrate agar (Simmons)	Oxoid CM155
Cooked meat broth*	Southern Group Laboratory
CLED	Oxoid CM301
Desoxycholate citrate agar	Oxoid CM3
DNAase agar	Oxoid CM321
Dorset's egg medium	Southern Group Laboratory
Fildes extract	Oxoid SR 46
Fletcher's medium (Bacto leptospira)	Difco
Isosensitest agar	Oxoid CM471
Loeffler's medium	Southern Group Laboratory
Löwenstein–Jensen medium	Southern Group Laboratory
MacConkey's bile salt agar	Oxoid CM76
Nutrient agar	Oxoid CM3
Peptone water (Tryptone)	Oxoid L42
Pyruvate egg (Stonebrink's medium)	Southern Group Laboratory
Sabouraud's dextrose agar	Oxoid CM41
Selenite F	Southern Group Laboratory
Sugar slopes for Neisseria	Difco
TCBS (for cholera isolation)	Oxoid CM333
Trichomonas medium	Oxoid
Wilkins–Chalgren supplemented agar	Oxoid CM691
Wilson and Blair's bismuth sulphite agar	Oxoid CM201
XLD	Oxoid CM469

Identification tests

Staphylococcal toxin
Although coagulase and DNAase production are closely related to pathogenicity they may occasionally be absent when it would appear from clinical evidence that the strain is pathogenic. A test for alpha toxin (rabbit red cells haemolysin) production may then be helpful.

Method
Incubate a subculture of the staphylococcus in 0.5 ml nutrient broth in air containing 30% CO_2 for 48 hours and then centrifuge. Deliver into a test tube three reagents – the supernatant fluid, saline (0.1 ml) and 2% suspension in saline of thrice-washed rabbit red cells (0.2 ml); and into a control tube the same volumes of supernatant fluid and red cells but 0.1 ml of staphylococcal antitoxin (antihaemolysin) instead of the saline. Incubate both tubes in the 37°C waterbath for 1 hour and leave them for 18 hours on the bench. When alpha toxin is present it will lyse the cells in the first tube but will be neutralized in the control tube, in which the cells will remain intact.

*The prepared broth should contain finely divided meat at least 2.5 cm in depth.

Plate test for nitrate reduction (Cook, 1950)

Soak sheets of Ford 428 Mill blotting paper in warm 40% potassium nitrate (Analar) solution. Dry in the incubator, cut in strips about 16 mm wide and autoclave at 10 p.s.i. for 10 minutes. Stab cultures to be tested on either side of a blood agar plate, place the strip between them and incubate overnight. Include positive and negative controls. (Stab far from each other but not more than 1 cm from the strip. Do not attempt to test more than two unknown strains and two controls per plate.)

Results

Greenish-brown discoloration round the inoculated area indicates a positive test and is due to oxidation of haemoglobin to methaemoglobin by nitrites.

Oxidase test (Kovacs, 1956, modified)
Reagent
p-aminodimethylamine oxalate (Difco). Weigh 0.2 g into each of a series of 30-ml (1 oz) screw-capped bottles and store at 4°C. Add 20 ml distilled water to a bottle when the test is required. The solution can be used repeatedly during the day and is then discarded.

Method

Moisten a strip of blotting paper with the reagent and place it on a microscope slide or a Petri dish. Smear it with a little growth from an overnight culture on solid medium, using a glass rod or platinum loop to avoid traces of iron oxide. When oxidation occurs, indophenol is produced and a deep pinkish-purple colour is seen on the paper. No change is seen when the test is negative. Positive (*Ps. aeruginosa*) and negative (*Esch. coli*) controls should be included.

Specimens for diagnostic tests

In general, specimens for culture should be received in the laboratory as soon as possible after sampling. With the exception of cerebrospinal fluid, which should be incubated, specimens are best refrigerated or left at room temperature in a cool dark place if immediate transmission is impossible. When delayed more than a few hours, transport medium and a special swab should be employed (page 311). When culture of tubercle bacilli in addition to pyogenic bacteria is required, send a liquid specimen, which can be divided, or exceptionally, two swabs.

When antibiotic treatment is contemplated, all samples required for culture must be collected before the first dose is given.

1. *Sore throat.* A swab from the tonsils or pharynx should be cultured on the day of sampling (pages 55 *et seq.*). When delay is unavoidable, swabs in transport medium should be used (page 311).

2. *Streptococcal and diphtheria carriers.* Nose and throat swabs are required. The nasal swab should be rubbed gently on the mucosa of both anterior nares. Note that these organisms are penicillin sensitive; samples

taken after treatment are unlikely to be positive. Other antibiotics may also kill them.

3. *Meningococcal carriers* (page 60). A nasopharyngeal swab must be seeded immediately on warm blood agar or be sent in transport medium (page 311). The suspected carrier should attend the laboratory whenever possible.

4. *Whooping cough* (page 61). Nasopharyngeal or per nasal swabs are seeded directly onto Bordet–Gengou or charcoal medium. The inoculated medium is then returned to the laboratory as soon as possible. Alternatively, the swab may be placed in blood agar transport-enrichment medium (page 61). In Britain the medium is not often required; therefore telephone the laboratory to arrange preparation of freshly poured plates *before* the specimen is taken.

5. *Staph. aureus carriers* (page 290). A nasal swab only is required in the first instance. For exclusion of carriage the patient should attend the laboratory for swabbing of all carrier sites.

6. *Enteric fever*
(a) First week. Blood culture (page 25). The sample of blood is best taken by a member of the laboratory staff before treatment is given. A sample of clotted blood is taken at the same time for serological tests later (page 9).

Faeces culture (page 69). A small sample of faeces containing any abnormal material such as pus or mucus is sent in a screw-capped container (blood in the stool will dilute the bacterial content and should be avoided). It should be cultured on the day on which it was voided.

Urine culture (page 37). A clean mid-stream specimen is sent in sterile screw-capped bottles for culture on the day of voiding.

(b) Second and subsequent weeks. Blood culture. A positive result becomes progressively less likely.

Faeces culture and urine culture (see (a) above). In the absence of treatment, a positive result is to be expected from faeces.

Agglutination tests. 5–10 ml of clotted blood is required (page 9).

7. *Dysentery*. Faeces or rectal swabs must be received on the day of sampling. Swabs must not be allowed to dry; transport medium can be employed (page 311). Stools for amoebae should be passed into a warm bedpan and must arrrive still warm. The laboratory staff should be warned that a specimen is on its way.

8. *Pyrexia of unknown origin* (fever lasting 3 days with no localizing signs)
(a) Viruses can be successfully cultured only at the onset of infection. Therefore send a throat swab in virus transport medium, a sample of faeces and, when indicated, a sample of urine and transmit them to the virus laboratory without delay. A sample of clotted blood and the patient's clinical details are also required.

(b) Blood culture: this is the most important investigation and blood must be taken before antimicrobial treatment. For patients already treated, antimicrobials should be withdrawn for at least 24 hours in order to take a satisfactory sample. When this is considered to be unjustifiable there is little hope of a positive result.

(c) Clotted blood: 5–10 ml should be collected at the time of blood culture and sent for serological tests. Another sample will usually be required 7–14 days later.

(d) Urine: a clean mid-stream sample in a sterile container is required. Suprapubic aspiration of urine may be necessary (see page 37).

(e) Faeces culture: several grams of faeces in a screw-capped container is required. A heat-treated or disposable bedpan should be used for collection (to prevent possible contamination by a pathogen from another patient) but the container need not be sterile. A large sample will be needed for parasitology (see page 171). Rectal swabs are not satisfactory.

9. *Tuberculosis*. Samples of sputum are sent for microscopic examination on 6 consecutive days. They can be collected separately, refrigerated or kept in a cool place, and sent together. The containers must never previously have been used for the purpose or else they must be specially treated, they need not be sterile (see page 9).

Samples of sputum or any other discharge for *culture* of tubercle bacilli must be received on the day of sampling and should be sent in a sterile container.

Gastric washings must either be received within a few hours or be neutralized and refrigerated.

Laryngeal swabs should be received on the day of sampling or the patient should be sent to the laboratory (page 151).

10. *Pleural effusion*. For complete examination, two samples are required: one in a sterile bottle for culture, the other (200 ml if possible) in a sterile jar containing citrate for examination and culture of tubercle bacilli (page 149).

11. *Pus and infected tissue* should arrive as soon as possible after sampling. Biopsy specimens for culture should be placed in a sterile screw-capped bottle *without added fluid*. When actinomycosis or tuberculosis is suspected and no biopsy is made, and when sampling discharge from a sinus, the whole inner dressing sent in a large sterile jar is more suitable than a swab.

12. *Meningitis*. Cerebrospinal fluid should be taken with a dry-sterilized puncture needle using extremely careful aseptic precautions. It should arrive while still warm or be incubated (page 9).

13. *Conjunctivitis*. Swabs should be seeded at the bedside or the patient should be sent to the laboratory (page 83). When neither of these conditions can be met, transport medium must be used (page 311).

14. *Puerperal sepsis*. Cervical swabs are either cultured within half an hour or are specially prepared and placed in transport medium (page 311). Blood for culture should be taken *before* antibiotic treatment is given (page 27).

15. *Genital infections*. The most reliable method is to take discharge direct from the cervix or urethra with a small disposable plastic loop and spread it directly on selective medium which is incubated forthwith. Failing this, urethra and cervix are sampled with specially prepared swabs

which are placed in transport medium (pages 78 *et seq.*). Fluid from a chancre is collected as described on page 81. It should be examined as soon as possible. Blood for serological tests (5–10 ml) is delivered into a sterile bottle and allowed to clot.

16. *Leptospirosis.* Fresh blood and alkaline urine, still warm, are examined under dark-ground illumination for spirochaetes and are inoculated into animals and into fluid media for culture (page 41). In the second week of the disease 5–10 ml clotted blood is sent for agglutination tests. Spirochaetes are unlikely to be demonstrable in the urine before the second week.

17. *Acute lung infection.* Samples of sputum for bacterial culture should be received on the day of collection (pages 64 *et seq.*). If virus infection is suspected, throat washings, taken by gargling virus transport medium, should be sent frozen at $-70°C$ (in a thermos flask containing solid CO_2). (See also 19, below.)

18. *Body fluids for antibiotic assay* should be transmitted to the laboratory as soon as possible. A note of the time and amount of the last dose given before sampling is essential. Note also any other antibacterial drugs recently received. (See pages 233 *et seq.*)

19. *Virus infection.* Serological tests are available for most common virus infections, with the exception of the enteroviruses. Infection by enteroviruses (i.e. poliomyelitis, ECHO and coxsackie) can be confirmed serologically only after successful isolation of the virus.

Herpesvirus infections can be rapidly detected by examination of vesicle fluid by electron microscopy. Fluid is collected from a fresh vesicle by puncturing the lesion with a sterile needle and applying a clean glass microscope slide. The fluid is allowed to dry before sending the slide to the laboratory. Prior arrangement with the laboratory is usually required.

Rapid diagnosis of respiratory syncytial virus, influenza and parainfluenza viruses is possible by direct immunofluorescence of virus seen in nasopharyngeal aspirates.

When virus isolation is required, telephone the laboratory for advice before taking a specimen. A sample of clotted blood should be sent with the culture specimen. If isolation succeeds, a second specimen of blood will be needed to demonstrate either a rise or a fall of antibody titre, which is important in assessing the significance of isolation.

The reader is referred to *Microbial Disease* by Tyrell *et al.* (1979) for a more detailed account of specimen collection.

References

Barber, M. and Kuper, S.W.A. (1951) *Journal of Pathology and Bacteriology* 63, 65

Brown, V.I. and Lowbury, E.J.L. (1965) *Journal of Clinical Pathology* 18, 752

Burt, R. and Phillips, K.D. (1977) *Journal of Clinical Pathology* 30, 1082

Cook, G.T. (1948) *Journal of Pathology and Bacteriology* 60, 171

Cook, G.T. (1950) *Journal of Clinical Pathology* 3, 359

Gargan, R.A. and Phillips, I. (1978) *Journal of Clinical Pathology* 31, 426

Greaves, P.G., Sharp, G. and Macrae, A.D. (1979) *Lancet* i, 551

Hodge, W., Ciak, J. and Tramont, C. (1978) *Journal of Clinical Microbiology* **7**, 102

Kligler, I.J. (1918) *Journal of Experimental Medicine* **28**, 319

Kovacs, N. (1956) *Nature* **178**, 703

Maitland, H.B. and Martyn, G. (1948) *Journal of Pathology and Bacteriology* **60**, 553

Marks, J. and Thomas, C.H.H. (1958) *Monthly Bulletin of the MOH and PHLS* **17**, 194

Miles, A.A. and Misra, S.S. (1938) *Journal of Hygiene Cambridge* **38**, 732

Mitchison, D.A., Allen, B.W. and Lambert, R.A. (1973) *Journal of Clinical Pathology* **26**, 250

Phillips, I., Humphrey, D., Middleton, A. and Nicol, C.S. (1972) *British Journal of Venereal Disease* **48**, 287

Public Health Laboratory Service Monograph No. 7 (1974) *The Preservation of Bacteria*. By S.P. Lapage and K.F. Redway. HM Stationery Office, London

Regan, J. and Lowe, F. (1977) *Journal of Clinical Microbiology* **6**, 303

Rosenblatt, J.E., Fallon, A. and Finegold, S.M. (1973) *Applied Microbiology* **25**, 77

Skinner, A. and Wise, R. (1977) *Journal of Clinical Pathology* **30**, 1030

Stamp, Lord (1947) *Journal of General Microbiology* **1**, 251

Stokes, E.J. and Ridgway, G.L. (1980) *Clinical Bacteriology*, 5th edn. Edward Arnold, London

Tyrrell, D.A.J., Phillips, I., Goodwin, C.S., Blowers, R. (1979) *Microbial Disease: the use of the laboratory in diagnosis, therapy and control*. Edward Arnold, London

von Haebler, T. and Miles, A.A. (1938) *Journal of Pathology and Bacteriology* **46**, 245

Watt, B., Collee, J.G. and Brown, R. (1974) *Journal of Medical Microbiology* **7**, 315

Appendix

Addresses of Suppliers mentioned in the text

(All addresses are in England unless otherwise indicated)

Abbott (Diagnostics Division)	Wokingham RG11 2QZ
Alpha Laboratories	Eastleigh, Hampshire S05 4NU
Ames Co.	see Miles Laboratories Ltd
API Laboratory Products Ltd	Grafton Way, Basingstoke, Hampshire
Assab Ltd	Epsom, Surrey
Baird and Tatlock Ltd	Romford, RM1 1MA
BDH Biochemical Reagents	Poole, Dorset BH12 4NN
Becton Dickinson UK Ltd	Wembley HA9 0PS
Berna (diphtheria antitoxin)	Regent Laboratories, London NW10
Bio-Rad Laboratories Ltd	Caxton Way, Watford, WD1 8RP
Boots Celltech	Slough, S11 4ET
Cambridge Biomedical Ltd	obtainable from Alpha Laboratories
Chance Propper Ltd	Warley, Worcs, B66 1NZ
Clinical Sciences Inc.	for UK agents, see Diamed Diagnostics Ltd
Denley Ltd	Billingshurst, RH14 9SJ
Diamed Diagnostics Ltd	Liverpool, L7 3JQ
Difco	PO Box 14B, East Molesey, Surrey
Don Whitley Scientific Ltd	Shipley, West Yorks, BD17 5JS
Endecotts Ltd	London SW 19
EL KAY	Galway, Eire
Flow Laboratories Ltd	PO Box 17, Irvine, KA12 8NB, Scotland
General Diagnostics Warner & Co.	Eastleigh, SO5 3ZQ
Genzyme Biochemicals Ltd	Sandling Road, Maidstone, ME14 2LE
Gibco Biocult Ltd	Paisley, PA3 4PE, Scotland
Gurr Products for Microbiology	see BDH
Henley, C.A. and Co.	Victoria Road, Buckhurst Hill, Essex

325

Immutech Ltd	Fishponds Road, Wokingham RG11 2QA
Lab M	Salford, M6 6PB
LIP Ltd	Shipley, BD17 7AS
Mast Laboratories Ltd	Merseyside, L10 1EA
Medical Wire & Equipment Ltd	Corsham, SN13 9RT
Mercia Diagnostics Ltd	West Byfleet, KT14 6RA
Miles Laboratories	Stoke Poges, Slough, SL2 4LY
Oxoid Ltd	Basingstoke, RG24 0PW
Phadebact, from Pharmacia Ltd	Milton Keynes, MK9 3HP
Schott Glass Ltd	Stafford, ST16 3EL
Servier Laboratories Ltd	Perivale, UB6 7PW
Seward Laboratories	London SE1 9UG
Southern Group Laboratory	Hither Green Hospital, London SE13 6RU
Southern Syringe Services Ltd	London N14 6JB
Sterilin Ltd	Teddington, Middlesex
Syva Co.	Maidenhead, SL6 1RD
Tissue Culture Services	Slough, SL1 2QL
Wellcome Diagnostics Ltd	London SE13 6TL
Whatman Biochemicals Ltd	Springfield Mill, Maidstone, Kent ME14 2LE
UKEQAS	Division of Microbiological Standards and Quality Control, Central Public Health Laboratory, London NW9 5HT
DMRQ	Division of Microbiological Reagents and, Quality Control, Public Health Laboratory, Service, Colindale, London

Index

Index

211-22